I0883239

Deep Learning Applications in Medical Imaging

Sanjay Saxena
International Institute of Information Technology, India

Sudip Paul
North-Eastern Hill University, India

A volume in the Advances in Medical Technologies and Clinical Practice (AMTCP) Book Series

IGI Global
PUBLISHER of TIMELY KNOWLEDGE

Published in the United States of America by
IGI Global
Medical Information Science Reference (an imprint of IGI Global)
701 E. Chocolate Avenue
Hershey PA, USA 17033
Tel: 717-533-8845
Fax: 717-533-8661
E-mail: cust@igi-global.com
Web site: http://www.igi-global.com

Copyright © 2021 by IGI Global. All rights reserved. No part of this publication may be reproduced, stored or distributed in any form or by any means, electronic or mechanical, including photocopying, without written permission from the publisher.
Product or company names used in this set are for identification purposes only. Inclusion of the names of the products or companies does not indicate a claim of ownership by IGI Global of the trademark or registered trademark.

Library of Congress Cataloging-in-Publication Data

Names: Saxena, Sanjay, 1986- editor. | Paul, Sudip, 1984- editor.
Title: Deep learning applications in medical imaging / Sanjay Saxena and Sudip Paul, editors.
Description: Hershey, PA : Medical Information Science Reference, [2021] | Includes bibliographical references and index. | Summary: "This book explores the application deep learning in medical imaging"-- Provided by publisher.
Identifiers: LCCN 2020008476 (print) | LCCN 2020008477 (ebook) | ISBN 9781799850717 (hardcover) | ISBN 9781799850724 (ebook)
Subjects: MESH: Diagnostic Imaging | Deep Learning | Medical Informatics Applications | Image Processing, Computer-Assisted
Classification: LCC RC78.7.D53 (print) | LCC RC78.7.D53 (ebook) | NLM WN 180 | DDC 616.07/54--dc23
LC record available at https://lccn.loc.gov/2020008476
LC ebook record available at https://lccn.loc.gov/2020008477

This book is published in the IGI Global book series Advances in Medical Technologies and Clinical Practice (AMTCP) (ISSN: 2327-9354; eISSN: 2327-9370)

British Cataloguing in Publication Data
A Cataloguing in Publication record for this book is available from the British Library.

All work contributed to this book is new, previously-unpublished material.
The views expressed in this book are those of the authors, but not necessarily of the publisher.

For electronic access to this publication, please contact: eresources@igi-global.com.

Advances in Medical Technologies and Clinical Practice (AMTCP) Book Series

ISSN:2327-9354
EISSN:2327-9370

Editor-in-Chief: Srikanta Patnaik, SOA University, India & Priti Das, S.C.B. Medical College, India

MISSION

Medical technological innovation continues to provide avenues of research for faster and safer diagnosis and treatments for patients. Practitioners must stay up to date with these latest advancements to provide the best care for nursing and clinical practices.

The **Advances in Medical Technologies and Clinical Practice (AMTCP) Book Series** brings together the most recent research on the latest technology used in areas of nursing informatics, clinical technology, biomedicine, diagnostic technologies, and more. Researchers, students, and practitioners in this field will benefit from this fundamental coverage on the use of technology in clinical practices.

COVERAGE

- Medical Imaging
- Clinical High-Performance Computing
- Biomechanics
- Biomedical Applications
- E-Health
- Telemedicine
- Clinical Nutrition
- Nutrition
- Biometrics
- Neural Engineering

IGI Global is currently accepting manuscripts for publication within this series. To submit a proposal for a volume in this series, please contact our Acquisition Editors at Acquisitions@igi-global.com or visit: http://www.igi-global.com/publish/.

The Advances in Medical Technologies and Clinical Practice (AMTCP) Book Series (ISSN 2327-9354) is published by IGI Global, 701 E. Chocolate Avenue, Hershey, PA 17033-1240, USA, www.igi-global.com. This series is composed of titles available for purchase individually; each title is edited to be contextually exclusive from any other title within the series. For pricing and ordering information please visit http://www.igi-global.com/book-series/advances-medical-technologies-clinical-practice/73682. Postmaster: Send all address changes to above address. Copyright © 2021 IGI Global. All rights, including translation in other languages reserved by the publisher. No part of this series may be reproduced or used in any form or by any means – graphics, electronic, or mechanical, including photocopying, recording, taping, or information and retrieval systems – without written permission from the publisher, except for non commercial, educational use, including classroom teaching purposes. The views expressed in this series are those of the authors, but not necessarily of IGI Global.

Titles in this Series

For a list of additional titles in this series, please visit:
http://www.igi-global.com/book-series/advances-medical-technologies-clinical-practice/73682

Expert Approaches to Health IT Tools in Clinical Practice
Ramgopal Kashyap (Amity University, Raipur, India)
Medical Information Science Reference • © 2021 • 300pp • H/C (ISBN: 9781799840510) • US $245.00

Opportunities and Challenges in Digital Healthcare Innovation
Kamaljeet Sandhu (University of New England, Australia)
Medical Information Science Reference • © 2020 • 261pp • H/C (ISBN: 9781799832744) • US $285.00

Mathematical Models of Infectious Diseases and Social Issues
Nita H. Shah (Department of Mathematics, Gujarat University, Ahmedabad, India) and Mandeep Mittal (Department of Mathematics, Amity Institute of Applied Sciences, Amity University, Noida, India)
Medical Information Science Reference • © 2020 • 316pp • H/C (ISBN: 9781799837411) • US $245.00

Nano-Strategies for Combatting Antimicrobial Resistance and Cancer
Muthupandian Saravanan (Mekelle University, Ethiopia) Venkatraman Gopinath (University of Malaya, Malaysia) and Karthik Deekonda (Monash University, Sunway Campus, India)
Medical Information Science Reference • © 2020 • 300pp • H/C (ISBN: 9781799850496) • US $285.00

Exploring the Role of ICTs in Healthy Aging
David Mendes (Universidade de Évora, Portugal) César Fonseca (Universidade de Évora, Portugal) Manuel José Lopes (Universidade de Évora, Portugal) José García-Alonso (Universidad de Extremadura, Spain) and Juan Manuel Murillo (Universidad de Extremadura, Spain)
Medical Information Science Reference • © 2020 • 292pp • H/C (ISBN: 9781799819370) • US $285.00

For an entire list of titles in this series, please visit:
http://www.igi-global.com/book-series/advances-medical-technologies-clinical-practice/73682

IGI Global
PUBLISHER of TIMELY KNOWLEDGE

701 East Chocolate Avenue, Hershey, PA 17033, USA
Tel: 717-533-8845 x100 • Fax: 717-533-8661
E-Mail: cust@igi-global.com • www.igi-global.com

Table of Contents

Detailed Table of Contents

number of parameters used in the operations of the convolution layer while increasing the efficiency of the representation. The authors present a deep architecture for classification with improved performance. The main objective of this architecture is to improve the main performances of the network thanks to a new design based on CONVblock. The proposal is evaluated on a classification database: CIFAR-10 and MNIST. The experimental results demonstrate the effectiveness of the proposed method. This architecture offers an error of 1.4% on CIFAR-10 and 0.055% on MNIST.

This work is focused on lung cancer prediction using machine learning technique. Lung cancer is one of the widespread diseases due to the growth of irregular cell in both the lungs as a result of which this irregular cell starts growing into tumour, and this tumour can be cancerous as well as non-cancerous. In the traditional approach CT scan images has been used based on the report image segmentation has been done to remove the noise so that a clear picture can be generated to detect the location of tumor. Once the location is known then classification or clustering approach can be used to predict the stage of cancer. Previously supervised machine learning algorithm has been used to predict lung cancer. In this work a prediction model is proposed that is based on the median filter, watershed segmentation, and then feature extraction has done like texture and region. And on the extracted feature classification technique was applied for prediction of cancer.

Diabetic retinopathy (DR) is a disease related to eye correlated with long-standing diabetes. It is a leading cause of blindness among working adults. Detection of this condition in the early stage is critical for good prognosis. Present day detection of DR normally requires digital fundus image or images generated using optical coherence tomography (OCT). As OCT are high-priced, diagnosis of DR using fundus image will benefit for the patient and the ophthalmologists. Manual inspection of morphological changes in blood vessels, microaneurysms, exudates, hemorrhages, and macula are time consuming and tedious tasks. So, designing a computer-aided system helps in analyzing the morphological changes and identifying the DR. This chapter reviews the applications of machine learning and deep learning algorithms for detection of nonproliferative diabetic retinopathy by analyzing fundus images.

Deep learning (DL) and artificial intelligence (AI) are emerging tools in the healthcare sector for medical diagnostics. This chapter elaborates on general reasons for the popularity of computational techniques such as deep learning and machine learning (ML) applications in the medical image processing domain. The initial part of this chapter focuses on reviewing the fundamental concepts of DL algorithms, competence with machine learning, need in healthcare, applications, and challenges in medical image processing. Doing so allows understanding the reasons for the construction of all of them and offers a different view on various domains in the medical sector. The tools and technology required for DL, selection, implementation, optimization, and testing are discussed with respect to an application of cancer detection. Thus, this chapter gives an overall vision of deep learning concepts related to biomedical research.

Machine learning is a technique of parsing data, learning from that data, and then applying what has been learned to make informed decisions. Deep learning is actually a subset of machine learning. It technically is machine learning and functions in the same way, but it has different capabilities. The main difference between deep and machine learning is, machine learning models become well progressively, but the model still needs some guidance. If a machine learning model returns an inaccurate prediction, then the programmer needs to fix that problem explicitly, but in the case of deep learning, the model does it by itself. Automatic car driving system is a good example of deep learning. On other hand, Artificial Intelligence is a different thing from machine learning and deep learning. Deep learning and machine learning both are the subsets of AI.

Foreword

I am happy to write a forward to this book titled *Deep Learning Applications in Medical Imaging*.

I have known Prof. Sanjay Saxena for many years. I had the opportunity of being the co-guide for a couple of research scholars. He is a keen researcher in the field of applying computational method to medical images. I am happy to note that he is collaborating with other researchers in authoring this book.

Medical imaging is used for both diagnosis and therapeutic purposes, making it one of our most powerful resources available to effectively care for our patients. X-Rays machines were invented in 1895, couple of millennia preceding today. The first time ultrasound was used for clinical reasons was in 1956. It was used in Glasgow by an Obstetrician named Ian Donald and an engineer named Tom Brown. These two men developed the first prototype system for ultrasound, but it wasn't perfected until the end of the 1950s.

Computed Tomography (CT) imaging, also known as "CAT scanning" (Computed Axial Tomography) was invented in 1972 by British engineer Godfrey Hounsfield of EMI Laboratories, England and by South Africa-born physicist Allan Cormack of Tufts University, Massachusetts. Hounsfield and Cormack were later awarded the Nobel Peace Prize for their contributions to medicine and science.

Raymond Vahan Damadian is an American physician, medical practitioner, and inventor of the first MR (Magnetic Resonance) Scanning Machine. Damadian discovered that tumors and normal tissue can be distinguished in vivo by nuclear magnetic resonance (NMR) because of their prolonged relaxation times, both T1 (spin-lattice relaxation) or T2 (spin-spin relaxation). Damadian was the first to perform a full body scan of a human being in 1977 to diagnose cancer. Damadian invented an apparatus and method to use NMR safely and accurately to scan the human body, a method now well known as magnetic resonance imaging (MRI).

There are more medical images such as Elastography, Photoacoustic imaging, Echocardiography, Functional near-infrared spectroscopy, Magnetic Particle Imaging, and Nuclear Medicine.

While traditionally the analysis and interpretation of the images was done by specialized experts in the concerned discipline, attempts are being made to analyze and interpret these images computationally.

Digital image processing allows the use of much more complex algorithms, and hence, can offer both more sophisticated performance at simple tasks, and the implementation of methods which would be impossible by analogue means.

In particular, digital image processing is a concrete application of, and a practical technology based on:

- Classification
- Feature extraction
- Multi-scale signal analysis
- Pattern recognition
- Projection

As the data sciences and machine learning techniques develop, medical images present an interesting domain to apply these techniques to perform more accurate analysis of the medical images. This book aims to document the state-of-the-art techniques for analysis of medical images using latest machine learning techniques. This book will be helpful for researchers and medical practitioners.

I hope that the book will provide enough material for budding researchers to kick-start their journey. Also, I hope that practitioners who are medical doctors will find confidence in the automated analysis of medical images to be more productive.

Gopal Krishna Nayak
International Institute of Information Technology, Bhubaneswar, India

Preface

Medical imaging is the process of generating pictorial depictions of the interior of a body for medical intervention and clinical analysis such as CT (Computed Tomography), MRI (Magnetic Resonance Imaging), PET (Positron Emission Tomography), X Rays and many more. Medical Image processing, the set of procedure is one of the major contributions towards society in the field of medical imaging modalities and its analysis. Broadly it consists image acquisition, image enhancement, image segmentation, feature extraction and pattern recognition of medical images.

In the recent years, CAD (Computer aided diagnostic) has drawn attention as of the researchers of its importance. We know that, computers are empowered to think by evolving acumen by learning. Machine learning which is the subset of Artificial Intelligence provides significant tools and techniques for analyzing data whether it medical or something else. Further, machine learning can make appropriate predictions and can learn itself. There are several kind of machine learning techniques such as supervised, unsupervised and reinforcement learning they are useful as per the requirement. Deep learning which is the subset of machine learning provides and efficient way to take the process a step further by enabling independent learning in a more continuous and manageable way. It is providing exciting solutions for medical image processing and its analysis problems and is seen as a main technique for future applications.

We are considering the current scenario of the machine and deep learning in healthcare engineering. Several giants' companies are investing too much on this for example Google has developed a machine learning algorithm to help identify cancer tumors on a mammogram. Stanford uses deep learning algorithms to identify skin cancer. An article recently reported the results of a deep machine learning algorithm capable of diagnosing diabetic retinopathy in retinal images. Machine learning places another arrow in the vibration of clinical decision making.

However, machine learning is suitable for some processes better than others. Algorithms can provide direct benefits to scientific disciplines with processes that can be reproduced or standardized. Also, those who have large drawing datasets, such as radiology, cardiology, and pathology, are strong candidates. Machine learning can be trained to see images, identify abnormalities, and point to areas that need attention, thereby increasing the accuracy of all these processes. Long-term, machine learning will be beneficial for family practitioners or internists at the bedside. Machine learning can offer objective opinions to improve efficiency, reliability and accuracy.

This book organized in eleven chapters; it comprises essential chapters written by researchers from prestigious laboratories/ educational institution. A brief description of each of the chapters in this section given below:

Chapter 1 discusses about the Conventional and Non-Conventional Artificial Neural Network's Techniques, Architectures, Algorithms, and Application in Medical Diagnostics. This chapter provides detailed working view of ANN, covering its various architectures and design techniques in brief. A detailed analysis and summary of medical diagnostics applications using various ANN techniques will be leveraged. Imbalanced data is one the major problem with medical data. This chapter briefs on the various methods to handle imbalanced data. Finally, future directions and potential current challenges are suggested for additional applications in neural networks.

Chapter 2 summaries the most popular deep learning-based image segmentation techniques and discusses their capabilities, and basic advantages and limitations in the domain of medical imaging. It also explains the recent innovation in deep learning brought revolutionary advances in computer vision. Image segmentation is one such area where deep learning shows its capacity and improves the performance by a larger margin than its successor.

Chapter 3 focuses on the fundamentals of machine learning algorithms for image analysis in the cardiovascular system, by evaluating the need for Machine Learning in this field and examining the potential obstacles and challenges of implementation in the context of three common imaging modalities used in cardiovascular medicine. For cardiovascular imaging, machine learning guarantees to be a transformative tool that can address many unmet needs for patient-specific management, accurate prediction of disease progression, and the tracking of identifiable biomarkers of disease processes.

Chapter 4 presents about the CONVblock of Convolutional Neural Network. The reduction in the size of convolution filters has been shown to be effective in image classification models. They make it possible to reduce the calculation and the number of parameters used in the operations of the convolution layer while increasing the efficiency of the representation. Further, a deep architecture for classification with improved performance has been presented. The main objective of this architecture is to improve the main performances of the network thanks to a new design based on CONVblock.

Chapter 5 focuses on Lungs cancer prediction using machine learning technique. Lungs cancer is one of the widespread diseases due to the growth of irregular cell in both the lungs as a result of which this irregular cell start growing into tumor and this tumor can be cancerous as well as non-cancerous. In the traditional approach CT scan images has been used based on the report image segmentation has been done to remove the noise so that a clear picture can be generated to detect the location of tumor. Once the location is known then classification or clustering approach can be used to predict the stage of cancer. Previously supervised machine learning algorithm has been used to predict lung cancer. In this chapter a prediction model is also proposed which is based on the median filter, watershed segmentation and then feature extraction has done like texture and region. And on the extracted feature classification technique was applied for prediction of cancer.

Chapter 6 discusses about Diabetic Retinopathy (DR). This chapter reviews the applications of machine learning and deep learning algorithms for detection of no proliferative DR by analyzing of fundus images. This is a disease related to eye correlated with long-standing diabetes. It is a leading cause of blindness among working adults. Detection of this condition in the early stage is critical for good prognosis. Presence of high blood sugar level for a long period of time destroys the nerves and blood vessels leading cardiac diseases and blindness. So, detection & treatment of DR in the early stage will prevent its development or progression. Clinically, DR can be divided into non proliferative diabetic retinopathy (NPDR) and proliferative diabetic retinopathy (PDR). In NPDR, the blood vessels inside the retina are weakened. Tiny bulges in the blood vessels, known as microaneurysms, may also leak fluid into the retina. This leakage may additionally lead to swelling of the macula. NPDR are again categorized into mild, moderate & sever. PDR is the advanced form of the DR characterized by growth of the new blood vessels as the vasoproliferative factors produced by retina begin to trigger. These blood vessels are fragile and abnormal in nature. Present days detection of DR normally requires digital fundus image or images generated using Optical coherence tomography (OCT). As OCT are high-priced, diagnosis of DR using fundus image will benefit for the patient and the ophthalmologists. Manual inspection of morphological changes in blood vessels, microaneurysms, exudates, hemorrhages, and macula are time consuming and tedious task. So, designing of a computer-aided system helps in analyzing the morphological changes and identifying the DR.

Chapter 7 gives an overall vision of deep learning concepts related to biomedical research. Further, this chapter elaborates on general reasons for the popularity of computational techniques such as deep learning, Machine learning (ML) applications in the medical image processing domain. The initial part of this chapter focuses on reviewing the fundamental concepts of DL algorithms, competence with Machine Learning, need in healthcare, applications and challenges in medical image processing.

Doing so allows us to understand the reasons for the construction of All of them serve a different purpose and offer a different view on various domains in the medical sector. The tools and technology required for DL, selection, Implementation, optimization, testing is discussed with respect to an application of cancer detection.

Chapter 8 focuses on the discussion of basic concepts of AI, ML in DL in Healthcare analysis. Which we will provide the overall pictures of CAD based on AI, ML and DL in Medical Field.

Chapter 9 represents the malaria parasites detection using Deep Neural Network. Malaria is a dreadful infectious disease caused by the bite of female Anopheles mosquito, by the protozoan parasites of the genus Plasmodium. It's being an epidemic disease, demands its rapid and accurate diagnosis for proper intervention. Microscopic test on the thick and thin blood smear to detect the malaria and counts the infected cells is the gold standard for diagnosis of this disease. An automation process in the form of computer-aided diagnosis is much needed as it plays a vital role in fully or semi-automated diagnosis of diseases based on medical image information. Deep learning has vast ranging applications and its application in the healthcare industry always fascinating. This chapter is to build a convolutional neural network to expertly detect the presence of malaria parasitized cells in the thin blood smear. The model as small and computationally efficient to obtain the highest level of accuracy as possible has constructed.

Chapter 10 gives the description about the generated Tuberculosis (TB) detection model using CXR (Chest Radiograph) image. TB is a communal disease with high death and disease rates worldwide. CXR is commonly used in diagnostic solutions for lung TB. Automatic computer-aided solutions to identify TB using CXRs can advance the efficiency of the diagnostic of TB. By identifying open issues include how detect the lung region automatically, and what are the features can identify a given CXR image is infected or normal are considered using three public datasets such as Schengen, Montgomery Country (MC), and JSRT set. The possible textural features of a lung object are obtained from the first order and second order Gray Level co-occurrence Matrix (GLCM) statistical features. The performance of the proposed model was evaluated using accuracy, sensitivity and specificity and the model achieved AUC 91%, 62%, 71%, and 81% on Schengen, JSRT, MC and Combined dataset.

The objective of this book is to provide the information of several machine learning techniques and specifically deep learning in the field of medical imaging. Further, this book will provide relevant theoretical frameworks and the latest empirical research findings in the area. The comprehensive review of deep learning-based algorithms in medical image processing problems will be the key feature of this book.

The target audience of this book will be composed of professionals, researchers and students working in the field of health care engineering, medical imaging technology, its handling, applications of machine and deep learning. Further, this book may be recommended as the curriculum of graduate students, post graduate students in computer engineering, biomedical engineering and electrical engineering based on artificial intelligence, machine learning and its applications in medical imaging.

The editors wish you a pleasant reading.

Acknowledgment

As nothing can be accomplished by oneself, this work is also not an exception. Though only our name appears on the cover, a great many people have contributed to this work. We would like to have some space to acknowledge them that frequently fade into the background. We would like to acknowledge the help of all the people involved in this project and, more specifically, to the authors and reviewers that took part in the review process. Without their support, this book would not have become a reality.

First, the editors would like to thank each author for their contribution. Our sincere gratitude goes to the chapters' authors who contributed their time and expertise to this book. Second, the editors wish to acknowledge the valuable contributions of the reviewers regarding the improvement of quality, coherence, and content presentation of chapters. Most of the authors also served as referees; we highly appreciate their double task.

Further, we want to express our deepest gratitude to all staffs of IGI Global, USA, Prof. Gopal Krishna Nayak, Director, IIIT Bhubaneswar, India and NEHU administration to complete this project. We am also thankful to all friends and colleagues whose significant contributions were evident in this book publication in accumulating information and discussion on various issues related to the subject under study. They have been very supportive and have encouraged us through every step.

We also want to mention our entire family for their immense support, eternal love and prayers. This work is possible because of their all-time moral support.

Last but not the least, all praises to Almighty God, who is the source of wisdom. We thank Him for the eternal love and for giving me this opportunity to edit this book.

Chapter 1
Conventional and Non-Conventional ANNs in Medical Diagnostics:
A Tutorial Survey of Architectures, Algorithms, and Application

Asha G. Karegowda
Siddaganga Institute of Technology, India

Devika G.
https://orcid.org/0000-0002-2509-2867
Government Engineering College, K. R. Pet, India

ABSTRACT

Computer technology advancements in recent days have offered professionals in different fields the ability to gather data, process information, store, and retrieve at a faster rate and make effective decisions. The large collection of data among all various applications including medical diagnosis has paved the need to employ advanced artificial neural networks (ANN). This chapter provides a detailed working view of ANN, covering its various architectures and design techniques in brief. A detailed analysis and summary of medical diagnostics applications using various ANN techniques will be leveraged. Imbalanced data is the major problem with medical data. This chapter briefs on the various methods to handle imbalanced data. Finally, future directions and potential current challenges are suggested for additional applications in neural networks.

DOI: 10.4018/978-1-7998-5071-7.ch001

Copyright © 2021, IGI Global. Copying or distributing in print or electronic forms without written permission of IGI Global is prohibited.

INTRODUCTION

In recent time's artificial neural networks (ANNs) has become a popular and helpful model for classification, clustering, pattern recognition and prediction in many disciplines including medical. ANNs are one category of the of machine learning (ML) and has become relatively competitive to conventional regression and statistical models regarding usefulness (Dave, 2014). Currently, artificial intelligence, information security, big data, cloud computing, internet, and forensic science are all hotspots and exciting topics of information and communication technology (ICT). ANNs full applications can be evaluated with respect to data analysis factors such as accuracy, processing speed, latency, performance, fault tolerance, volume, scalability and convergence (He, 2009; Muzoffair, 2018). The great potential of ANNs is the high-speed processing provided in a massive parallel implementation and this has heightened the need for research in this domain (Izebudien, 2014). ANNs can be developed and used for image recognition, natural language processing and so on. Nowadays, ANNs are mostly used for universal function approximation in numerical paradigms because of their excellent properties of self-learning, adaptivity, fault tolerance, nonlinearity, and advancement in input to an output mapping (Wang, 2018). In (Raval, 2016) usage of machine learning techniques for medical diagnosis analysis of disease considering reports of lab and symptoms for acute analysis is considered.

Scope of the Work

ANN for medical diagnosis is an active research area currently, and researcher's estimates to it to be more widely used in biomedical systems for next few decades as its result are restricted to linear form. ANN will identify disease by learning method without using details of how to recognize the disease, hence it doesn't require any algorithm to identify disease.

ANNs has significant advantages over statistical models, when both are relatively compared. In ANN models, there are no assumptions about data properties or data distribution. Therefore, ANNs are more useful in practical application. Also, unlike some statistical models that require certain hypothesis for testing, ANN models do not require any hypothesis. ANNs are very flexible, data reduction models, encompassing nonlinear regression models, discriminant models, and more fault tolerant. That is, they can handle incomplete and noisy data; and can solve non-linear problems, Also, trained ANNs, can generalize at high speed and make predictions. Furthermore, ANNs are scalable when relatively compared to support vector machine, extreme learning machine, and random forest. ANN processing is promising in several areas of medical analysis such as glucose monitoring (Catalogna, 2012), blood disorders (Raval,2018), diagnosis of various health related issues related to heart (Mihaela,

Figure 1. Number of research work on ANN year wise from 1996-2019
(Source Google)

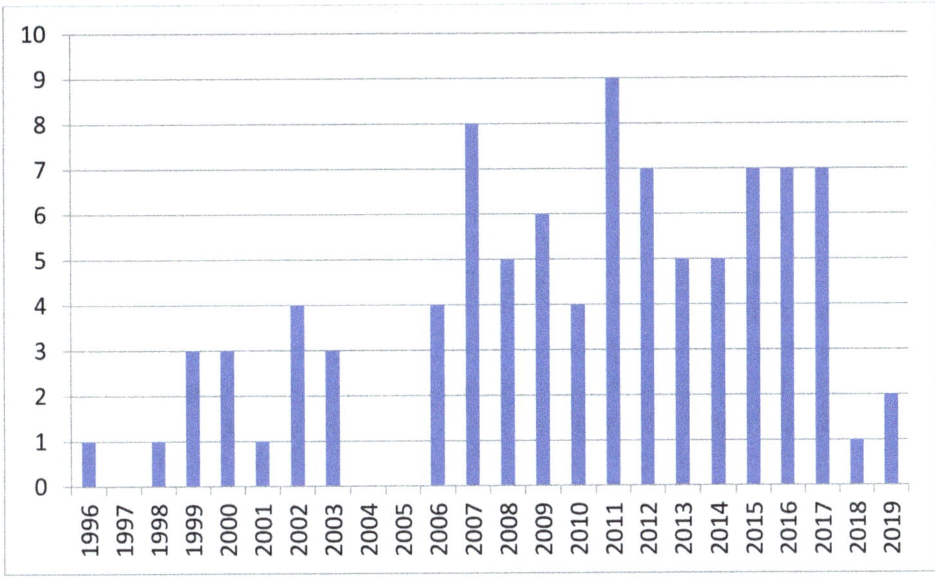

2019), eyes (Xiangyu Chen, 2015), kidney(Yafeng Ren, 2019), liver(Amitha, 2019), lung(Mehdi, 2018), brain(Ali, 2018) and many more. The number of research works on ANN carried out in period 1996-2019 indicated in figure 1.

ANN Overview

Artificial Neural Networks are the computational models that are inspired by the human brain. Many of the recent advancements have been made in the field of Artificial Intelligence, including Voice Recognition, Image Recognition, Robotics using Artificial Neural Networks. Artificial Neural Networks can be viewed as weighted directed graphs in which artificial neurons are nodes, and directed edges with weights are connections between neuron outputs and neuron inputs. The Artificial Neural Network receives information from the external world in the form of pattern and image in vector form. These inputs are mathematically designated by the notation x(n) for n number of inputs. Each input is multiplied by its corresponding weights. Typically weight represents the strength of the interconnection between neurons inside the Neural Network. Activation function decides, whether a neuron should be activated or not by calculating weighted sum and further adding bias to introduce non-linearity into the output of a neuron. The weighted inputs are all summed up inside the computing unit (artificial neuron). To limit the response to arrive at the desired value, the threshold value is set up. For this, the sum is passed through an activation function. The activation function is set to the transfer function used to get the desired output. There are linear as well as the nonlinear activation function. Some of the commonly used activation functions are: binary, sigmoidal (linear), tan hyperbolic sigmoidal functions (nonlinear), RELU(Rectified linear unit) and Softmax. The most common activation function's Plot and Equation are listed in Table 1.

- **Binary:** The output has only two values either 0 or 1. For this, the threshold value is set up. If the net weighted input is greater than 1, an output is assumed one otherwise zero.
- **Sigmoidal:** It is 'S' shape curve, specifically used for models where one need to predict the probability as an output since it's range is from (0 to 1).
- **Tan Hyperbolic:** This function has a 'S' shaped curve. It is considered to be stronger tan sigmoid function. The range of tanh function is from (-1 to 1). It is also called as scaled sigmoid function. It is mainly used for binary classification problems. Both tanh and logistic sigmoid activation functions are used in feed-forward nets.
- **ReLU(Rectified linear unit)**: It signifies the pixel-wise function which is nonlinear in nature given by g(x) = max(0,x) i.e. it return x for all positive values, and zero for all negative values. . ReLU is the most commonly used activation function in neural networks, especially in CNNs acting as a layer wise down-sampling nonlinear function. The advantage of ReLU is it t doesn't have the vanishing gradient problem as seen in activation functions like sigmoid or tanh. One of the matter of concern with ReLUs is that all the negative values become zero immediately which drops the ability of the model to fit or train from the data properly.
- **Softmax:** Softmax is often used in Convolutional neural networks, to map the non-normalized output of a network to a probability distribution over predicted output classes. It is used for multi-classification in logistic regression model. The range will 0 to 1, and the sum of all the probabilities will be equal to one; which not be the case for sigmoidal function. If the softmax function used for multi-classification model it returns the probabilities of each class; with the highest probability for the target class.

A neural network can be "shallow", in the sense it has an input layer, few number of hidden layer followed by an output layer. A Deep Neural Network (DNN) has many layers of neurons between the input and the output layer.

Table 1. Most common activation function's

Name	Plot	Equation	Output Value
Binary	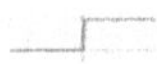	$f(x)=\begin{cases}0\ for\ x<0\\1\ for\ x>0\end{cases}$	0/1
Sigmoidal	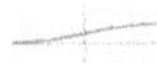	$f(x)=\dfrac{1}{1+e^{x}}$	0-1
Tanh	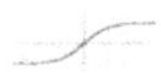	$f(x)=\tanh(x)=\dfrac{2}{1+e^{-2x}}-1$	-1 -1
Rectified Linear unit (ReLu)	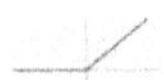	$f(x)=\begin{cases}0\ for\ x<0\\x\ for\ x>0\end{cases}$	Positive value with in x
Softmax	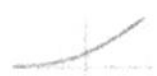	$f(x)=\log_{e}\left(1+e^{x}\right)$	0-1

Contributions

Inspired by research focus of neural network in reshaping medical field, this work concentrates on its efforts in medical diagnostics. Neural network technique has reshaped the research landscape of medical field in almost all aspects such as algorithm designs, training/test data sets, application scenarios and even the evaluation protocols. Therefore, it is of great significance to review the breakthrough and rapid development process in recent years. Numerous survey work on medical diagnostics activates have been carried on (Litjens, 2017; Bolboca,2019), and also its subdomains. Most of these surveys summarize and compare adverse set of techniques related to specific technique (Razzak, 2017). Our paper distinguishes itself from earlier surveys from the following perspectives:

- We focus on ANN applications (in particular DNN) for medical diagnosis
- We discuss cutting-edge ANN techniques from the perspective of applications (focusing on their applicability to this area, whilst giving less attention to conventional models that may be out-of-date).
- Various method to handle imbalance data is addressed.
- A systematic review on the evolution of the network architectures and loss functions for deep FR.

- We analyze similarities between existing problems and those specific to medical diagnosis; based on this analysis we provide insights into both best ANN architecture selection strategies and adaptation approaches, so as to exploit the characteristics of ANN by conducting analysis and management tasks.
- Highlights will be provided with challenges and future directions for the successful and fruitful usage for various applications.

Artificial Neural Network Techniques

The artificial neural networks techniques can be broadly classified as follows:

Classification Neural Network

A Neural Network can be trained to classify given pattern or dataset into predefined class. The most common and state of art method is the one which uses Feed forward Networks. The ANN can be categorized based on learning strategies employed: supervised and unsupervised. In first learning method the network is trained in presence of input and output patterns. The input weights will be adjusted until desired output value reaches expected output value. The self-organizing map or other techniques will be devised in unsupervised learning method. The network has to calculate its own representation of input value by calculating acceptable connection weights. The values can be found by clustering input data and with features inherent problem.

Prediction Neural Network

A Neural Network can be trained to produce outputs that are expected from a given input for example: Stock market prediction. The usage of neural network for prediction will make it able to learn from examples only and that after their learning is finished, the algorithms are able to catch hidden and strongly non-linear dependencies. This can identify significant characters even in presence of noise in the training set. The neural network prediction can be classified based on criteria to predict as i) data that we have for teaching prediction and for prediction and ii) what we want to predict - value or trend. The first method is applicable for case when exact value or more values of a variable are needed for prediction and further is applicable for time series based.

Clustering Neural Network

The Neural network can be used to identify unique features of the data and classify them into different categories without any prior knowledge of the data. The commonly used clustering techniques in neural network are,

- Competitive networks
- Adaptive Resonance Theory Networks
- Kohonen Self-Organizing Maps.

Association Neural Network

A Neural Network can be trained to remember the particular pattern so that when the noise pattern is presented to the network, the network associates it with the closest one in the memory or discard it. E.g., Hopfield Networks which performs recognition, classification, and clustering, etc. the pattern based association support to store different patterns and at the time of giving an output, it will produce one of the stored patterns by matching them with the given input pattern,

Optimization Neural Network

The optimization problem will minimize or maximize certain objective function/s. The problem to be optimized are not linear or polynomial. ANN will resolve the problems of heuristic based and expects precise output. Neural networks approximate the objective function in optimization problems to make it possible to apply other techniques such as non-linear regression to resolve the problem to resolve an optimization problem. The derivate of the new objective function should be polynomial, so that the solution of the optimization problem can be calculated.

Pattern Recognition Neural Network

The neural network is trained to associate input and output patters for pattern recognition. The network is used to train; it identifies input pattern and tries to output for associated pattern. The networks comes to life when a pattern that has no output associated with it, is given as an input. In this case, the network gives the output that corresponds to a taught input pattern that is least different from the given pattern. During training, the network is trained to associate outputs within input patterns. When the network is used, it identifies the input pattern and tries to output the associated output pattern. The power of neural networks comes to life when a pattern that has no output associated with it, is given. In this case, the network gives the output that corresponds to a taught input pattern that is least different from the given pattern. Pattern recognition could be used for a design of proper learning algorithm, while learning algorithm could be used to enhance the result of pattern recognition.

Artificial Neural Network Architectures

A neural network can be "shallow", in the sense it has an input layer, few number of hidden layer followed by an output layer. A Deep Neural Network (DNN) has many layers of neurons between the input and the output layer.

Shallow Neural Network

This form of neural network as name suggests consist of less depth usually of only one or very few hidden layer as against many hidden layers in deep neural network. The number neurons in hidden layer may vary. The figure 2 indicates a shallow neural network of one input, hidden and output layer. The commonly used shallow neural networks such as feed forward, radial basis function, wavelet and time delay neural network are described below.

Figure 2. Shallow Neural Network

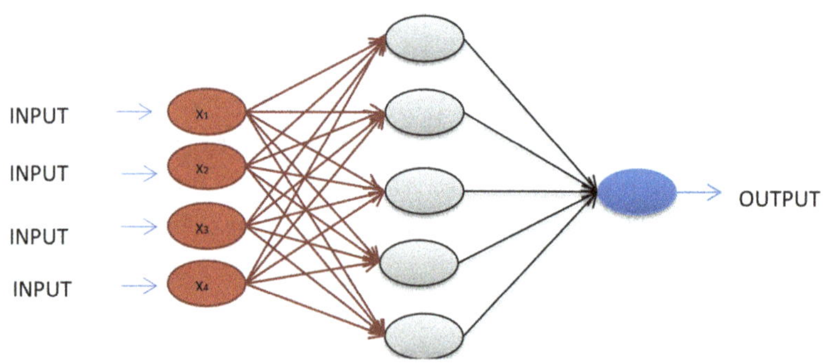

Feed-Forward Neural Networks

This type of neural network is common among practical applications. The architectural design includes one input, output and hidden layers which will compute series of transformations to change similarities between cases. The activation function for neurons a non-linear functioin will be applied.

Radial Basis Function Neural Networks

The model includes three-layer neural network one input, one hidden and one output layer. The hidden layer uses radial basis function as activation function. Radial basis function are real valued function gives outputs based on only Euclidean distance from origin or center to inputs and maximum frequently used function is Gaussian function. (Buliali, Hariadi, Saikhu, & Mamase, 2016). These networks are similar to the feed-forward Neural Network except radial basis function is used as the activation function of these neurons. The radial basis function is indicated in figure 3(a).

Wavelet Neural Networks

This model combines concept of wavelet theory and ANN. The wavelet neural network consists of only single input, hidden and output layer. The activation function in hidden layer is replaced with wavelet function. The structure of wavelet neural network is shown in figure 3(b). The wavelet model is applicable in time series prediction and signal processing (Yang & Hu, 2016).

Time Delay Neural Network

This model is defined as multilayer neural network with delayed input or states utilized through time shifting approach. A simple delayed neural network example is shown in figure 3(c). The neurons in hidden layer receive input value at time t as given from inputs tl and t2. It is possible to use delay in other layers also.

Deep Neural Network

The form of neural network usually consists of multiple hidden layers when compared against shallow neural network.

Recurrent NN (RNN)

RNN are well-made ML techniques for their quality in different fields of activity like signal processing, natural language processing and speech recognition. CNN considers only the current input while RNN considers the current input in addition to previously received inputs. The internal memory of RNN is used to store the previous input as shown in figure 4. CNN is apt for spatial data such as images, whereas RNN is apt for temporal data/sequential data. RNN use their internal memory to process arbitrary sequences of input temporal data. CNN contemplates only the present input while RNN considers both the present and recent past inputs. This is possible since RNN has its internal memory. The two variants of RNN long-short

Figure 3. (a) Radial Basis neural network (b) Wavelet Neural Network (c) Time delay based neural network

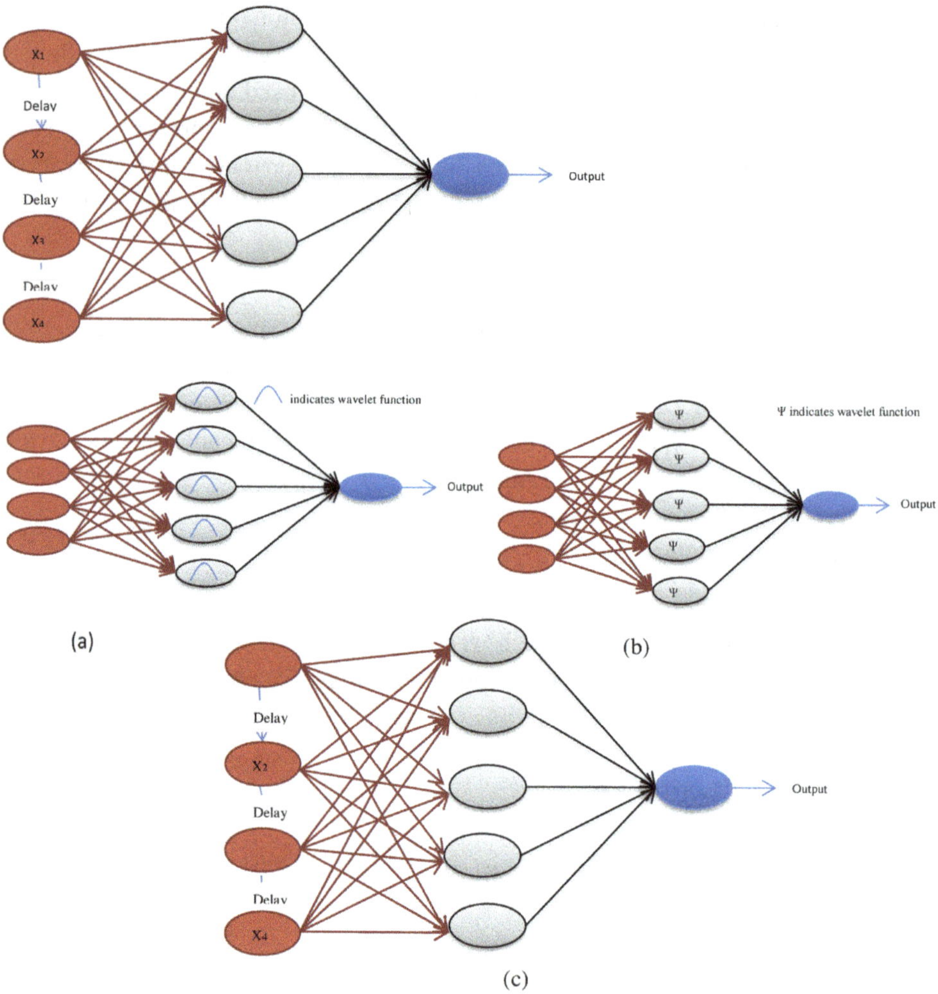

term memory (LSTM) and gated recurrent unit (GRU)(Kamilaris, 2018; Lecun, 1995;Tseng, 2018) are shown in figure 4(a).

Long Short-Term Memory Neural Network (LSTM)

The type of Neural Network in which memory cell is incorporated into hidden layer neurons is called LSTM network. LSTM is extension of RNN. RNN has problem with vanishing and exploding gradients which is solved by LSTM. LSTM has three gates: forget gate, read /input gate and write/output gate. If forget gate is active the

Figure 4. Typical construction of (a) RNN (b) LSTM

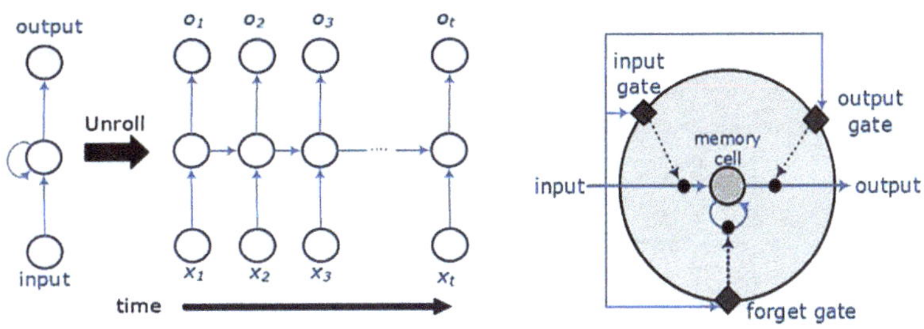

neuron writes its data to itself. If forget gate is turned off by sending a 0, then neuron forgets its last content. If write gate is set to 1, then connected neurons can write to that neuron. When read gate is set to 1, the connected neurons can reads the content of neuron. The figure 4(b) depicts the structure of LSTM. The main difference between RNN and LSTM units is that LSTM utilize forget gates to actively control the cell states and ensure not to degrade. The gates can use sigmoid or tanh as their activation function. Activation functions cause the problem of vanishing gradient during back propagation in the training phase of other models using them (Deng, 2014;Tseng, 2018).

Convolutional Neural Network

These networks have large number of hidden layers compared to conventional ANN and are primarily used for image, video, and audio processing. The typical CNN architecture includes exchange layer by connecting one or more fully connected layers at the end as next of convolution and pooling layers. For specific application, these fully connected layers will be replaced with global average pooling layer. In some cases, in order to optimize performance, the CNN will additionally include batch normalization and dropout in addition to learning stages as regulatory layers. The performance of CNN is totally based on the arrangement of different components in its new architecture. The CNN sequencing to classify handwritten digits is shown in figure 5 (a)(towardsdatascience.com). The CNN can be categorized based on features such as spatial exploitation, depth, multi-path, width, feature map exploitation, channel boosting, and attention as depicted in Figure 5(b) (khan, 2016).

Transfer Learning method (TL) is used when pre-trained models require processing. In such case, the model will be reused as of starting point for an operations reused as the starting point. For example if CNN trained on one dataset, then according to training remove or retain on last layers. The training models are applied to recognize different higher level features. The training time will be reduced

Figure 5a. Typical CNN example for character identification

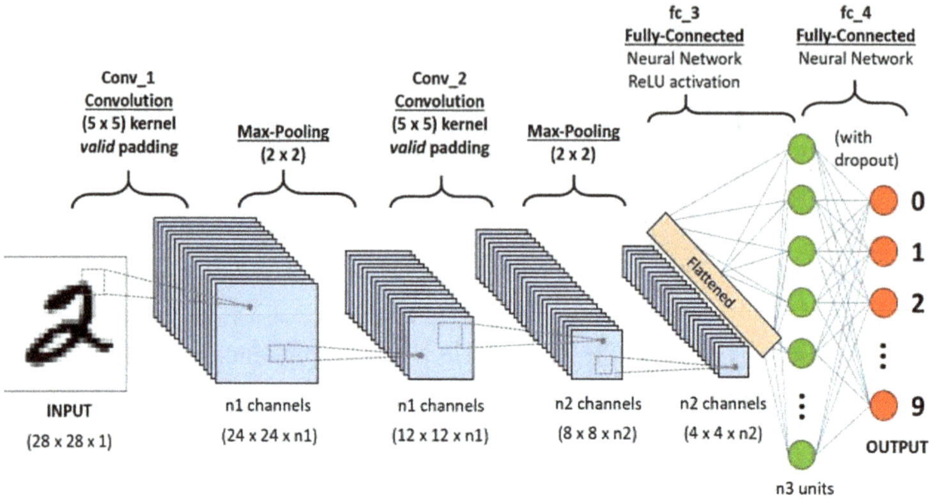

Figure 5b. Classification of CNN

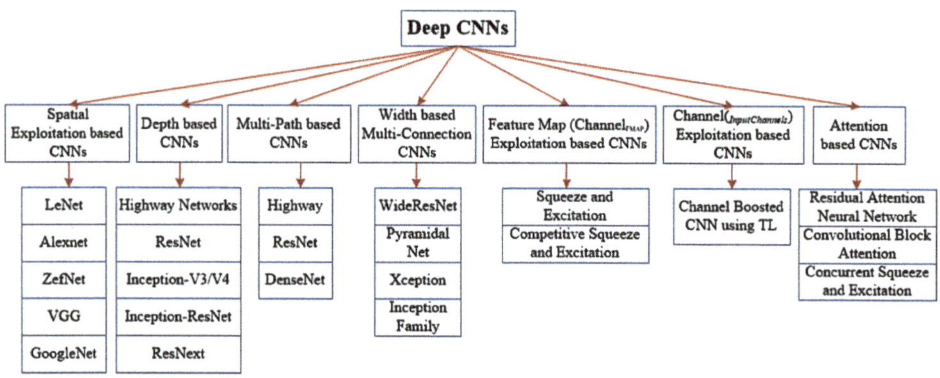

Figure 5c. Transfer learning method (left); Dropouts (right)
(Nitish, 2014)

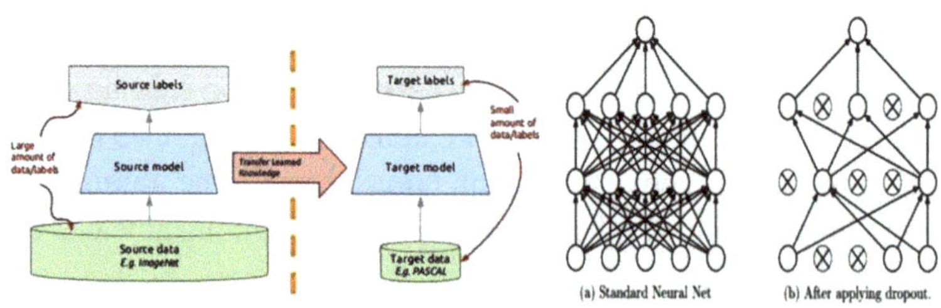

Figure 5d. Max pooling example (left); Batch Normalization (right)
(source: https://medium.com)

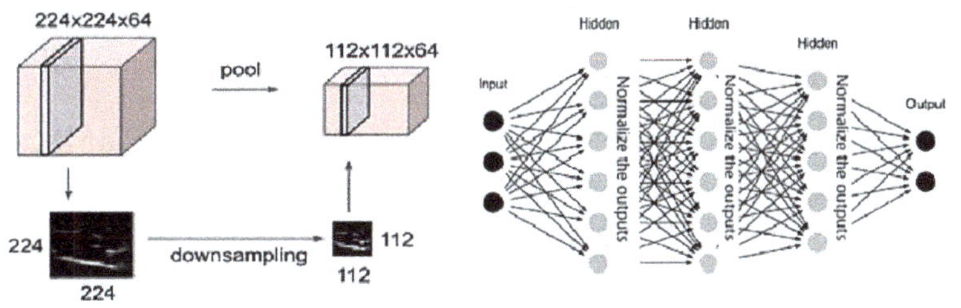

in transfer learning. It is helpful tool when enough data or training takes too much resource. The transfer learning is shown in figure 5(c)(Ruder, 2017).

In **Dropout address** (DA) problem of CNN where neurons are dropped or ignored randomly during training process. Larger the network it slows to use, making it difficult to deal with overfitting by combining predictions of many different large deep networks at training time. In dropout randomly dropped units from the neural network will prevents units from adapting much for training. This method normally improves performance of neural networks on supervised learning. The improved dropout method is presented in figure 5(d).

Max Pooling (MP) method involves discretization sample-based process. Its main objective is to down-sample input representation by minimizing its dimensionality and features contained in sub-regions case (**Sutskever, 2017**). This will provide an abstraction form of representation by reducing computational cost with reduction in number of parameters to learn and provide basic conversions invariance to its original representations. This method is suitable when applied with maximum filter without overlapping in subset regions of its original representations. A max pool example is shown in figure 5(e).

Batch Normalization (BN) is a process to routinely standardize (making mean as 0 and standard deviation as one) the activations and gradients proliferating through a network. In simple words the batch Normalization layer can be included in network model so as to standardize raw input variables or the outputs of a hidden layer with the objective of accelerating the training of deep learning neural networks and get improved results. The sample batch normalization process is given in figure 5(f).

Deep Auto Encoders

It is a method used to train input and output applying unsupervised neural network technique. It consists of one input, output and hidden layer. A hidden layer defines code to represent input. The two main operational parts of auto encoders are encode and decode functions. The encoding is done at input initially, and subsequently decoders construct code to rebuild the original input. Normally auto encoders produce an approximately same copy of input according to training data.

Deep Belief Network

This model is formed by multiple Restricted Boltzmann machines (RBM) layers. The probability distribution over the input are made with undirected connections layers. The first layer will be input layer, next layer is hidden layer and from there output will be forwarded to RBM to reconstruct the inputs. The output of one RBM will be forwarded to next RBM as input. The multiples layers of RBM can be grouped as stacks also. Normally deep belief network is used to construct supervised models. The figure 6 shows as example model of deep belief network.

Figure 6a. Example model of Deep Belief Network

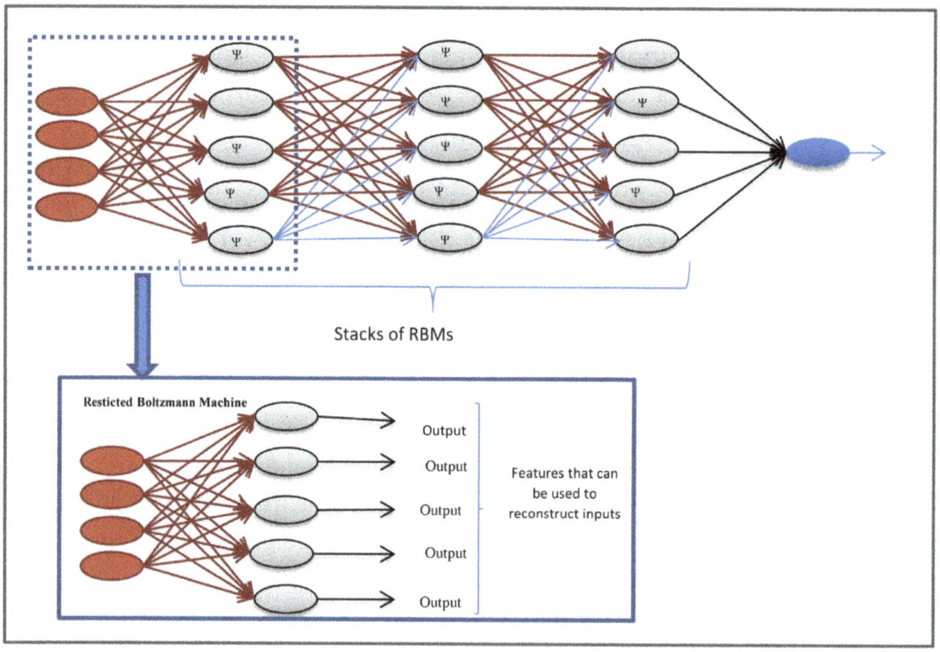

Multilayer Perceptron Neural Network

These networks use more than one hidden layer of neurons, unlike single layer perceptron. These are also known as Deep Feedforward Neural Networks.

Recurrent Neural Network

It is a type of Neural Network in which hidden layer neurons have self-connection. Recurrent Neural Networks possess memory. At any instance, hidden layer neuron receives activation from the lower layer as well as its previous activation value.

Gated Recurrent Unit (GRU)

In order to assist the computation and implementation of LSTM model, the neuron GRU was introduced. GRU uses update and reset gates the GRU to carry forward information over many time periods in order to influence a future time period. That value is stored in memory for a certain amount of time and at a critical point pulling that value out and using it with current state to update at next future data. GRU requires less number of parameters hence need less memory, less training time (hence fast) compared to LSTM. Figure 6 (b) depicts LSTM with i, f and o as input, forget and output. C and ~C denote memory and the new memory cell content. Figure 6 (c) shows r and z i.e. Reset and Update gate for GRU, h and ~ h are the activation and the candidate activation. Both LSTM and GRU are preferred for time series data for forecasting. GRU use less training parameters and therefore needs less memory, execute faster and train faster than LSTM's whereas LSTM is more accurate on dataset using longer sequence.

Figure 6b. Variants of RNN. LSTM (left); GRu (right)

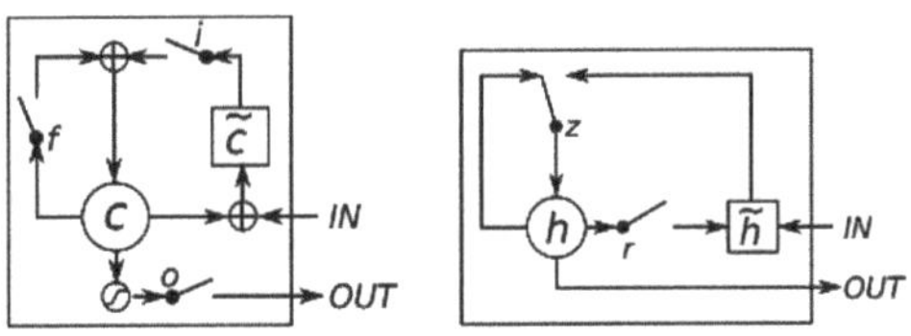

Other Neural Network

Hopfield Network

A fully interconnected network of neurons in each neuron is connected to every other neuron. The network is trained with input pattern by setting a value of neurons to the desired pattern. Then its weights are computed. The weights are not changed. Once trained for one or more patterns, the network will converge to the learned patterns. It is different from other Neural Networks.

Modular Neural Network

It is the combined structure of different types of the neural network like multilayer perceptron, Hopfield Network, Recurrent Neural Network, etc. which are incorporated as a single module into the network to perform independent subtask of whole complete Neural Networks.

Physical Neural Network

In this type of Artificial Neural Network, electrically adjustable resistance material is used to emulate the function of synapse instead of software simulations performed in the neural network.

Hardware Architecture for Neural Networks

Two types of methods are used for implementing hardware for Neural Networks.

- Software simulation in conventional computer
- Special hardware solution for decreasing execution time.

When Neural Networks are used with a fewer number of processing units and weights, software simulation is performed on the computer directly. E.g., voice recognition, etc.

APPLICATIONS OF DEEP LEARNING FOR MEDICAL DIAGNOSTICS

The design of the conventional ANN and steps involved for the purpose of medical diagnosis include: Initially patient's data to predict the diagnosis of a certain disease needs to be collected then target disease is predicted. The features are analyzed properly with selection of related attributes which provide the information needed to distinguish the different health conditions of the patient. This condition can be further analyzed with specific tools to allow the elimination of factors that provide redundant information or those that contribute only to the noise. The literature survey during 2015 and later reveal that researchers are adopting Deep learning medical diagnosis over conventional ANN methods. In deep learning models, data is filtered through a series of multiple layers, with each proceeding layer providing the output to the next successive layer. Deep learning models provide more accurate after processing huge amount of data and have the capability of learning from previous results to further enhance their ability to make correlations and connections between the unstructured data, identify the abnormalities in medical images with minimum involvement of human beings.

Compared to conventional ANN, the deep learning requires less preprocessing of data as it has self ahs the caliber to take care of many of the filtering and normalization tasks, feature extraction which was the tasks of the programmers in conventional ANN.

Deep learning has been applied for diagnosis of various health issues which include: Alzheimer's disease, diabetic retinopathy, lung cancer, liver cancer, heart related problem, fall event of elderly, benign and malignant detection in thyroid, and many more. This section covers few of the recent papers published pertaining to use of Deep learning for diagnosis of various health issues and compared its performance with conventional machine learning algorithms. The major steps of conventional method in diagnosis of medical images include image processing, segmentation followed by feature extraction; these steps are taken care by deep learning in automated fashion.

Alzheimer's disease (AD), is the most common form of dementia and is the major concern since it an irretrievable, progressive brain ailment marked by a deterioration in cognitive functioning with very poor disease modifying treatment. In this study(Siqu,2014), authors have designed a deep learning architecture, with stacked auto-encoders and a softmax regression layer as output layer, for diagnosis of AD and its prodromal stage, Mild Cognitive Impairment (MCI). The proposed method is semi-supervised which can be trained using unlabelled training samples, which are easy to obtain of less cost. Overall Results obtained are better with overall accuracy and the overall specificity of 47.42% and 83.75% respectively when compared with single-kernel SVM (SK-SVM) and multi-kernel SVM (MK-SVM) (using radial basis function (RBF) kernel) which used 'one against all' approach to classify four-class classification problem.

Most of the researchers have applied machine learning for predicting the current stage of Alzheimer's disease. Authors in (Xin Hong, 2019), have proposed Long short-term memory (LSTM) which is able to connect previous information to the present task using temporal relation between features and the next stage of Alzheimer's Disease. The work is carried out using (PET, CT and MRI)images from AD Neuroimaging Initiative (ADNI) database. The data pre-processing step includes reclassifying (eight categories are reclassified into three categories according to the stages of the disease: AD, NC, and MCI), data interpolation (for filling missing data), data normalization, data serialization, and time step preprocess. The proposed model, as depicted in figure 7 has 3 layers: the Pre-Fully Connected with fully connected layer and ReLU function; Cells Layer with one LSTM layer and a Dropout Wrapper; and the Post-Fully Connected Layer with one fully connected layer and a softmax layer. During the model training, the state of AD for next 6 months is predicted using pre-processed sequential data with time steps as input to the model. The proposed model outperform the performance of the following three work carried out by other researchers: (a) Discriminative Self-representation Sparse Regression for feature selection with SVM classifier (b) Random Forest (RF) for feature selection and Deep Neural Network (DNN) as classifier and (c) CNN along with PCA-LASSO for feature selection and SVM as classifier.

Figure 7. Alzheimer's disease prediction model with LSTM
(Xin Hong 2019)

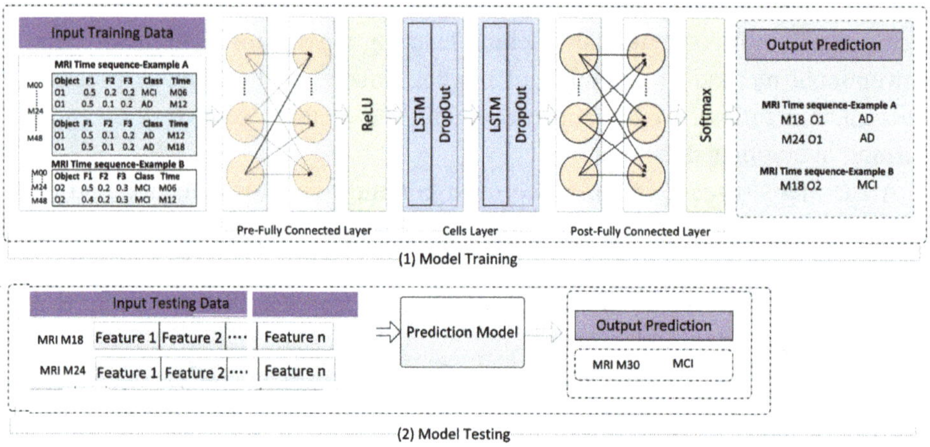

In, (Mehdi Fatan, 2018), authors have proposed CNN architecture with 3 convolution layers(to extract high order feature), 2 max-pooling layers, a full-connected layer, and a binary soft-max as depicted in figure 8 for Lung Cancer diagnostic. The fully-connected layer results in output of 10 dimensions which are passed to fully connected layer containing 2 softmax units, which indicates the probability of presence of lung cancer or not. Cross-entropy is used as the loss function of training model which is computed using multinomial logistic regression. The performance is measured using specificity, sensitivity, and F1 score on (Kaggle Data Science Bowl 2017) KDSB17 data set having CT scan images of non-cancer and cancer patients. The results obtained were better than those obtained by some of the high-ranked methods in Kaggle competition.

In (Goran,2019), authors have applied DNN for lung cancer detection. Two piles of images were done so as to create positives and negatives samples to train and test the network, but the groups in each pile were created so that Deep Neural Network would focus on recognizing same slice (angle) images of lung. The groups

Figure 8. Proposed CNN architecture for lung cancer detection
(Mehdi Fatan 2018)

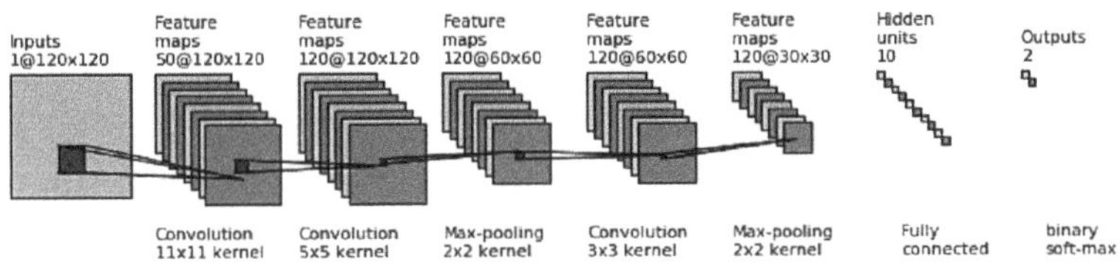

were created using K-means algorithm based on slice group. The Neural Network was adopted with additional layers to create the Deep Neural Network. The inner layers are composed of one convolution layer, max pooling layer, followed by double convolution layers (two convolutions) and an additional max pooling. The first convolution layer does the initial segmentation of the images and the interconnection of the nodes followed by max-pooling layer so as to avoid over-fitting. The second and the third convolution were used to make a more thorough search to obtain more precise information of where the cancer might be. They divided the images into small parts so that they can focus on (isolate) a certain part of the image and use that (smaller) image to search for a pattern. In the convolution function, they used sharpening and edge detection filters so as get images with sharp edges. They tested their proposed work on lung cancer images from Tx stages 2, 3 and 4 and determining at which Tx stage one can detect the possibility of lung cancer.

Authors in (Amitha Das, 2019), have used watershed Gaussian segmentation to CT image to extract the liver, followed by Gaussina mixure model to segment the cancer tissue in liver. Then the statistical, textural and geometrical feature are extracted from segmented cancer tissue in liver and provided as input to DNN to classify it as HEM, HCC and MET types of liver tumor. Work was carried out on 225 CT images with 75 cases each of hemangioma(HEM), hepatocellular carcinoma(HCC) and metastatic carcinoma(MET) types of cancer as shown in figure 11. Work is compared with other conventional classifiers like Naïve bayes, MLP, SVM, KNN, AdaBoost, J48, Random forest. The performance of proposed method is best with accuracy of 98.38%, sensitivity of 100%, specificity of 97.72%, Jaccard index of 95% and dice similarity coefficient (DSC) of 97.43%.

In (Tarek M, 2017), authors have applied deep network for diagnosing focal liver diseases. Firstly, level set method is used followed by Fuzzy -c-means clustering for segmentation of liver lesions. Then stacked sparse auto-encoder is used to extract the high-level features from the segmented images, which is input to the softmax layer for finally diagnosing the three focal liver diseases along with the normal liver. The Proposed work achieved accuracy, sensitivity and specificity of 97.2%, 98% and

Figure 9. Deep learning model proposed by (Amitha Das, 2019) for liver cancer detection

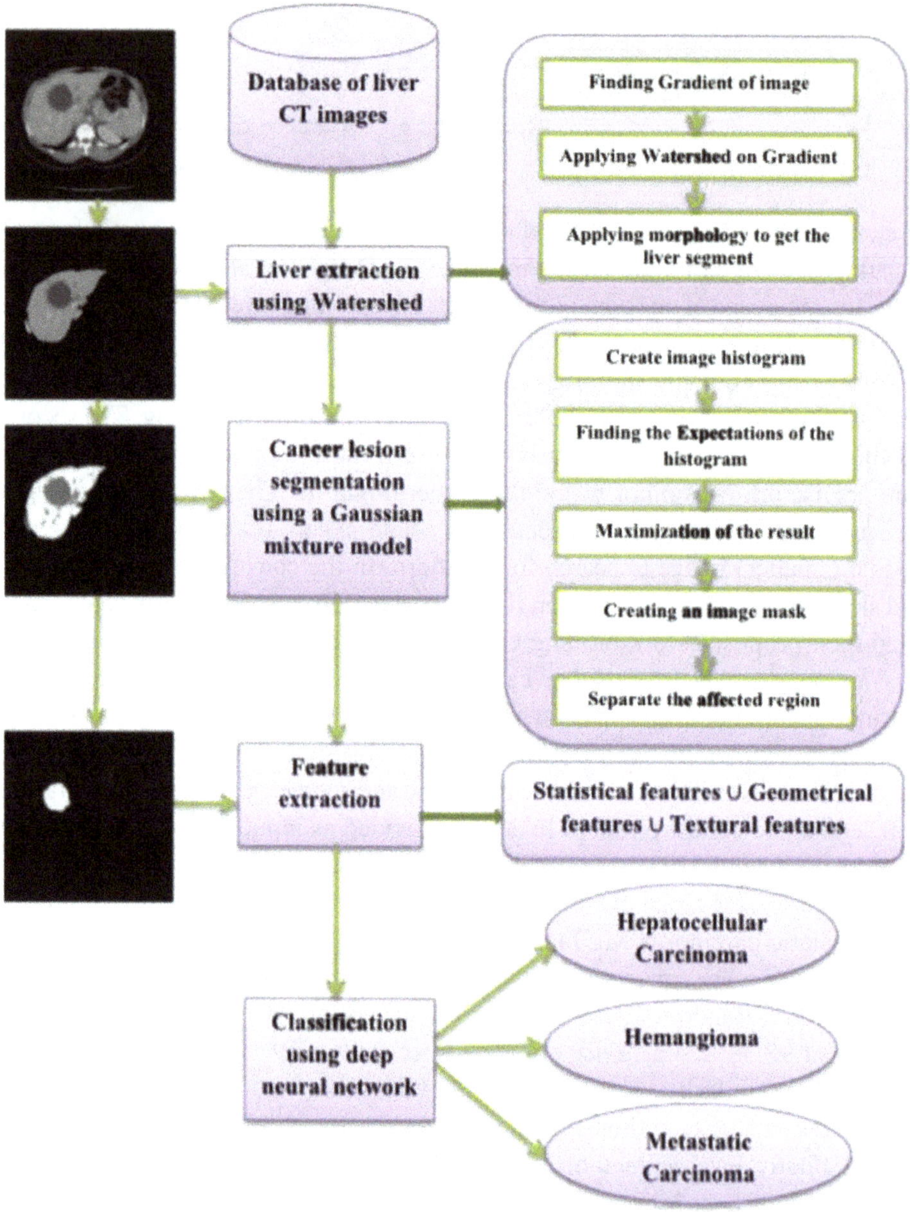

95.7% respectively. The performance was better when compared with 3 traditional machine methods: multi-SVM, KNN, and Naïve Bayes.

(Yang Yu, 2018) have used 100 liver section of images of TAA-induced fibrotic rat using Second Harmonic Generation (SHG) microscopy with automatic feature extraction was carried out by deep learning-based algorithms using the convolution and max pooling layers. The input of AlexNet-CNN was replaced liver fibrosis assessment using SHG image. The 7 hidden layers was made up of 5 convolution layers (with intermediate max pool layer) and 2 fully connected layers i.e. the layer 6 and 7 are 4096-dimension fully connected layers where the input matrix is transformed into a vector for Softmax activation function through General MATRIX Vector Multiply (GEMV) approach. The final output layer has 5 nodes representing outcomes corresponding to the 5 liver fibrosis stages from F0 to F4 using the Metavir scoring (shown in figure 10) . Four conventional algorithms: ANN, MLR, SVM and RF for scoring of liver fibrosis were used using the morphology and textural features of collagen fibers. The proposed fully automated method results were similar to conventional methods. The authors appreciate the deep learning-based approach as a better compared to conventional methods because of two reasons: (a) it automatically finds features and calculates the weight of each feature and (b) transfer learning is helps to deal with the limited dataset.

Figure 10. AlexNet-CNN for predicting 5 liver fibrosis stages from F0 to F4
(Yang Yu, 2018)

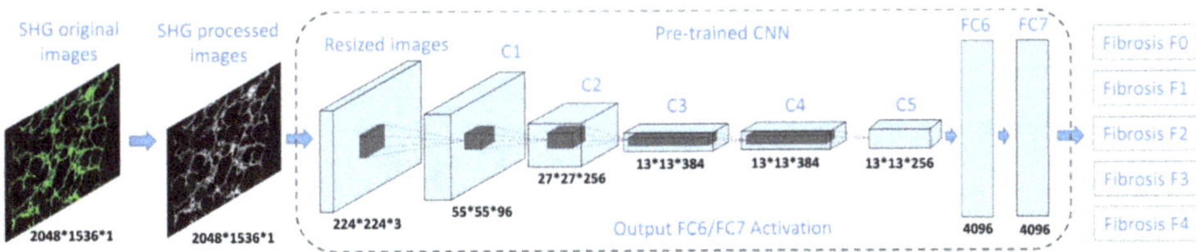

In (Seokmin, 2019), authors have used deep learning framework to differentiate 3 subtypes of renal cell carcinoma: clear cell, papillary, and chromophobe using computed tomography (CT) images. A total of 169 renal cancer cases dataset was acquired with each with three phases: (a) before injection of contrast agent; (b) one minute after the injection and (c) 5 minute after the injection. Radiologists marked the region of interest(ROI). The three-phase input images linearly combined and fed to the GoogLeNet after removal of two auxiliary classifiers to classify the 3 types of renal cell carcinoma. Because transfer learning followed by fine-tuning gives better results, the proposed network by initialized by ImageNet pertaining mode and then fine-tuned using RCC images. They obtained 0.85 accuracy, 0.64–0.98 sensitivity and 0.83-0.93 specificity.

The objective of the work as proposed by (Yafeng Ren, 2019), was given a patient who has been diagnosed with hypertension, predict the probability of the person to suffer from kidney disease. Authors have attempted to study kidney disease prediction in hypertension patients by using a hybrid neural network (shown in figure 12) which incorporates Bidirectional Long Short-Term Memory (BiLSTM) and Autoencoder networks to fully capture the information in Electronic Health Records (EHR). They worked on EHR dataset with 35,332 records from hypertension patients to achieve an accuracy of 89.7%. The textual features from EHR are learnt by BiLSTM and Autoencoder network capturing important numerical cues using numerical indicators from HER.

Figure 11. Bidirectional Long Short-Term Memory (BiLSTM) and Autoencoder networks Model for predicting the probability of person to suffer from kidney disease (Yafeng Ren, 2019)

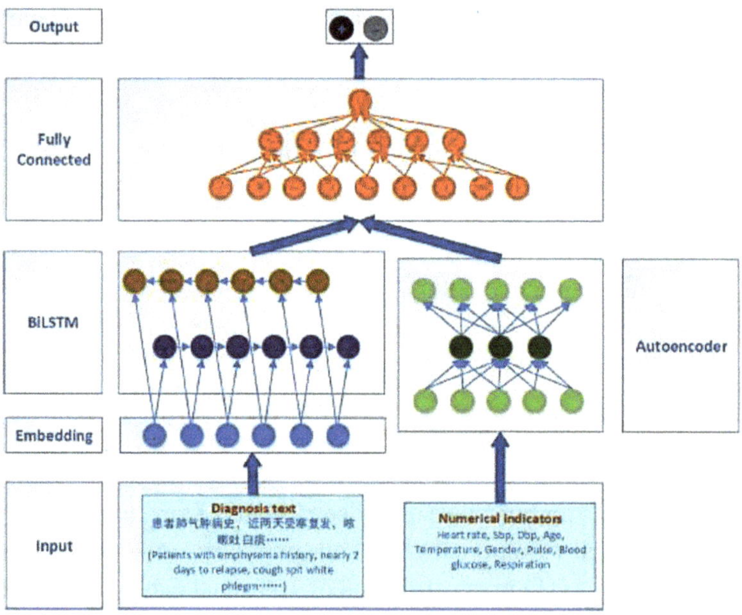

In (Ali, 2018), authors have used CNN (with convolution and maxpooling layers) for extracting hidden features which is fed as input to Extreme Learning Machines (ELM) with radial base function as a kernel function to classify three types of brain tumors including meningioma, glioma and pituitary tumors in T1-weighted contrast-enhanced MRI (CE-MRI) images. Results are compared with traditional classifier which include Support Vector Machine, Radial Base Function, MLP, Stacking, and XGBoost classifiers. The proposes method resulted in an accuracy of 93.68%.

In, (Deepak, 2019), authors focus on a 3-class classification problem to differentiate among glioma, meningioma and pituitary tumors, which form three prominent types of brain tumor. The proposed classification system adopts the concept of deep transfer learning and uses a pre-trained GoogLeNet to extract features from brain MRI images. The fully connected (FC) layer in the original GoogLeNet was replaced by a new FC layer with an output size. The transfer learned model has a softmax classifier layer, which can classify image data from figshare into three tumor classes. The pretrained GoogLeNet provided the low level features and FC of the the modified GoogLeNet was used to study the high-level features specific to the target domain using fighshare dataset as shown in figure 12. The deep CNN features (provided by GoogLeNet) were tested using SVM and K-nearest neighbors classifiers in addition to softmax classifier within deep CNN. The classification accuracy of the deep transfer learned (standalone) was found to be 92.3±0.7% and that of SVM and KNN as 97.8±0.2% and 98.0±0.4%. respectively.

Figure 12. Deep learning architecture proposed by (Deepak, 2019) for tumor detection

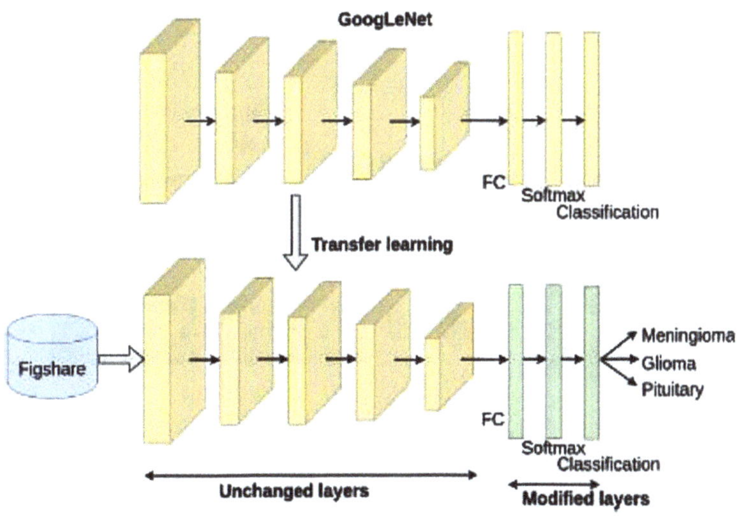

The proposed work for work multi-grade brain tumor classification system (Figure 14) is carried out in three steps: (a) the tumor regions from the dataset are segmented through a InputCascadeCNN CNN model (which contains two streams:

Figure 13. InputCascadeCNN architecture for brain tumor segmentation through two way CNN
(Muhammad Sajjad, 2019)

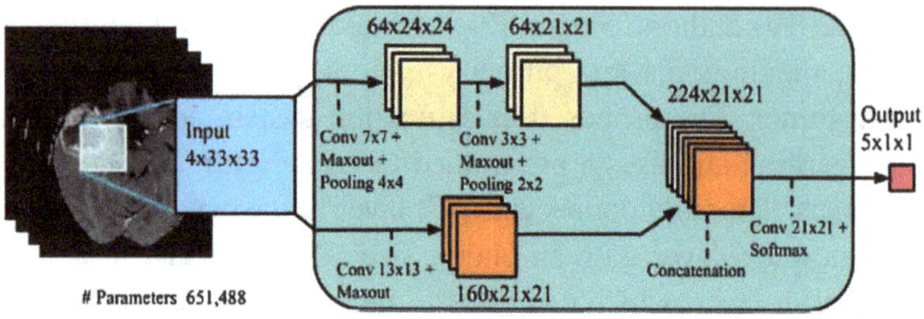

one with 7 × 7 accessible fields for extracting local features and another with 13 × 13 accessible fields for extracting global features) (figure 15), (b) the segmented data is further augmented (using techniques: rotation, flipping, skewness, and shears for geometric transformations invariance, Gaussian blur, sharpening, edge detection, and emboss) to increase the number of data samples, and (c) a pre-trained

Figure 14. Proposed 1-D CNN architecture for beat classification and visualization of the class discriminative sequences in the input heartbeats
(Mihaela, 2019)

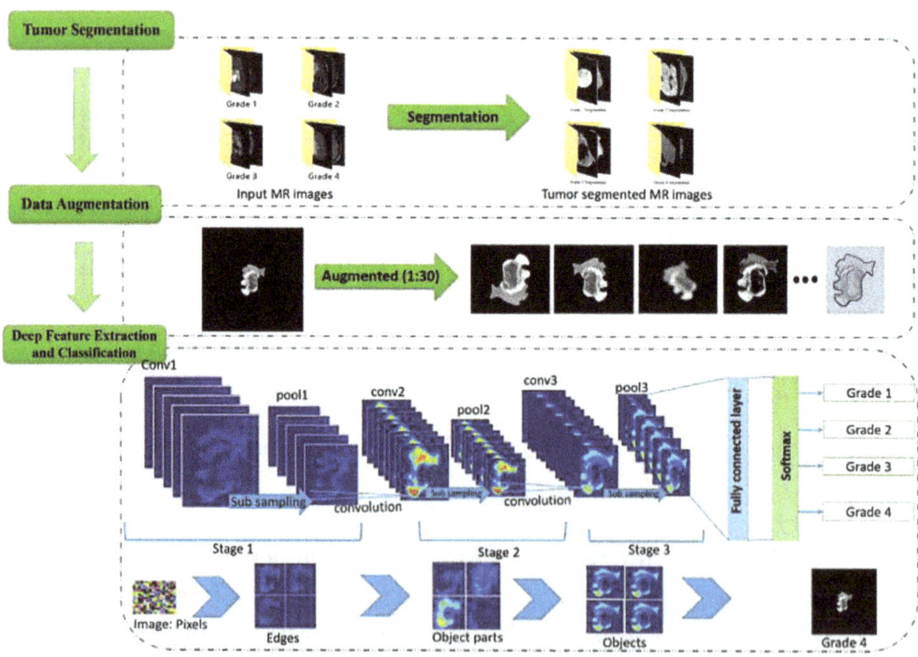

VGG-19 CNN model is fine-tuned trained on MR brain images for final prediction of four grades of tumor (Muhammad Sajjad, 2019) . Proposed method achieved an Sensitivity, Specificity and Accuracy of 88.41%, 96.12% and 94.58% respectively.

Figure 15. CNN assisted multi-grade tumor segmentation and classification framework (Muhammad Sajjad, 2019)

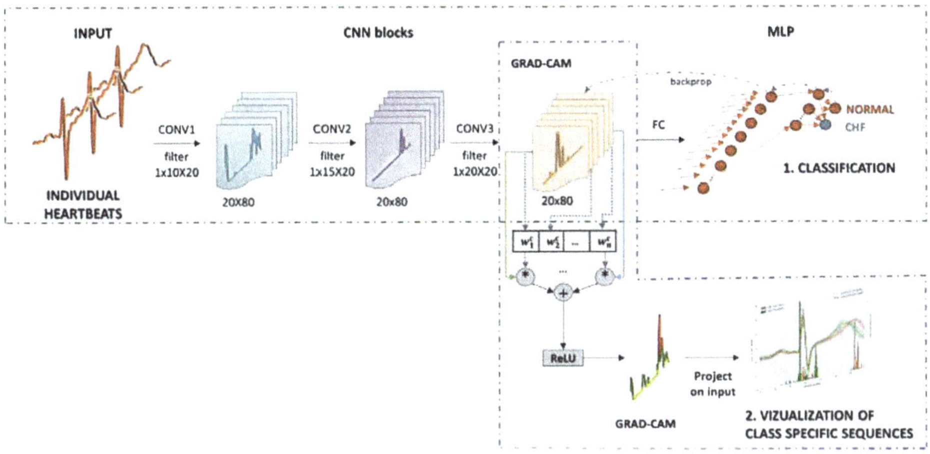

In (Mihaela, 2019), authors have presented CNN model for identifying Congestive Heart Failure(CHF) using raw electrocardiogram(ECG) heartbeat only. CHF is a pathophysiological ailment accountable for the let-down of the heart in pumping blood in the body. They used publicly available ECG BIDMC datasets (Beth Israel Deaconess Medical Center) which includes data related to 490,505 heart-beats. Each heartbeat was labeled with a binary value of 0 or 1 corresponding to healthy or suffering from CHF, respectively. They obtained cent per cent accuracy in detection of CHF by identifying heart beat sequences and ECG's morphological characteristics. Proposed 1-D CNN classifier is depicted in figure 16 is used for feature extraction, and the MLP module for the classification of the raw ECG heartbeats. Work is compared with few of the conventional method on similar kind of dataset in literature study which include: CART based on HRV features; Linear discriminant analysis and Bayesian classifier based on HRV features; k-NN based on HRV features; Non-equilibrium decision-tree, support vector machine classifier based on dynamics of 5-minute short-term HRV measures, SVN and k-NNN on-standard HRV features; and one deep learning method: Raw, 2 seconds ECG based CNN. The performance was measured in terms of accuracy, sensitivity and specificity. The proposed work is different in two aspects: (a) previous work have used raw ECG signals, whereas CNN was applied with HRV features and hence results in better prediction of detecting CHF. (b) They also claim that with advanced machine learning approaches it was first attempt to reveal which morphological characteristics of the ECG beats are the most important to efficiently detect CHF.

Falls are also one of the major health concern in particular for elderly person, since it is the second leading cause of accidental or unintentional injury deaths as mentioned by world health organization(WHO). Authors (Ahemed, 2018), have proposed a robust fall detection system which can serve as an assistive device for detecting and alerting fall incidents by means of an end-to-end deep machine learning model designed using both convolutional and recurrent neural networks. Work is carried out on UR Fall Detection Dataset which has a activities distributed as: falls from standing and sitting on a chair, daily activities such as walking, sitting down, squatting and picking-up an object and sequences with fall-like activities such as lying on wooden sofa and lying on the floor. The visual features from the input sequence of depth frames are extracted by deep convolutional network: ResNet (residual learning network). On top of ResNet lies the Long Short-Term-Memory (LSTM) recurrent neural network module. The LSTM is to learn temporal dynamics which is fed to fully connected layer (logistic regression layer) for recognition of occurrence of a fall event as shown in figure 17. The proposed ConvLSTM is robust enough to focus on human body movements, and overlook static scene objects and outperforms to similar kind of work carried out using SVM.

Figure 16. Hybrid convolutional and recurrent neural networks for fall activity recognition
(Ahemed, 2018)

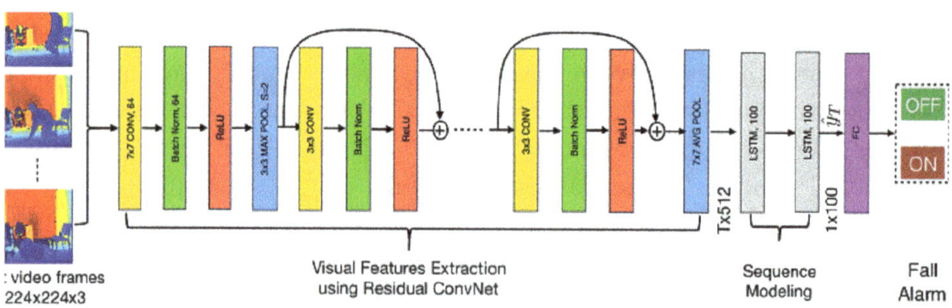

Glaucoma is one of the common causes of blindness, which is caused by progressive damage of the the optic nerve. Authors (Xiangyu Chen, 2015) have used deep learning architecture with 4 convolutional layers and 2 fully connected layers (with dropout layers) for glaucoma detection. To reduce the over fitting problem, response-normalization (using Rectified Linear Units (ReLUs)) layers follow the first and second convolutional layers; followed by Max Pooling layer. In addition both dropout is used to avid over fitting problem and data augmentation to increase the diversity of data set. Work is carried out on SRIGA and SCES datasets. The ROI image is used as the input of the proposed deep Convolutional Neural Network. The area under the curve (AUC) values of 0:831 and 0:887 is obtained for ORIGA and SCES are, respectively using the proposed method for glaucoma detection.

HANDLING IMBALANCED CLASS PROBLEM IN MEDICAL DATASETS

Imbalanced dataset has comparatively less number of observations belonging to one class than those belonging to the other classes. In medical domain, the major problem is imbalanced dataset since pathologic findings are by and large unusual. In addition the dataset may be very small or very large to fit in RAM, may have missing data which affects the performance of the classifier. The three common approaches to handle imbalanced data are:

- Over sampling: Replicate the dataset examples belonging to under- represented class. The drawback is, there is hike in the likelihood of overfitting because of replication of examples of under-represented class.
- Under sampling: Eliminate the percentage of dataset examples belonging to most represented class. The drawback is, discarding potentially useful information which could of importance for building the classifier model.
- Generate synthetic data: Generate new synthetic dataset examples from the under-represented class. The problem of over fitting which occurred in over sampling can be avoided, since a subset of data from the minority class is selected and not replicated but used to generated new synthetic dataset similar to data of minority class.

In addition to the above three methods other methods used for handling imbalanced data using ensemble methods; which modify the classification algorithms to make them apt for imbalanced data sets.

For deep learning, one of the major challenges is insufficient training data which usually leads to overfitting. Few of the techniques commonly adopted by deep learning to overcome the overfitting because of insufficient target data is to include techniques like dropout, transfer learning, and data augmentation.

Data Augmentation

Data augmentation techniques seek to expand the amount of training data automatically by applying automatic transformations to images using various traditional conventional techniques to list a few: horizontal image flips, cropping, translations, rotation, and advanced method which include elastic distortion, tilting, and theme adjustments. Most of the traditional data augmentation techniques usually produce highly correlated image training data. Few of the commonly used augmentation methods include:

- **Color augmentation**: Very simple color augmentations include isolating a single color channel such as R, G, or B followed by and adding 2 zero matrices from the other color channels. In addition, the RGB values can be easily modified by increasing or decreasing the brightness of the image.One more method under color augmentation involves deriving the color histogram followed by changing the intensity values in these histograms.
- **Translation**: In translation method, one can shift the images left, right, up, or down and henceforth to retain the spatial dimension after post augmentation, the remaining spaces are either padded with 0s or 255 or with random or Gaussian noise.
- **Rotation**: Rotation augmentations are carried out by rotating the image right or left on an axis Between 1° and 359°.
- **Noise injection**: It helps to construct CNN to learn more robust features by injecting a matrix of random values usually drawn from a Gaussian distribution.
- **Cropping**: Cropping images involves either cropping the central patch of each image or apply random cropping to provide effect of translation. The difference between cropping and translation is that the former reduces the size of input image whereas the special dimension is preserved in translation.
- **Flipping**: apply flipping either to horizontal or vertical axis and is most easy method to implement augmentation.
- **Mixing images**: Mixing images by averaging their pixel values is a very counterintuitive approach to Data Augmentation which may seem not useful to human observer; use of for used GANs to produce mixed images in the training data not only reduced training time but also enhanced the diversity of GAN samples(Daojun Liang et al.,2018)

In addition among the new upcoming methods GAN based data augmentation is becoming popular to generate synthetic images.

- **GAN based data augmentation**: GANs has two sub-models: the generator model which is trained to generated new (synthetic) instances and the discriminator model decides whether each instance is synthetic/fake/ generated or real one from the domain. The two models are trained together in adversarial; awaiting the discriminator model accepts the plausible instances generated by generator model.

(Hoo et.al., 2018) have applied GAN to generate synthetic brain images with tumor using Alzheimer's Disease Neuroimaging Initiative (ADNI) and Multimodal Brain Tumor Image Segmentation Benchmark: (BRATS) datasets. Since the ADNI data set does not contain tumor information, authors trained the pix2pix model to segment normal brain anatomy from the T1-weighted images of the ADNI data set. The segmentation of neural anatomy, in combination with tumor segmentations provided by the BRATS data set, provide a complete segmentation of the brain with tumor. The GAN is trained to generate synthetic images by merging brain anatomy label (obtained from ADNI dataset) and tumor label separately (from BRATS dataset), by either altering the tumor characteristics such as size, location of the existing brain

Figure 17. GAN based synthetic brain image with tumor
(Hoo et.al., 2018)

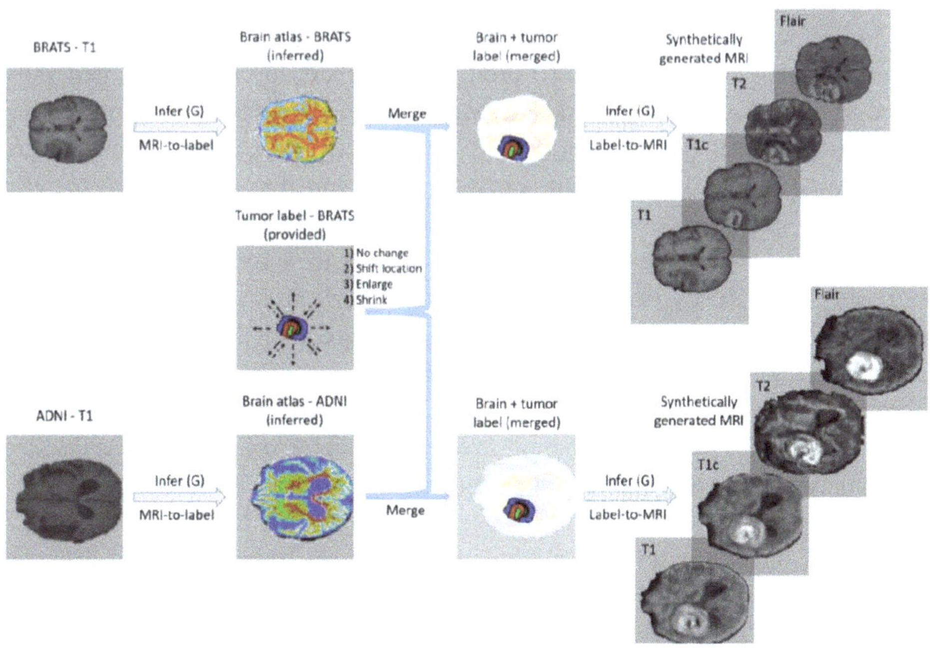

and tumor label set, or place tumor label on an otherwise tumor-free brain label. The process of generating synthetic brain images with tumor is illustrated in figure 18.

(Darius et al., 2019) adopted GAN trained on real human embryo cell images to generate a synthetic dataset of one-, two-, and four-cell embryo images. They have manipulated the size, position, and number of the artificially generated embryo cell images and used these images to train and validate other embryo image processing algorithms, to compensate when there is lack of availability or less number of real embryo images for training neural networks.

Dropout

Dropout is one the solution to avoid over fit a training data of small size by randomly dropping out nodes (i.e. ignoring few neurons chosen randomly) during training (Nitish Srivastava et al., 2014). The neurons may develop co-dependency amongst each other during training which limits the individual power of each neuron progressing to over-fitting of training data. (Xin Hong,2019), have proposed Long short-term memory (LSTM) to predict the next stage of Alzheimer's Disease using dropout concept. Dropout is used to avid over fitting problem for glaucoma detection (Xiangyu Chen, 2015).

Transfer Learning

When we have limited set of data which in not sufficient to train deep neural network then transfer learning is one of the solution. In transfer learning, training of neural network happens in two phases: (i) pre-training, where the network is generally trained on a large-scale benchmark dataset (to extract general features) representing a wide diversity of labels/categories (e.g., ImageNet); and (ii) fine-tuning, where the pre-trained network of first phase is further fine-tuned to extract more specific feature. In context to medical domain, the pre-trained weights of first phase are fine tuned in second phase for specific medical task for interpreting chest x-rays, diagnosing eye diseases, early detection of Alzheimer's disease and so on. The two main benefits of transfer learning are: fast training in second phase, since the model readily uses high level features obtained as part of pre-training phase; and one can manage model with less number of medical data for training in second phase.

Few of the rules of thumb to be followed for transfer learning, based on the size and similarity of the target data with trained dataset are as follows:

- Size of target dataset is small and similar to base training dataset. Transfer learning can has its impact in this case. The last layer of trained dataset is replaced by the fully connected layer depending on the number of class labels of target dataset. The weights of pre-trained phase are freeze and only the new fully connected layer is trained with the target dataset.

- Size of target dataset is small and dissimilar to base training dataset. Transfer learning can has its impact in this case. The last layer of trained dataset is replaced by the fully connected layer depending on the number of class labels of target dataset. Remove most of the pre-trained layers i.e. retain less number of pre-trained layers and freeze the weights of retained pre-trained layers. The new fully connected layer is trained with the target dataset.
- Size of target dataset is large and dissimilar to base training dataset. Transfer learning should not be applied, since the high features extracted by the pre-trained layers are of not much use for classification of target dataset; instead train the ConvNet from scratch using target dataset.

As explained in application section, (Yang Yu, 2018) developed an automated feature classification and liver fibrosis scoring using a transfer learning-based deep learning network, AlexNet-Convolutional Neural Networks (CNN). (Tarek M, 2017), authors have applied deep network with transfer learning for diagnosing focal liver diseases. (Deepak, 2019), adopts the concept of deep transfer learning and uses a pre-trained GoogLeNet to extract features from brain MRI images to differentiate among glioma, meningioma and pituitary tumors.

Medulloblastoma is one of the most common types of malignant brain tumors (Angel et al., 2018) have applied transfer learning for medulloblastoma tumor differentiation using two CNN models trained on natural and histopathology images for visual feature extraction. The first model is a 16 layer deep CNN: Visual Geometry

Figure 18. IBCa-CNN and VGG-CNN based transfer learning for medulloblastoma tumor differentiation
(Angel et al., 2018)

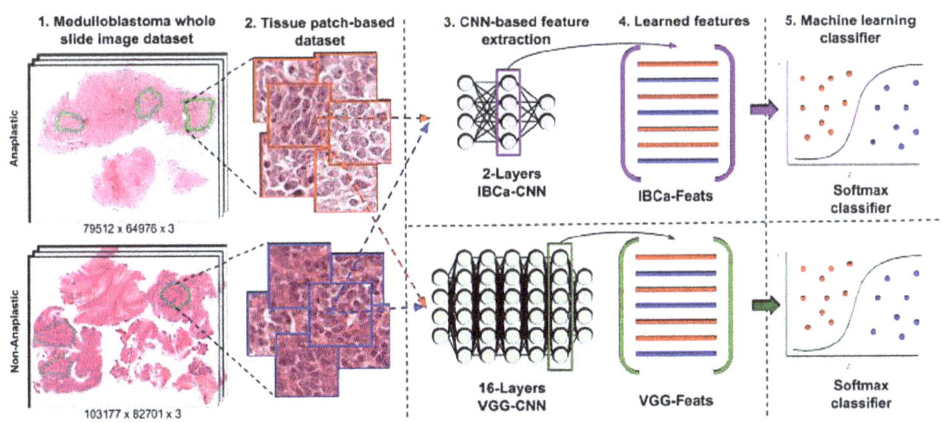

Group (VGG) CNN trained ImageNet dataset. The second one is a 2-layer CNN (IBCa-CNN) trained for classifying breast cancer tumor. The new target dataset is medulloblastoma tumor diffrentiation with set of patches related to anaplastic and non-anaplastic class. Both CNNs are used as visual feature extractors of histopathology image are used separately for training softmax classifier to classify anaplastic and non-anaplastic medulloblastoma tumor (figure 19). IBCa-CNN feature resulted in enhanced accuracy of 89.8% compared to 76.6% accuracy of VGG-CNN. Thus transfer learning trained on histopathology images can be applied for classification task on different imbalanced target data.

General Medical Diagnosis Scheme

From the literature reviewed, few of important steps to model neural network for diagnosis can be stated as follows:

- **Image data transformation:** The past and current studies indicate that it is unnecessary to transform or change data not normally or usually distributed that reveal non-regular periodic development or variant i.e. conventional data augmentation is not much use for medical field. Instead the modification of heteroscedasticity and trends in data are helpful in addition to, data normalization, GAN based transformation are of much use for medical domain for creating synthesized data to handle privacy issues in medical domain as well as for imbalanced data
- **Input model identification:** Input variables can be determined with the support of a priori knowledge, using a stepwise model-building method, transfer learning or analytical method like cross-correlation technique.
- **Network geometry choice**: One hidden layer may be enough as adequate in most network practical uses. However, mathematical expression could determine the upper bound of number of hidden nodes and hidden layer nodes required to approximate continuous function. Except, if non-convergent techniques, like cross-validation, the connection between the quantity of training and the quantity of hidden layer units likewise should be considered. The relationship can be investigated with the guide of the rules given in some literature.
- **Design of phased step for model development:** Researchers can focus on network characteristic at variable specification phase. Also, it is useful to conduct trials in determining required local minimum in the error surface, and oscillations in the R.
- **Training for different neural network operations:** Forecasting with continuous training, with different step sizes taken in weight space. These

steps can be useful when selecting appropriate network parameters like (transfer function, momentum, epoch size, learning rate, and error) and how many training samples in the network for a case study.

- **Validation of model.** The validation of model is necessary for standardization and practical scenarios of ANNs for optimization of performance.

CHALLENGES AND FUTURE DIRECTION DISCUSSIONS

This section will provide details regarding known and unexposed problems of ANN in medical domain and suitable improvements that are to be included in future in order to develop better system design comparatively. The advanced ANN is powerful tool to help physicians for medical diagnosis as second opinion. The major advantages includes: ability to process large amount of data, reduce likelihood of overlooking relevant information, and reduce diagnosis time, automated feature identification for medical diagnosis.

Challenges

- **Lack of large training data sets:** the images used for medical diagnosis are developed or predicted, and for some diseases availability of dataset is more and rest absolute. Even for existing relevant annotations labeling for these images will not be included and in few cases turning reports into accurate annotations or structures labels in an automated manner requires sophisticated text-mining methods.
- **Classification and segmentation:** the medical data or images collected will be presented as binary task for either classification or segmentation. But this task is complex as both classes are normally with high heterogeneity.
- **Handling class imbalance:** Even this problem is currently found to be depending on task at hand. This issue can be solved with application of proper deep learning systems like transfer learning and data augmentation.
- **Standardization:** there is no standard policy and regulations in design of compatible devices or technologies for medical domain. In medical context, many vendors exist, they manufacture range of devices and new vendors join the race leading to interoperability issues. So, immediate actions are to be taken in this direction to provide knowledge to medical experts to handle diversity in medical domain.
- **Necessity to build medical care platforms:** A platform with a service oriented approach has to be taken so that service can be taken considering different application package interfaces together with platform, libraries and

appropriate frameworks should be built. By this, effort medical care software developers and designers will be able to collaborated and construct documents, codes, classes, message templates, and other useful data in an effective and efficient manner. So, that further issues based on disease accessibility will be easier and useful.

- **Development of interactive app:** Regular updates on healthcare apps based on recent advances with inclusion of neural network like concepts with reach audience of interest at faster rate.
- **Require translation of technology:** still efforts are needed to move from legacy system to new medical diagnostic based approaches. Meanwhile there is a need to ensure backward compatibility and flexibility in the integration of existing devices.
- **New disease and disorders:** Continuous monitoring efforts are required from research and development activities to identify new type of diseases and disorders. The early detection will be bone for many individuals for long been an important task.
- **Data protection steps to be strengthened:** The data under analysis or being diagnosed requires protection from illicit access. Hence, stern polices and technical measures have to be devised at organization and Government level. The optimal security algorithms can also be developed between protection, detection, and reaction services to prevent various attacks, threats, and vulnerabilities.

Future Directions

This research essentially requires many areas in need of further investigation. Further research is required in the following areas:

- A greater focus on adaptive dynamic programming (ADP) could produce interesting findings that account more for significant contributions in the area of brain research and computational intelligence.
- Emerging topic in engineering and computer science include parameter adjustment technique in machine learning algorithms. The successful use of algorithms optimization in adjusting network variables should be well studied.
- Further investigation into the applications of reinforcement-learning, unsupervised, semi-supervised methods to the deep neural network for complex and multi-complex systems.
- Future research should concentrate on the use of intelligent analysis such as neural network models, back propagation neural networks, probabilistic

neural network, supervised associating networks, multi-layer perceptron neural network architectures, learning vector quantization, multi-layer neural network, and hybrid neural network models, since they promise better performance in the for diverse challenges of life-science applications.

- Since the use of inferential statistics and neural networks can be more predictive in data analysis. Hence, the predictive approach can also be another focus in the study of the subject in particular using recurrent networks (e.g. LSTM) because in many cases prediction of health related issues is more significant than just diagnosis.
- Research is required for implementation of DL algorithms interfacing with mobile gadgets. As recently, DL chips idea emerged that is attracting research interest.
- Public awareness training on artificial network neural models should continue regularly, especially on the need for providing useful information using empirical analysis and digital data.
- More investigation is required in the stability analysis of deep NN because, in recent times, the DNNs stability analysis has become a hot topic for research focus due to its advantages in many industrial sectors.
- With the new trend in big data technique, DL would be useful where large amounts of un-supervised data are applied. It would be interesting to construct DL models that can learn from fewer training data, particularly for visual and speech recognition systems.
- Further research should focus on the use of DNNs to nonlinear networked control systems. More understanding of complicated dynamics would help us establish how to obtain better performances in control, and filtering capability effectively and efficiently.
- The governments and institutions need to provide funds to carry out research in diverse application of neural networks for success, especially in this era of modern education, technology advancement, industrial growth, economic challenges, artificial intelligence development, and information and communication revolution.

CONCLUSION

This chapter reviews various techniques, architectures of both conventional and nonconventional ANN in general. Few of the conventional ANN have proved to be equally good with those of the nonconventional ANN in terms of accuracy. But the very fact that the nonconventional ANN are robust enough to handle noisy input and identify features autonomously, are few of key reasons for its popularity over conventional ANN methods. The chapter covers applications of Deep learning on various medical cases. One of the major drawbacks of CNN is that they need huge training data. In medical domain, the major problem is imbalanced dataset since pathologic findings are by and large unusual. Various methods to handle this imbalanced data are briefed with medical domain case studies. However, despite of wide application of ANN in modern diagnosis, they must be considered only as a tool to facilitate the final decision of a clinician, who is ultimately responsible for critical evaluation of the both conventional and nonconventional ANN diagnosis. Lastly the challenges and future scope of ANN for medical domain is discussed.

REFERENCES

Abobakr, Hossny, Abdelkader, & Nahavandi. (2018). *RGB-D Fall Detection via Deep Residual Convolutional LSTM Networks*. IEEE.

Altunay, Telatar, Erogul, & Aydur. (2009). A New Approach to urinary system dynamics problems: Evaluation and classification of uroflowmeter signals using artificial neural networks. *Expert Systems with Applications*, *36*(3), 4891–4895.

Ameer. (2019). Brain tumor classification using deep CNN features via transfer learning. *Computers in Biology and Medicine*, *111*, 103345. PMID:31279167

Angel, Arevalo, Judkins, Madabhushi, & Gonzalez. (n.d.). A method for Medulloblastoma Tumor Differentiation based on Convolutional Neural Networks and Transfer Learning. *Conference: Proc. SPIE 9681, 11th International Symposium on Medical Information Processing and Analysis*. DOI: 10.1117/12.2208825

Bakator & Radosav. (2018). Deep Learning and Medical Diagnosis: A Review of Literature. *Multimodal Technologies and Interact, 2*, 47. doi:10.3390/mti2030047

Bolboca. (2019). *Medical diagnosis tests: a test anatomy, phases and statistical treatment of data*. Hindawi.

Catalogna, Cohen, Fishman, Halpern, Nevo, & Ben-Jacob. (2012). ANN based controller for gloucose monitoring during, clamp test. *PLoS One*, *7*, e44587.

Cetiner, Sari, & Aburas. (2009). Recognition of dengue disease patterns using artificial neural networks. *Proceedings of the 5th International Advanced Technologies Symposium (IATS'09)*, 359–362.

Chen, Xu, Wong, Wong, & Liu. (2015). Glaucoma Detection based on Deep Convolutional Neural Network. *2015 37th Annual International Conference of the IEEE Engineering in Medicine and Biology Society (EMBC)*. Doi:10.1109/EMBC.2015.7318462

Daojun, Feng, Tian, & Peter. (2018). Understanding mixup training methods. *IEEE Access, 6*, 58774- 58783.

Das, Acharya, Panda, & Sabut. (2019). Deep learning based liver cancer detection using watershed transform and Gaussian mixture model techniques. *Cognitive Systems Research*, *54*, 165–175.

Das, Turkoglu, & Sengur. (2009). Effective diagnosis of heart disease through neural networks ensembles. *Expert Systems with Applications*, *36*(4), 7675–7680.

Dirvanauskas, Maskeli, Raudonis, Damaševiˇcius, & Scherer. (2019). *HEMIGEN: Human Embryo Image Generator Based on Generative Adversarial Networks Sensors*. Academic Press.

Dutta. (2014). Neural network-based models for software effort estimation: a review. *Artif. Intell. Rev., 42*(2), 295-307.

Francisco, Manuel, Antonio, & Daniel. (2008). A robust model of the neuronal regulator of the lower urinary tract based on artificial neural networks. *Neurocomputing*, *71*(4-6), 743–754.

Gil, Johnsson, Garicia Chemizo, Paya, & Fernandez. (2009). Application of Artificial Neural Networks in the Diagnosis of Urological Dysfunctions. *Expert Systems with Applications*, *36*(3), 5754–5760.

Han, Hwang, & Lee. (2019). The Classification of Renal Cancer in 3-Phase CT Images Using a Deep Learning Method. *Journal of Digital Imaging*, *32*, 638–643. doi:10.100710278-019-00230-2]

Hassan, Elmogy, & Sallam. (2017). Diagnosis of Focal Liver Diseases Based on Deep Learning Technique for Ultrasound Images. *Arabian Journal for Science and Engineering*. Advance online publication. doi:10.100713369-016-2387-9]

He & Garcia. (2009). Learning from imbalanced data. *IEEE Trans. Knowl. Data Eng., 21*(9), 1263-1284.

Heckerling, Canaris, Flach, Tape, Wigton, & Gerber. (2007). Predictors of urinary tract infection based on artificial neural networks and genetic algorithms. *International Journal of Medical Informatics*, *76*(4), 289–296. PMID:16469531

Hong, Lin, Yang, Zeng, Cai, Gou, & Yang. (2019). Predicting Alzheimer's Disease Using LSTM. *IEEE Access: Practical Innovations, Open Solutions*. Advance online publication. doi:10.1109/ACCESS.2019.2919385

Ibrahim, Taib, Abas, Guan, & Sulaiman. (2005). A novel dengue fever (DF) and dengue haemorrhagi fever (DHF) analysis using artificial neural network (ANN). *Computer Methods and Programs in Biomedicine*, *79*(3), 273–281. PMID:15925426

Izeboudjen, Larbes, & Farah. (2014). A new classification approach for neural networks hardware: from standards chips to embedded systems on chip. *Artif. Intell. Rev., 41*(4), 491-534.

Jakimovski & Davcev. (2019). Using Double Convolution Neural Network for Lung Cancer Stage Detection. *Applied Sciences (Basel, Switzerland)*, *9*, 427. doi:10.3390/app9030427]

Liu, Cai, Pujol, Kikinis, & Feng. (2014). *Early Diagnosis of Alzheimer's Disease with Deep Learning*. IEEE.

Moein, Monadjemi, & Moallem. (2009). A Novel Fuzzy-Neural Based Medical Diagnosis System. *International Journal of Biological & Medical Sciences*, *4*(3), 146–150.

Monadjemi & Moallem. (2008). Automatic Diagnosis of Particular Diseases Using a Fuzzy-Neural Approach. *International Review on Computers & Software*, *3*(4), 406–411.

Mozaffari, Emami, & Fathi. (2018). A comprehensive investigation into the performance, robustness, scalability and convergence of chaos-enhanced evolutionary algorithms with boundary constraints. *Artificial Intelligence Review*, ▪▪▪, 1–62.

Pashaei, S., & Jazayeri. (2018). Brain Tumor Classification via Convolutional Neural Network and Extreme Learning Machines. In *8th International Conference on Computer and Knowledge Engineering (ICCKE 2018)*. Ferdowsi University of Mashhad.

Pearce, Wong, Mirtskhulava, AlMajeed, Bakuria, & Gulua. (2016). Artificial Neural Network and Mobile Applications in Medical Diagnosis. *2015 17th UKSimAMSS International Conference on Modelling and Simulation*.

Porumb, Iadanza, Massarod, & Pecchia. (2020). A convolutional neural network approach to detect congestive heart failure. *Biomedical Signal Processing and Control*, *55*, 101597. doi:10.1016/j.bspc.2019.101597

Rachata, Charoenkwan, Yooyativong, Chamnongthal, Lursinsap, & Higuchi. (2008). Automatic prediction system of dengue haemorrhagic-fever outbreak risk by using entropy and artificial neural network. In *Proceedings of the International Symposium on Communications and Information Technologies*. IEEE.

Raval, Bhatt, Kumhar, Parikh, & Vyas. (2016). Medical diagnosis system using machine learning. *International Journal of Computer Science & Communication, 7*(1), 177–182.

Razzak, Naz, & Zaib. (2017). *Deep Learning for Medical Image Processing: Overview, Challenges and Future*. arXiv:1704.06825v1

Razzak, Naz, & Zaib. (2017). *Deep Learning for Medical Image Processing: Overview, Challenges and Future, DL for medical imaging*. Cornell university.

Ren, Fei, Liang, Ji, & Cheng. (2019). A hybrid neural network model for predicting kidney disease in hypertension patients based on electronic health records. *BMC Medical Informatics and Decision Making, 19*(Suppl 2), 51. doi:10.118612911-019-0765-4

Sajjad, Khan, Muhammad, Wu, Ullah, & Baik. (2019). Multi-grade brain tumor classification using deep CNN with extensive data augmentation. *Journal of Computational Science*, *30*, 174–182.

Serj, Lavi, Hoff, & Valls. (2018). *A Deep Convolutional Neural Network for Lung Cancer Diagnostic*. arXiv:1804.08170

Shin, Tenenholtz, Rogers, Schwarz, Senjem, Gunter, Andriole, & Michalski. (2018). *Medical Image Synthesis for Data Augmentation and Anonymization using Generative Adversarial Networks*. arXiv:1807.10225v2

Srivastava, Hinton, Krizhevsky, Salakhutdinov, & Sutskever. (2014). Dropout: a simple way to prevent neural networks from overfitting. *JMLR*.

van Ginneken & S´anchez. (2017). *A Survey on Deep Learning in Medical Image Analysis*. arXiv,1702.05747v2

Wang, He, & Liu. (2018). Intelligent optimal control with critic learning for a nonlinear overhead crane system. *IEEE Transact. Ind. Inf., 14*(7), 2932-2940.

Yu, Wang, Ng, Ma, Mo, Li, Fong, Xing, Song, Xie, Si, Wee, Welsch, So, & Yu. (2018). Deep learning enables automated scoring of liver fibrosis stages. *Scientific Reports*, *8*(16016). Advance online publication. doi:10.103841598-018-34300-2

Chapter 2
Deep Learning for Medical Image Segmentation

Kanchan Sarkar
Indian Institute of Technology, Bombay, India

Bohang Li
Peking University, China

ABSTRACT

Pixel accurate 2-D, 3-D medical image segmentation to identify abnormalities for further analysis is on high demand for computer-aided medical imaging applications. Various segmentation algorithms have been studied and applied in medical imaging for many years, but the problem remains challenging due to growing a large number of variety of applications starting from lung disease diagnosis based on x-ray images, nucleus detection, and segmentation based on microscopic pictures to kidney tumour segmentation. The recent innovation in deep learning brought revolutionary advances in computer vision. Image segmentation is one such area where deep learning shows its capacity and improves the performance by a larger margin than its successor. This chapter overviews the most popular deep learning-based image segmentation techniques and discusses their capabilities and basic advantages and limitations in the domain of medical imaging.

INTRODUCTION

Image segmentation is the process in computer vision to assign a label to each pixel in an image. Image segmentation splits the input image into different connected components based on some user-defined high-level semantics. Image segmentation

DOI: 10.4018/978-1-7998-5071-7.ch002

Copyright © 2021, IGI Global. Copying or distributing in print or electronic forms without written permission of IGI Global is prohibited.

and object detection have numerous applications in medical imaging. This chapter would explain different types of image segmentation and their application in the domain of medical imaging. The chapter would mainly highlight the important contribution of deep learning in image segmentation. In this chapter, the author discusses various state-of-the-art image segmentation techniques, different evaluation metrics and their application in medical imaging. This chapter also highlights popular open-source tools that use for medical image segmentation data labelling. The chapter ends with an implementation detail of instance segmentation for medical image.

In existing cutting-edge technology of image segmentation, pixel-level dense prediction can achieve an extremely good accuracy which is safe and convenient for medical image processing purposes. Currently, some medical diagnosis tasks are searching for image segmentation technique's support, for example, lung disease diagnosis based on X-ray images, nucleus detection, and segmentation based on microscopic pictures and kidney tumour segmentation. And even some techniques like U-Net and etc. are designed specifically for medical image segmentation usage. Meanwhile, to make deep learning-based segmentation and such AI technology much quicker apply in the medical field, there are quite of competitions are hosted publicly.

For the same purpose, this chapter has a brief overview of segmentation technology and the state of the art models for different subtasks. First, the authors give an explanation for image segmentation types, mainly for discriminating between traditional and deep learning-based methods. The authors focus on the illustration of different kinds of deep learning-based image segmentation models that are suitable for different scenarios in medical imaging.

Usually, it is not enough for real application by just segmenting the objects, for which the authors introduce in the 3rd section some post-processing techniques to refine the segmentation mask. For completeness, in the last two parts, the chapter describes how to augment your own custom dataset that helps to get better results and how to implement 2-3 classical image segmentation models that help you do some quick experiments with your own dataset.

So, this complete chapter overviews the most popular deep learning-based medical image segmentation techniques and discusses their capabilities, their use cases in a medical imaging application, data labelling, data augmentation, post-processing of segmented mask, and basic advantages and limitations.

IMAGE SEGMENTATION

Image segmentation is the process in computer vision to assign a label to each pixel in an image. Image segmentation splits the input image into different connected components based on some user-defined high-level semantics. Image segmentation and object detection have numerous applications in medical imaging. Here are a few use cases where image segmentation shows its capabilities in medical imaging which is not limited to lung disease diagnosis based on X-Ray images, nucleus detection and segmentation based on microscopic pictures, kidney tumour segmentation and many more. This section explains the different early traditional methods for image segmentation.

Thresholding

Thresholding is an early approach of segmentation where the image is segmented based on a threshold for each pixel intensity value. If the pixel intensity is greater than a pre-defined threshold it is considered as foreground pixel else belongs to background pixel. This method sometimes called ROI (Region of Interest) segmentation. Figure 1 is a typical grey level histogram of an image. At the pixel value "a" there is a deep valley on the histogram. The image can be segmented in background and foreground object based on the threshold value "a". Thresholding is an early and novice approach of segmentation that can not be applied to sophisticated segmentation i.e instance segmentation, semantic segmentation and, images with multiple objects.

Figure 1. ROI Segmentation

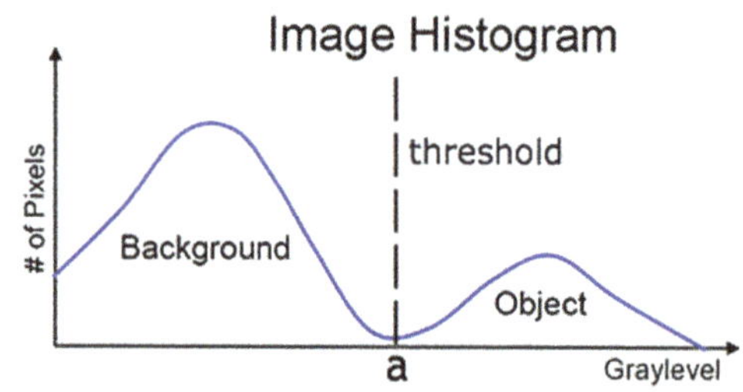

Clustering Method

K-Means is a very popular clustering algorithm that is used to partition an image into k different clusters. The algorithms start with an initial k cluster centers which are selected manually, randomly or based on some initial heuristics. Iteratively the image is partitioned and each pixel of the image is assigned to one cluster (out of k cluster) which has a minimum distance between the pixel and cluster centers. Normally euclidean distance is used to calculate the distance metric. Once each pixel is assigned to a particular cluster, the cluster centers are readjusted as the mean of all the pixels within the cluster. K-means try to minimize the intra-cluster distance and maximize inter-cluster centers distance. k-means is one of the early approaches of image segmentation which works well when the k is properly selected. The segmentation results may not be always optimal but the algorithm is guaranteed to converge. For the distance calculation k-means uses low-level feature i.e color, location, blob, texture, edges which is unable to capture high-level object-specific semantic information which sometimes results in bad quality segmentation.

Motion and Interactive Segmentation

Motion-based segmentation is a way to understand the changes in images to segment the object of interest. Given multiple images or multiple frames of a video, assuming the object of interest only moves, motion segmentation detects the background and do background subtraction comparing different pair of images to segment the object. Motion-based segmentation is a very simple approach that can be efficiently applied to video object segmentation where the camera is fixed and only the object moves. *(Jacqueline, 2009)* proposed an improved version of motion-based segmentation where they use a robot to poke each of the objects of interest to generate motion to segment the object in an iterative manner.

Compression Based Method

Image segmentation method can be posed as a compression problem where out of all the possible segmentation of an image the one that minimizes data based on some coding length is the best possible segmentation solution. Segmentation tries to find an object which has a pattern and regularity in structure. If the object is compress based on low-level features i.e texture, color, boundary shape the coding length would be minimal. Compression based segmentation generates multiple segmentation candidates, and model each of them as a probability distribution function. The coding length scheme encodes the boundary as Huffman coding and the texture of the object as lossy compression. Coding length scheme generates the number of bits required to encode each of the segmentation. Among all the possible solution the segmentation which requires less number of bits to represent is the best solution.

Edge Detection

Edge detection is well studied and very popular in image processing which finds the pixels with sharp intensity changes. The most popular edge detection methods are the Sobel edge detector and the Canny edge detector. There is a close relationship between edge and object boundaries in an image. Once the edges are properly detected that information can be used in image segmentation to increase efficiency and improve the segmentation quality. This method is called guided segmentation where the segmentation algorithm uses edge detection as prior information. (*Lindeberg,1997)* are some of the early approaches which use edge detection that detects straight and curves edges into an image segmentation algorithm.

Graph-Based Method

GrabCut *(Boykov, 2001)* is the most popular method in graph-based segmentation algorithms. GrabCut is also widely used for interactive image segmentation and segmentation data annotation where the user provides input for background, foreground, probable background and probable foreground pixels. GrabCut is a min-cut max-flow energy maximization method. The GrabCut uses a Gaussian Mixture model to find the color distributions of the foreground and background pixel based on the user input for background, foreground, probable background and probable foreground pixels. Because of the low-level color-dependent features, GrabCut may not always capture high-level semantic information of an object which results in bad quality segmentation. The implementation of GrabCut is available in most of the image processing framework i.e Matlab, OpenCV. Figure 2 is an example of

Figure 2. GrabCut - an iterative image segmentation
(Boykov, 2001)

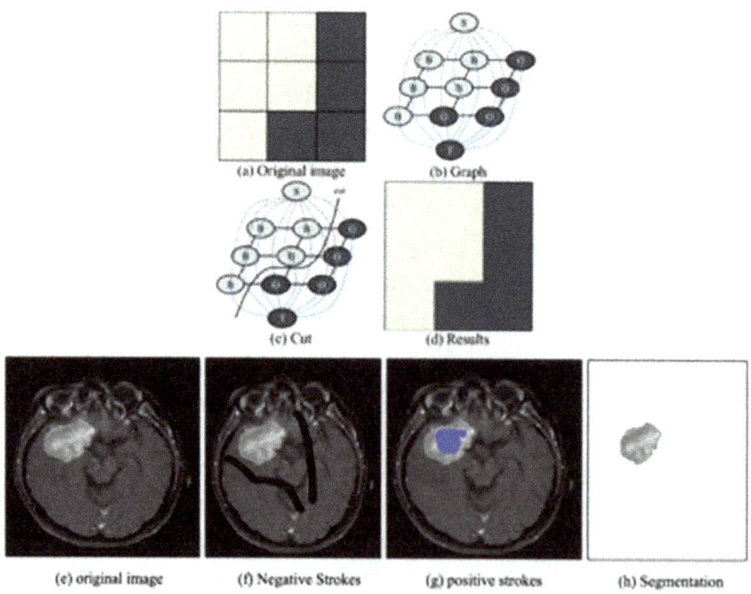

GrabCut Image segmentation where the user provides positive and negative brush for the object of interest.

Deep Learning-Based Method

The recent advances in deep learning show its capability in computer vision and AI. The deep learning-based method improves the quality of image segmentation in all applications. A Convolutional Neural Network (CNNs) is the basic building block for deep learning-based image segmentation. The next section describes most of the popular deep learning-based models for image segmentation.

DEEP LEARNING FOR IMAGE SEGMENTATION

This section describes the recent advances in deep learning and their application in medical image segmentation.

Convolutional Neural Network

Convolutional Neural Network(CNN) *(Krizhevsky, 2012)* has brought another round of prosperity to the field of computer vision since AlexNet *(Krizhevsky, 2012)* proposed in ImageNet Competition 2012. Today talking about deep learning technology in computer vision tasks is mainly based on CNN architecture.

For your convenience to have a better understanding of the next sections, this section gives a short brief about CNN. Generally speaking, CNN can be seen as a feature extractor, through which a model can automatically extract features from an image, rather than using traditional hand-crafted features. This kind of feature automatic extractor decreases the top-5 error rate dramatically from 28% to 6%, which proved learnable features is much more powerful than hand-crafted features like HOG (Histogram of the Oriented Gradient) etc. To make the best use of the powerful features in different tasks, CNN architecture can be described as follows,

1. CNN + classifier(softmax, sigmoid, SVM) for classification tasks.
2. CNN + classifier + regressor for object detection tasks.
3. CNN + pixel-level classifier for semantic segmentation tasks.
4. …

In detail, given a 3-channel(RGB) image, need to define a 3-channel kernel to do the convolutional computation, called convolution layer, in a sliding window with the input image. Then the model obtains a feature map which has a smaller size. For training to converge, there will be a ReLU (Rectified Linear Unit) layer following with convolution layer. After ReLU, there is a pooling layer for further downsampling which will make the feature map smaller again. Above 3 steps constitute the basic CNN operation group. Usually, those 3 steps are repeated to expand the depth of a neural network for better presentation capability. The final layer will be a fully connected layer to flatten the feature map from (N, W, H) to 1-d vector for the classifier in the next stage, where N denotes the number of channels in the last feature map. As shown in Figure 3, the CNN architecture converts an input image from a 3-channel matrix to 1-d feature vector.

Figure 3. CNN Architecture
(Alex, 2012)

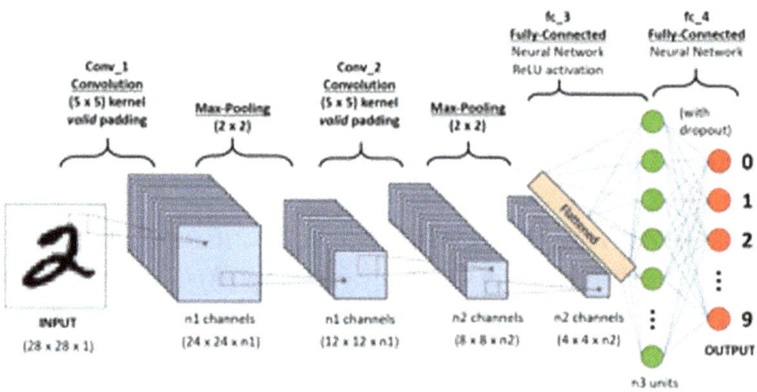

In general, there are 3 hyper-parameters to describe a convolutional neural network.

1. Depth
2. Width
3. Cardinality

Due to that CNN has been an entrance for different deep learning-based computer vision tasks, conventionally the CNN is called as a backbone. And with more and more research in CNN architecture, data scientists designed more and more advanced backbone networks by changing the networks' depth, width and cardinality for efficiency, precision and many other purposes.

Up to now, you should have a big picture of CNN architecture. Based on this, the following parts of this section you will learn more about backbone networks, classification, object detection and segmentation as well as the link between segmentation tasks and medical images processing field.

Convolutional Neural Network for Image Classification

As mentioned at the very beginning of this section, classification tasks can be seen as a foundation of deep learning-based computer vision field, either detection or segmentation models are all based on classification networks. And that is also the reason why these classification networks are called as a backbone network.

LeNet *(LeCun, 1998)*, developed by Yan Lecun in 1998, which for the first time introduced CNN into image classification and made a great success, has only 5 layers in-depth as shown in Fig 3.2. However, ResNet *(He, 2016)*, developed by Kaiming He in 2016 increased the depth to 152 layers as shown in Fig 3.3 and with a dramatic decrease in error rate.

It is not easy all the way to the current state-of-the-art model, data scientists take a lot of experiments, add a lot of new operations and even use some of the training tricks to get today's achievements. So it is very important to get some ideas about some extremely classical classification networks and how they are actually improved step by step.

Alex Net

Let's start with Alex Net *(Krizhevsky, 2012)* which is the championship of ImageNet Competition 2012. After LeNet, VGG *(Simonyan, 2014)* is another image classification model who astonished the world. Figure 4 is the architecture of LeNet.

Figure 4. LeNet-5
(Szegedy, 2015)

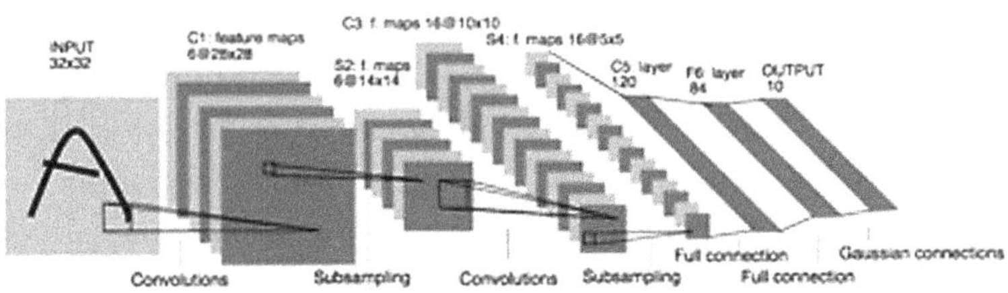

The AlexNet architecture is shown in Figure 5, as you can see, all of the operations are the combinations of convolutional computation, activate function and pooling,

Figure 5. AlexNet
(Krizhevsky, 2012)

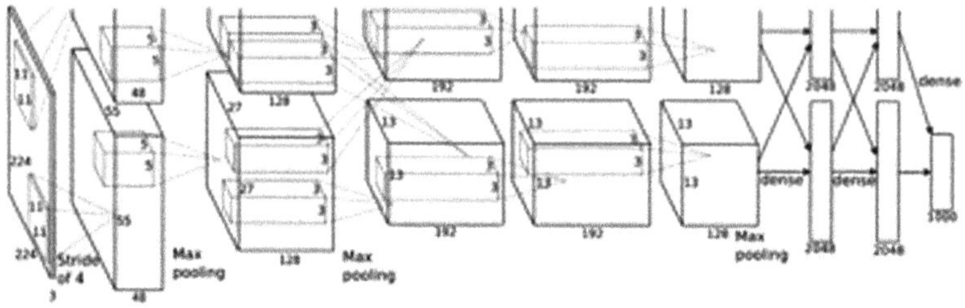

just like it has been discussed at the very beginning of this section. It constrained the input image size as 224*224*3, and first introduced ReLU function as an active method. In addition, it broadens LeNet from 84 to 2048 and depthen the LeNet from 5 layers to 8 layers.

VGG Net

VGG Net *(Simonyan, 2014)*, proposed by the University of Oxford, is the 2nd classification network in ILSVRC2014 Competition. The main architecture keeps similar with AlexNet, a stack of convolution layers including pooling layers and 3 fully connected(FC) layers. According to the different number of weights layers, there are VGG-11, VGG-13, VGG-16, VGG-19, the detailed structures are shown in Figure 6(note:conv-3-128 means 3*3 kernel conv layers with 128 channels). Among all VGG-16 and VGG-19 have the best performance in the paper's experiment. One thing that needs to be noticed is the author proved that a stack of 2 conv-3(3*3 kernel convolution layer) layers has an effective receptive field of conv-5, so that in VGG Net, all Conv layers are using 3*3 kernels.

GoogLeNet

GooLeNet *(Szegedy, 2015)*, a salute to LeNet, was proposed by Google in 2014. Basically, GooLeNet refers to a network family including Inception v1, Inception v2, Inception v3 and Inception v4. Due to the networks in this family are of high similarity in structure, this chapter introduces them into different sub-section. In general, these networks not only further deepen the network to much deeper layers(22 layers) but also firstly introduce 1*1 convolution, which can largely reduce the number of parameters, into the backbone network.

Figure 6. Structure of VGGNet
(Simonyan, 2014)

ConvNet Configuration					
A	A-LRN	B	C	D	E
11 weight layers	11 weight layers	13 weight layers	16 weight layers	16 weight layers	19 weight layers
input (224 × 224 RGB image)					
conv3-64	conv3-64 **LRN**	conv3-64 **conv3-64**	conv3-64 conv3-64	conv3-64 conv3-64	conv3-64 conv3-64
maxpool					
conv3-128	conv3-128	conv3-128 **conv3-128**	conv3-128 conv3-128	conv3-128 conv3-128	conv3-128 conv3-128
maxpool					
conv3-256 conv3-256	conv3-256 conv3-256	conv3-256 conv3-256	conv3-256 conv3-256 **conv1-256**	conv3-256 conv3-256 **conv3-256**	conv3-256 conv3-256 conv3-256 **conv3-256**
maxpool					
conv3-512 conv3-512	conv3-512 conv3-512	conv3-512 conv3-512	conv3-512 conv3-512 **conv1-512**	conv3-512 conv3-512 **conv3-512**	conv3-512 conv3-512 conv3-512 **conv3-512**
maxpool					
conv3-512 conv3-512	conv3-512 conv3-512	conv3-512 conv3-512	conv3-512 conv3-512 **conv1-512**	conv3-512 conv3-512 **conv3-512**	conv3-512 conv3-512 conv3-512 **conv3-512**
maxpool					
FC-4096					
FC-4096					
FC-1000					
soft-max					

Inception v1

GoogLeNet first proposed a module called Inception, which combines the results of convolution layers with different kernel size in the channel dimension. As shown in Figure 7, for a more powerful presentation of features, GoogLeNet introduces 1*1, 3*3 and 5*5 kernel size respectively. And in order to reduce the number of parameters, an extra layer of 1*1 convolution is added. By doing that, it can reduce ¾ parameters without any trade-off on accuracy(even increased by 0.6%). This kind of module is so named as Inception, because of the extra 1*1 convolution layer. The whole network consists of 9 repeated Inception module with 22 layers in depth.

Inception v2

GoogLeNet Inception v2 *(Ioffe, 2015)* network adopts almost the same architecture with Inception v1 while the modification lies mainly in normalization processing. In the previous version, they use dropout technology for regularization and prevention of

Figure 7. Inception Module
(Szegedy, 2015)

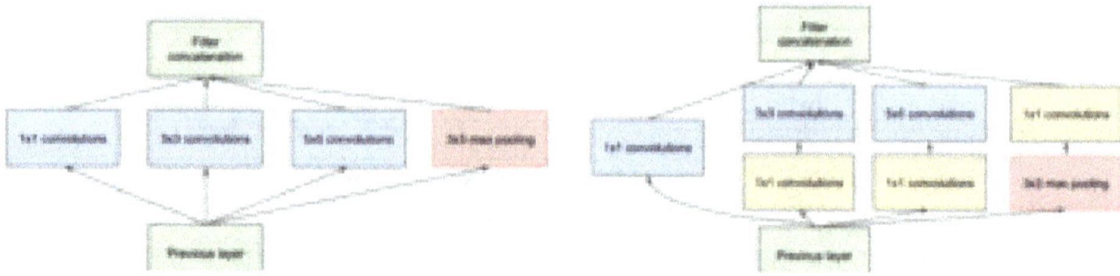

overfitting, however, in version 2, they use batch normalization instead as regulation and remove dropout operations.

Inception v3

Inception v3 *(Szegedy, 2016)* network continues to study along the 1*1 convolution line of thought, which can largely reduce the number of parameters without any bells and whistles, and first introduced convolution factorization to break down the n*n convolution into 1*n convolution and n*1 convolution as shown in Figure 8. By doing this, the network becomes more robust and lighter.

Figure 8. Inception v3 Convolution Factorization
(Szegedy, 2016)

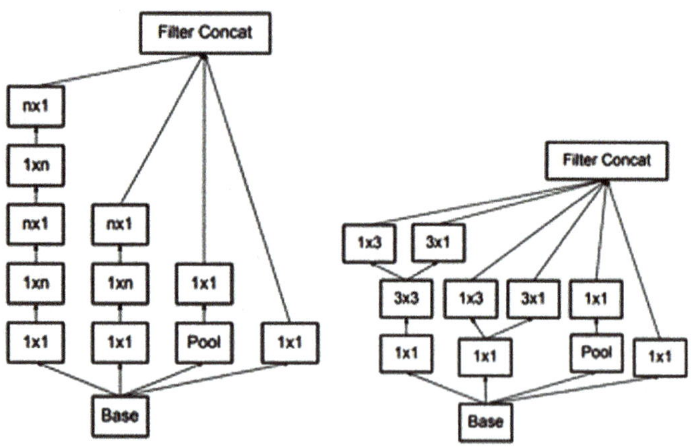

Figure 9. Inception v4 Inception-ResNet
(Szegedy, 2017)

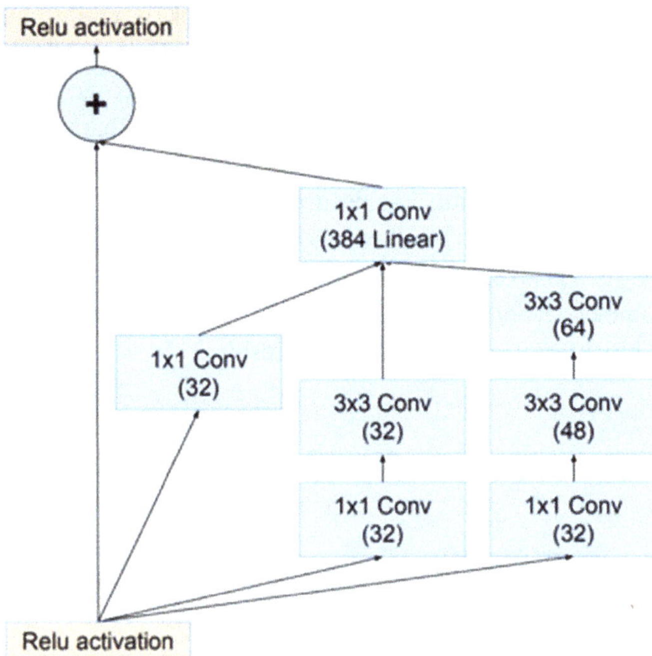

Inception v4

Inception v4 *(Szegedy, 2017)* borrows the idea from ResNet *(He, 2016)*, which is mentioned in 3.5.4. From an architecture perspective, it is a combination of GoogLeNet Inception and ResNet *(He, 2016)*, as shown in Figure 9. Compared with Figure 8, Inception v4 module just adds an extra shortcut between input and output.

Summary

In summary, GoogLeNet family mainly introduce:

1. 1*1 convolutional layer for reducing the number of parameters and deepen the network.
2. Batch normalization for regularization and better accuracy.
3. Convolution factorization for further reducing the number of parameters and deepen the network.
4. Different kernel size in the same convolution layer for broadening the network.

ResNet

ResNet *(He, 2016)*, proposed by Kaiming He, Facebook, is a milestone in the deep neural network. It dramatically increased the depth of the network from 22 layers to more than 100 layers with a booming performance in accuracy.

In the previous work, the bottleneck of network depth is that very deep network cannot be trained due to the vanishing of gradient and very high-level feature map contains very limited information. ResNet use residual block to solve the bottleneck, as shown in Fig 3.8, it connects the previous layer with the current layer so that each level feature map can also receive previous levels' information. Also, to decrease the number of parameters, it borrows the idea from GoogLeNet using 1*1 conv consist of a "bottleneck" block as an improvement of the residual block(left part of Figure 10).

Figure 10. Residual Block and Bottleneck Block in ResNet
(He, 2016)

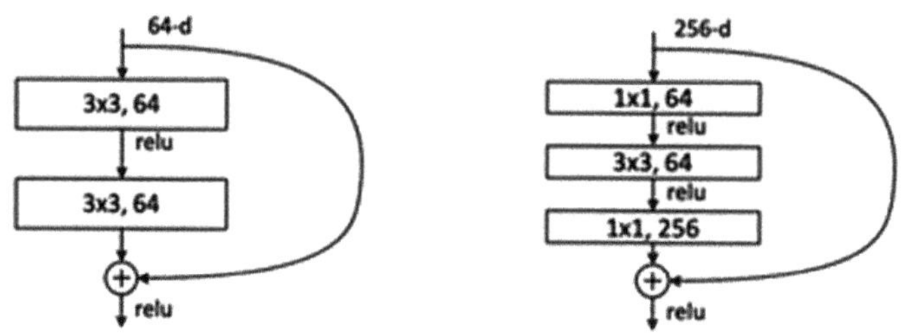

MobileNet

Some application scenarios have a strict time requirement, such as some medical diagnosis based on CT image classification and real-time cells detection, and using a large and heavy classification model like ResNet, VGG and etc, may cost too much computation time. An application needs a faster but with as less as possible loss on accuracy method. There comes MobileNet. MobileNet is a lightweight model trained on ImageNet dataset for deployment on edge devices.

Comparison of Backbone Networks

As shown in Table 1, towards different requirements on accuracy against efficiency, readers can choose deeper and densely connected classification networks, like ResNet family and VGG Net or lightweight networks like MobileNet and ShuffleNet.

Table 1. Comparison of backbone networks

Model	#Layes	Top-5 Error	#Params	Main Contribution
Alex Net*(Krizhevsky, 2012)*	5	84.70%	62M	Prove efficiency of CNN architect
VGG Net*(Simonyan, 2014)*	19	92.30%	138M	Multiple small kernels have the same effect compared with one large kernel.
GoogLeNet*(Szegedy, 2015)*	22	93.30%	6.4M	Broaden the width of the network and reduce the parameter quantity by 1*1 conv.
ResNet*(He, 2016)*	152	95.51%	60.3M	Deepen the network depth by using a residual network.
MobileNet	18	89.9%	4.2M	Usage separable convolutional neural network.

Object Detection

Object detection is an important type of computer vision tasks, also benefits from the flourish of deep learning. Object detection has a close bond with segmentation, for example, object detection is a key component of instance segmentation. So in this part, the authors give a brief introduction of object detection for better understanding of segmentation.

In general, detection algorithms are classified as one-stage methods and two-stage methods. Two-stage methods include a region proposal network and a detection network. In comparison, one-stage methods remove region proposal part and combine the function with the detection network.

Most of the backbone networks for detection task are the network for classification task but taking out the last fully connected layers, which readers can refer to the previous section "Convolutional Neural Network for Image Classification" for details.

Two-stage Detector

Two-stage detector follows an intuitive idea which is cropping out the different size of the region of interests(ROIs), and input the ROIs to a classifier to determine whether they contain expected objects, afterwards, using a regressor to regress more precise bounding boxes of detected objects as final outputs. The whole structure of the two-stage detector can be depicted as Figure 11, it can be summarized as a backbone network plus a proposal generator and detection network. In fact, you may simplify the structure as a proposal generator plus a classifier(remove the regressor of location), because to our best knowledge, the regressor here has a weak influence on the final results.

Figure 11. Two-Stage Detector Architecture
(Jiao, 2019)

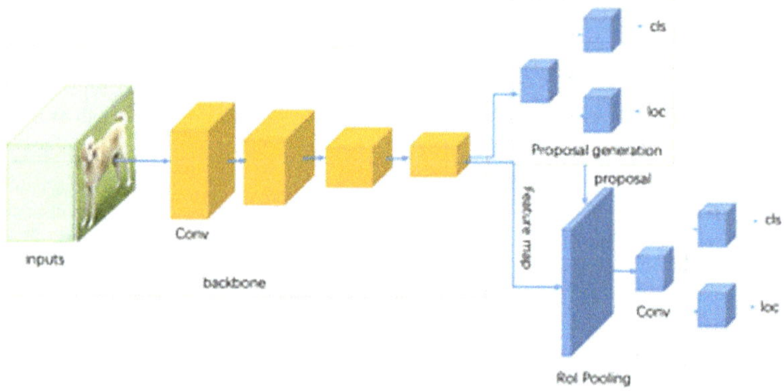

The most representative two-stage methods are the region R-CNN family, including R-CNN, Fast-RCNN and Faster-RCNN, etc,. This type of detectors have an impressive performance on accuracy, they still hold the state-of-the-art performance on most public detection datasets, the drawback, however, is that the speed is too slow to meet the real-time requirement. The typical speed of the two-stage method is about 5-10 frames per second(fps) while the real-time situation requires a speed of at least 25 fps.

Basically, researchers made many efforts on improving the speed performance. The foremost idea is to reduce the time consumption by sharing computation between proposal generator and classifier, as shown in Fig 3.9, which is exactly what R-CNN family did. Unfortunately, though the model is accelerated, it still cannot meet the real-time requirement. So the scientists switch the structure to a one-stage detector, see the details in the next part.

Here, as Table 2 shows, this section collects some experiments statistical data for different two-stage methods for you to conveniently select the proper method in your own application scenario.

Table 2. Statistics of Estimation for Two-stage Detectors

Model	mAP(VOC/COCO)	FPS
R-CNN	66.0%/NaN	0.02
Fast RCNN	70.0%/19.7%	0.5
Faster RCNN	73.2%/21.9%	7
Mask RCNN	NaN/39.8%	5

Note: Applications usually prefer two-stage models with higher FPS, because it is the bottleneck of the two-stage method.

One-stage Detector

As it has been discussed in the two-stage detection part, the most significant shortcoming of it is the slow speed which is mainly caused by the ROI proposal part. So the one-stage detection method is proposed to solve this problem.

One-stage methods remove the proposal generator thoroughly and use a regressor instead to directly predict the location, as shown in Figure 12, the structure can be depicted as a backbone network plus a location regressor and an object classifier. By this structural modification, a huge amount of computation is cut, through which a typical speed of one-stage detector can easily arrive 40-50 fps. However, this simplification also causes a decrease in accuracy. So for one-stage detector, the key point is to increase the accuracy performance.

Figure 12. One-Stage Detector Architecture
(Jiao, 2019)

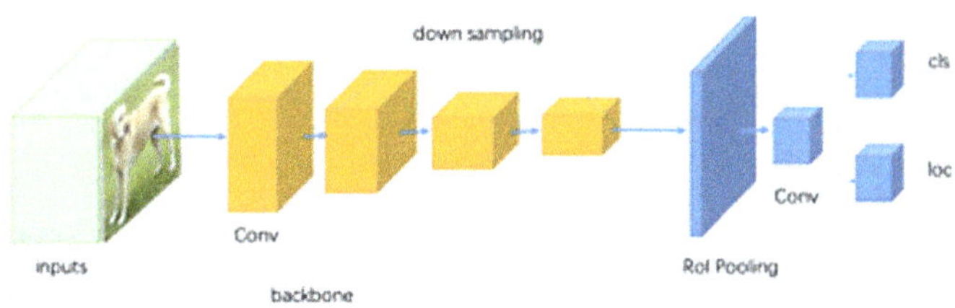

The most representative models in the one-stage detector are YOLO family, ***RetinaNet***, ***CenterNet***, etc. Researchers made efforts in improving the accuracy of this type of detector and achieved some milestones. Currently, the cutting-edge one-stage detectors even have comparable accuracy against two-stage methods. Due to this achievement, one-stage detectors are becoming a trend in the industry.

For the convenience of model selection, this section also summarizes some key parameters for estimation of one-stage detection models, as shown in Table 3.

Table 3. Statistics of Estimation for Two-stage Detectors

Model	mAP(VOC/COCO)	FPS
YOLO v1	63.4%/NaN	45
YOLO v2	78.6%/NaN	40
YOLO v3	NaN/21.6%	45
SSD513	81.6%/34.4%	19
RetinaNet	NaN/39.1%	11
CenterNet	NaN/45.1%	16
FCOS	NaN/42.8%	13

Note: Applications usually prefer one-stage models with higher mAP, because it is the bottleneck of one-stage method.

Other Detector

Other than two-stage detectors and one-stage detectors, recent years researchers also explored some other ideas like anchor-free detectors, deformable convnets and ***feature pyramid scale networks(FPN)***, as shown in Figure 13. Through all the newly proposed approaches, there is a trend of combination two-stage detectors with one-stage detectors.

Figure 13. Object Detection Development Timeline
(Jiao, 2019)

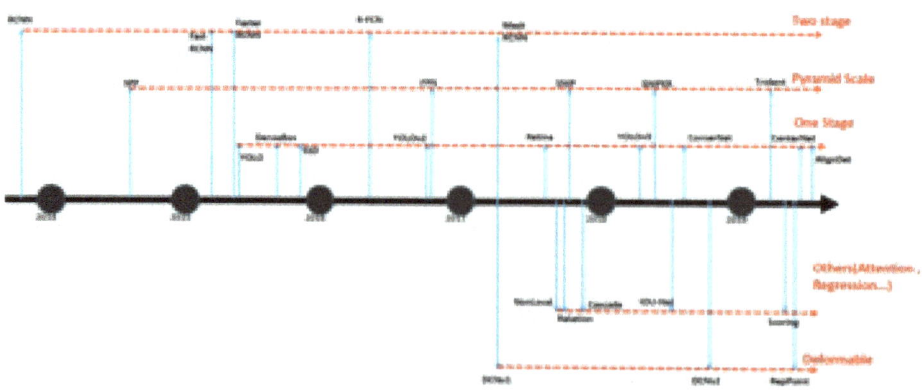

Semantic Segmentation

Semantic segmentation is a high-level computer vision task. Compared with image classification classify each image, this task aims to classify each pixel in an image. The labels of classification could be cells, nerves, blood vessels, etc., just to mention a few. As shown in Figure 14, given the input cells image(left), semantic segmentation model will segment all the cell objects with masks.

Figure 14. Cells Segmentation
(image from https://www.robots.ox.ac.uk/~vgg/research/cell_detection/)

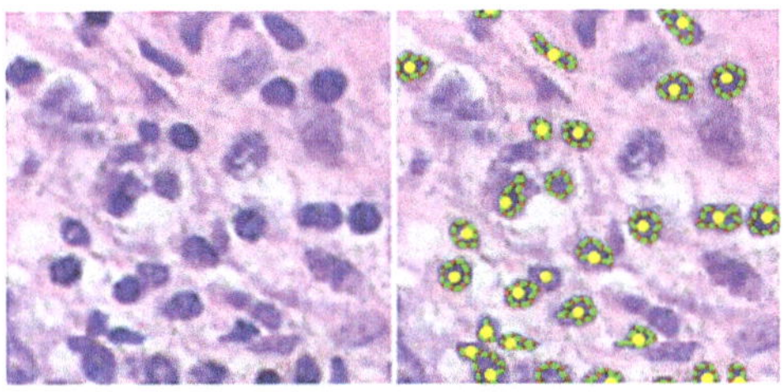

You can consider that the mask result is a dense prediction on pixels. For example, the cells' boundaries are decided by pixel classification result, pixels in the boundaries are predicted as a "cell" class, while pixels out of the boundaries are predicted as "background" class or "others" class. Usually, you can choose the categories according to the project requirement, supposing you need to distinguish between "red blood cell", "leukocyte", "platelet" and "vascular wall", your model has to tell which class it belongs to for each pixel. Then the model will output a dense prediction(matrix) as the segmentation result.

Traditional ways to deal with semantic segmentation mainly used hand-crafted features like color, grey-level segmentation and conditional random fields(CRF). Modern methods for semantic segmentation mainly based on deep learning. And in most of the cases this type of models follow a quite similar fashion which is encoder-decoder fashion. In this fashion, an encoder is usually a backbone network discussed in the previous parts for different levels feature extraction, and decoder is usually as an upsampling part to restore the size of feature map. Finally, the model will output the prediction based on the upsampled feature map.

The general architecture of semantic segmentation can be summarized as "encoder-decoder" fashion, but, in fact, there are many details in different models, which is the key point of improvement on performance. So this section discusses some details for some creative, insightful and classical models.

Fully Convolutional Network(FCN)

Semantic segmentation task needs pixel-level predictions. CNN models always used fully connected layer as the last layer until FCN was proposed. In 2015, Jonathan Long and Evan Shelhamer proposed FCN *(Long, 2015)*, replacing the fully connected layer with another convolutional layer, and used this architecture into semantic segmentation with the state-of-the-art result on public datasets. It is FCN that makes the pixel-level prediction, some also call it as a dense prediction, possible.

Figure 15. FCN architecture(left) and comparison between FCN and fully connected layer(right).
(Long, 2015)

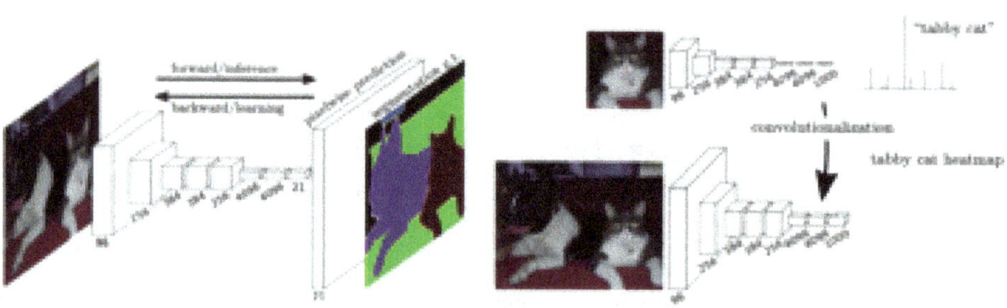

Figure 15 shows the FCN architecture and how FCN convert a fully convolutional layer into dense prediction. However, after layers of convolutional operations, the feature map becomes very small, even dense prediction cannot satisfy the segmentation accuracy demand. To address this, FCN provides different sizes of outputs. Typically, FCN includes FCN-8s, FCN-16s and FCN-32s, which means upsample the feature map 8 times, 16 times and 32 times respectively. As shown in Figure 16, intuitively, the FCN-8s includes more detailed information but less global information, while FCN-32s contains more global information but fewer details. So

Figure 16. Different versions of FCN(left) and their performances(right)
(Long, 2015).

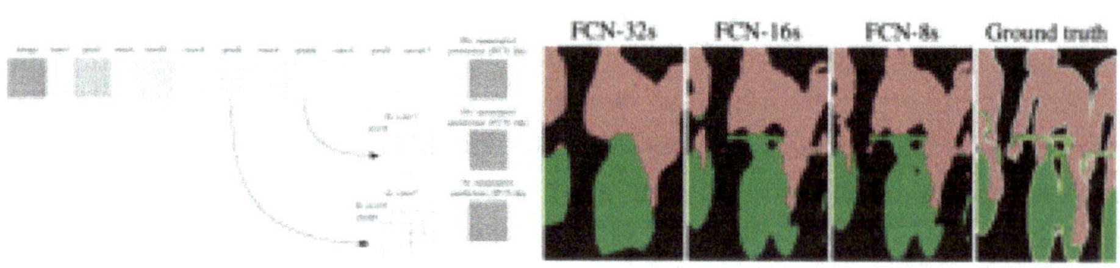

people usually directly use FCN-8s if they require both quality and efficiency or combine FCN-8s, FCN-16s and FCN-32s together to obtain the best segmentation quality while sacrificing some efficiency.

Based on the above introduction, FCN is the fundamental of semantic segmentation in the deep learning era. In the rest sections of semantic segmentation, FCN will always play a key role of those SOTA methods.

Apart from that, upsampling is also a key operator for FCN. There are different kinds of upsampling methods: nearest upsampling, bi-linear upsampling and lanzo upsampling. In most deep learning models, bi-linear upsampling is adopted but different methods have limited effect on the performance, according to experiments. And also, to further efficiently increase the receptive field of feature maps, some new convolutional techniques like deformable convolution and dilated convolution are adopted by recent SOTA models.

Feature Pyramid Network(FPN)

FPN *(Lin, 2017)* is another fundamental not only in semantic segmentation but also in other computer vision tasks like detection and face recognition. This is a feature map fusion method to solve size problems which happen when the model needs to recognize both large objects and small objects. Before FPN was proposed, lots

Figure 17. Feature Pyramid Networks
(Lin, 2017)

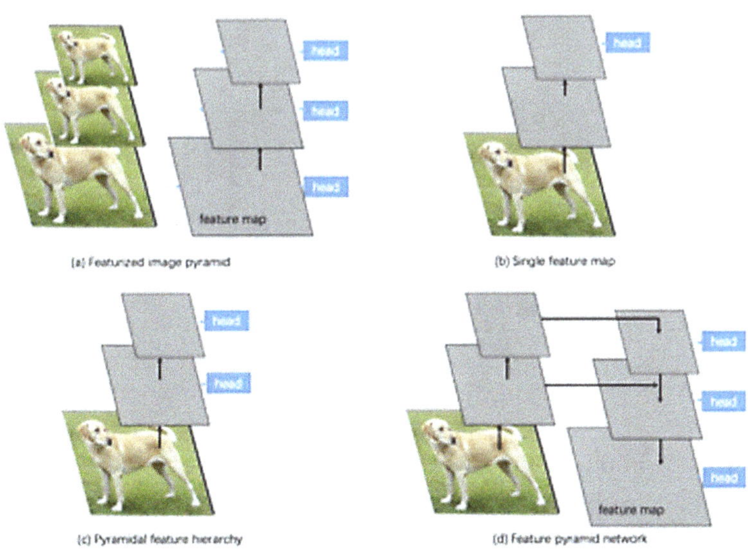

of deep learning models cannot well process different sizes of objects, especially small objects.

However, with FPN, as shown in Figure 17(d), different sizes of feature maps will be merged together as the final feature map, so the final feature map contains all sizes of information that can generate the most accurate prediction.

FPN can serve as a portable plug-in module to solve the size problem in lots of models, for example, the main idea in U-Net is combining FCN with FPN-like module and Mask-RCNN, for instance segmentation, also borrows the idea of FPN in its modification version. If you watch carefully, FPN ideas lay everywhere in the computer vision field.

U-Net

U-Net *(Ronneberger, 2015)* is a semantic segmentation model proposed in 2015. This model wins the ISBI Challenge, which concentrates on medical image segmentation. This model is a light-wise segmentation with an architecture shape similar to "U" as shown in Figure18.

Figure 18. U-Net architecture
(Ronneberger, 2015)

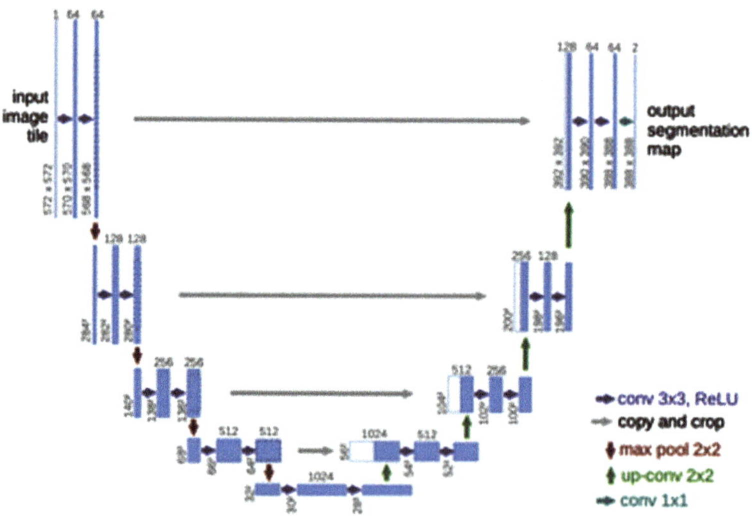

As mentioned in the previous section, U-Net is one of the earliest models that adopt the fully convolutional network in segmentation tasks and it also employs the feature map fusion method to solve the size problem. But unlike FPN's pixel-wise adding, U-Net adopts a channel-wise concatenating fusion method to make the output feature map even deeper. In the current research, there is no evidence that shows which fusion methods are better. So there are still improvement rooms for feature fusion parts.

Figure 19. U-Net performance on Cells segmentation
(ISBI Challenge)

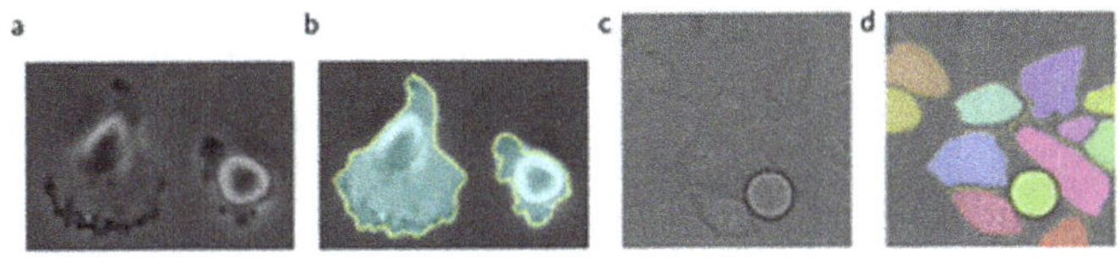

U-Net performs excellent in segmentation especially medical image segmentation. It has been widely used in Kaggle medical image segmentation competitions and even other segmentation tasks. It seems that since U-Net wins the ISBI Challenge, it has become the baseline model for other segmentation competitions. So if FCN and FPN are the fundamental modules of segmentation, then U-Net is the fundamental model of medical image segmentation. Since the theory of FCN and FPN have been already introduced above, U-Net should not be hard to understand.

Seg-Net

Apart from U-shape networks, there exists another fashion for segmentation architecture which is Encoder-Decoder fashion. Seg-Net (Badrinarayanan, 2017) is one of the representative networks for encoder-decoder.

Figure 20. Seg-Net encoder-decoder architecture
(Badrinarayanan, 2017)

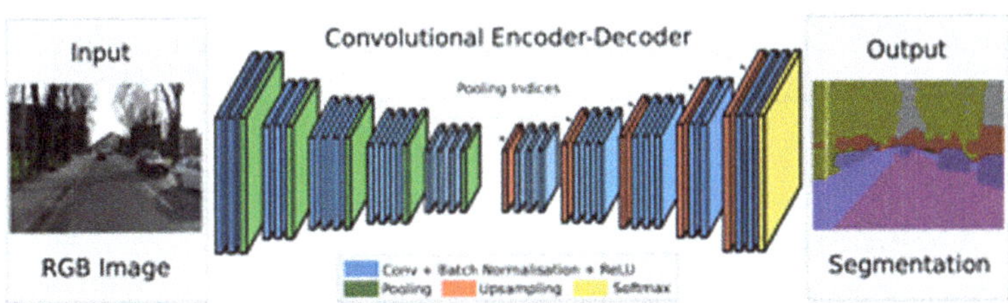

As shown in Figure 20, Seg-Net, proposed in 2015 by Vijay etc., contains an encoder and a decoder. The encoder part is in charge of feature extraction while the decoder part is responsible for feature map upsampling and feature fusion. Seg-Net designed their own encoder by 5 layers of convolutional operator plus batch normalization and relu activation function, while in recent papers researchers would like to directly use some stages of ResNet or VGG as an encoder. In terms of the decoder, Seg-Net adopts deconvolutional operator which is upsampling plus feature fusion and learnable convolutional layers. Actually, it is quite similar between FCN and encoder-decoder. The most important difference lies in the learnable convolutional layers. In FCN, after feature extraction, the feature maps are merged directly, but in encoder-decoder and U-shape networks after feature extraction(encoder) and upsampling, the feature maps will go through another convolutional layers which make the decoder part also learnable.

Above are about two mainstream architectures of semantic segmentation models. From the architecture aspect, there are no big differences between them, but a lot of tiny differences like convolutional operators, upsampling methods and decoder methods which are key factors that affect the model performances. That is also the reason why most recent segmentation models are based on the 2 baseline models to make some further modifications.

Instance Segmentation

Instance segmentation is another task in the computer vision field. Unlike semantic segmentation only takes class into consideration, instance segmentation has even higher requirements which need the model to distinguish not only the class but also the individuals belonging to the same classes. For example, semantic segmentation can only tell you "these are cells" or "these are viruses", but instance segmentation can tell you "these are cells and this is cell no.1, this is cell no.2...".

So how do the models work to satisfy the requirement? All of the techniques are introduced above. The answer is detection plus semantic segmentation. Currently, mask R-CNN (He, 2017) is the state-of-the-art instance segmentation model. It was proposed in 2017 by Kaiming He, etc. As shown in Figure 21, it contains a detection model plus a segmentation branch. In the detection part, faster-r CNN is adopted and in the segmentation branch, FCN is adopted.

Saliency Object Detection

Salient object detection aims to identify the most visually conspicuous objects in an image and segment the objects precisely. It is an important preprocessing step

Figure 21. Mask R-CNN architecture
(He, 2017)

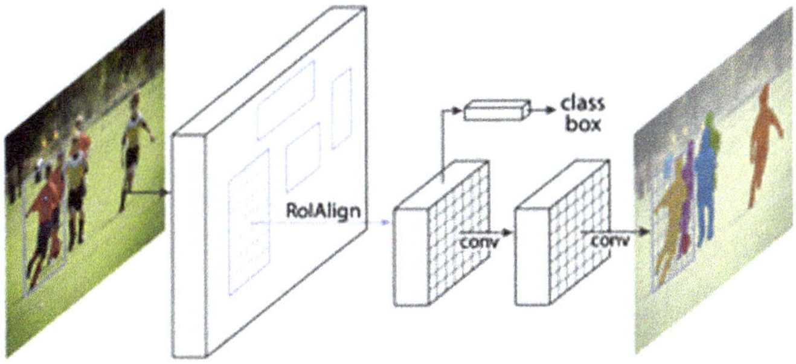

for various tasks such as image segmentation, image content understanding and visual tracking.

Currently, the architecture of saliency object detection methods are quite similar, as shown in Figure 21, it usually consists of a backbone part, feature fusion part and saliency inference part. The backbone network is in charge of feature map extraction. Feature fusion part, as its name, works for different levels of feature maps fusion for both accurate salient object recognition and precise mask prediction. Saliency inference part is mainly designed for the mask refinement, instance segmentation model like mask-rcnn can only generate coarse masks, so the post-processing part is needed to take care of the mask refinement.

Figure 22. Salient Object Detection General Framework
(Li, 2019)

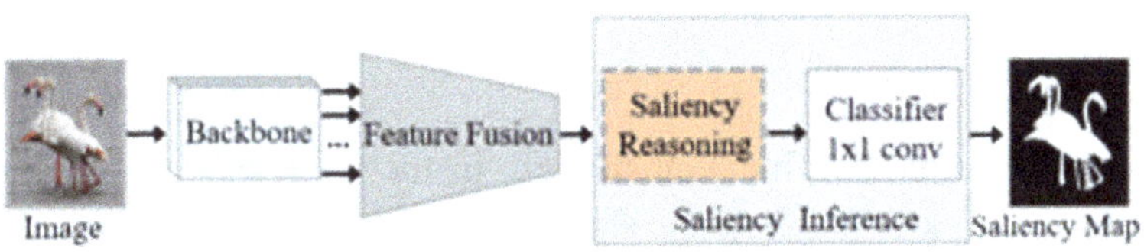

POST PROCESSING

Post-processing is a way to improve the quality of segmentation especially at the boundary where the segmentation mask is not good enough to use in real-world applications. There are a lot of post-processing methods to refine the generated mask using image processing and deep learning model. This section explains a few popular mask refinement algorithms i.e Deep GrabCut a deep learning-based model and the alpha matting based on image processing.

Deep GrabCut

GrabCut *(Boykov, 2001)* is a rectangle and/or curve-based interactive segmentation method. Deep GrabCut *(Ning, 2017)* is an extension of the GrabCut based on deep learning which uses soft rectangle as input. GrabCut requires the rectangle to properly encode the object of interest. Deep GrabCut removes the constraint on rectangle input. The rectangle may few pixels smaller or larger than the object to cover. Deep GrabCut converts the user-provided rectangles to a euclidian distance map and concatenates to the input image. Deep GrabCut trains a dense encoder-decoder network on the concatenated image to generate an object mask. This method can be used for class agnostic instance and semantic segmentation coupled with an object detection method. Figure 22 shows the basic architecture of Deep GrabCut.

Figure 23. Deep GrabCut
(Ning, 2017)

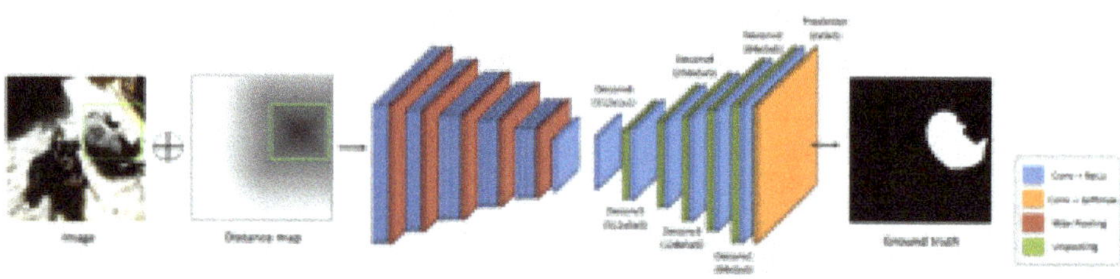

Alpha Matting

Alpha matting is a mask refinement process in the interactive image and video segmentation to smooth the boundaries of a foreground object. This method is called “Alpha Matting” because it adds an alpha channel to the RGB image where each pixel has a value between 0-255 for alpha transparency unlike the traditional segmentation which is a binary task that assigns either 0 or 1 as a label to each pixel. Alpha matting reassigns the pixel level to the foreground or background based on user input using a low-level color measurement feature to the neighbouring pixels. There are different methods for alpha matting. This section discusses the most popular alpha matting algorithm closed-form method, spectral based solution and one deep learning-based model deep alpha matting.

Closed-Form Solution

This method uses a closed-form solution *(Levin, 2008)* to the natural image matting. The closed-form solution is very popular for natural image matting in interactive image segmentation with very little user interaction. Closed-form alpha matting derives a quadratic cost function from the low-level color smoothing assumption between the foreground and background pixel. An analytic solution is possible for the derived cost function that finds a global optimal solution of the system of quadratic equations. This closed-form solution uses an eigenvalue decomposition method for the analytic solution. In Figure 23, a.) is the original image b) is the segmentation result after Mask R-CNN instance segmentation model. The generates segmentation quality is not good at the boundary. To smooth the results at boundary alpha matting can be used. Figure c) is the segmentation result after the closed-form solution which smooths the boundary.

Figure 24. Closed-form alpha matting. left: original image middle: after instance segmentation, right: smoothing after the closed-form matting

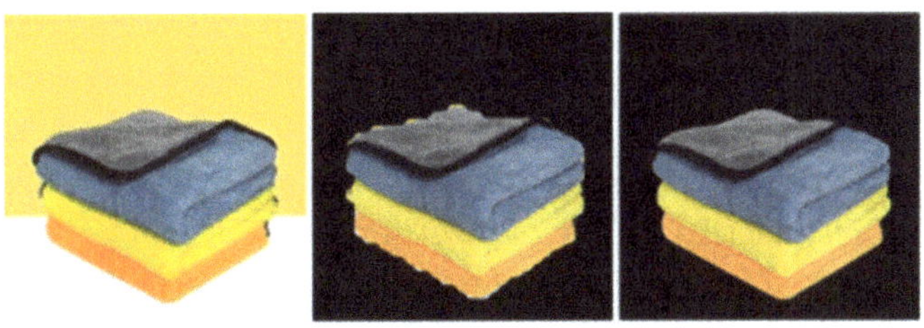

Deep Matting

Deep alpha matting *(Xu, 2017)* is an extension of the deep learning-based model to the matting problem and *(Xu, 2017)* first uses a deep learning-based model for this type of task. Deep alpha matting *(Xu, 2017)* propose a two-stage network for alpha matting consist of a deep encoder-decoder module and a refinement module. Deep alpha matting *(Xu, 2017)* Uses a fully convolutional neural network as a mask refinement module for alpha matting. The refinement module is an encoder-decoder architecture called residual refinement module (RRM) which takes the generated segmentation mask as input and produces a refined mask as output where each pixel has value in the range of 0 to 255 to generate smoothing effects at the boundary. Figure 24 is the architecture of the proposed model in Deep alpha matting *(Xu, 2017)*.

Figure 25. Deep Matting
(Xu, 2017)

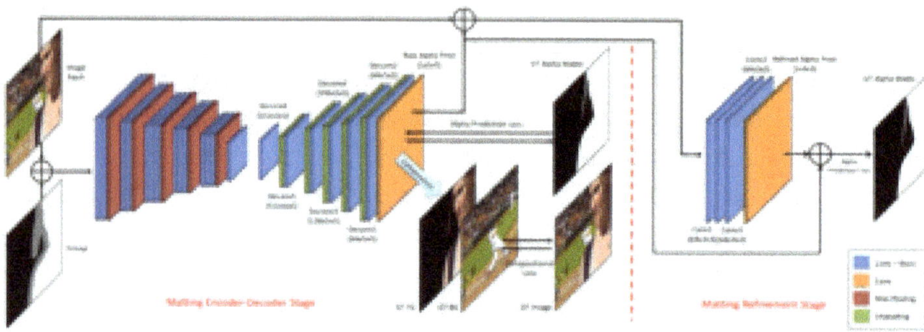

Spatial Propagation Network (SPN)

(Liu, 2017) propose Spatial Propagation Network (SPN) to learn the affinity matrix of an image. Affinity is a generic matrix which encodes pairwise similarity between pixels. Each pixel in an image is represented as a node in the affinity matrix. For image segmentation and object detection, the affinity matrix needs to learn high-level semantic information of the object of interest. *(Liu, 2017)* propose the way to learn this affinity matrix with high-level semantic information using a spatial propagation network. The proposed architecture uses a deep CNN network. SPN is trained using stochastic gradient descent (SGD) and the model is computationally efficient because of the linear structure of the recurrent network.

EVALUATION METRIC

To evaluate and benchmark different object detection and image segmentation model there is a need for proper evaluation metric. Average Precision (AP) is widely used for measuring accuracy of popular object detector i.e YOLOv3, Faster-RCNN and mAP (Mean Average Precision) for popular instance segmentation model Mask-RCNN.

Figure 26. Precision, Recall
(image from https://en.wikipedia.org/wiki/Precision_and_recall)

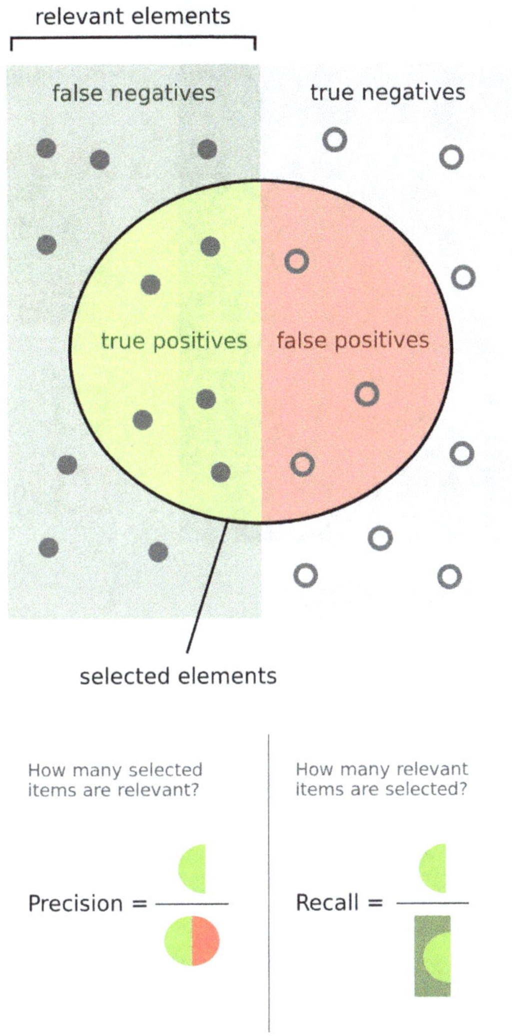

Precision and Recall

Precision measures how accurate the prediction is. Precision is the percentage of correct prediction out of total prediction. Precision is the ration of True Position (TP) and True Positive (TP) + False Positive (FP).

Recall measures how good the prediction is to find all the actual positive. Recall is the ratio of True Positive (TP) and True Positive (TP) + False Negative (FN). Figure 25 shows the precision and recall calculation from user prediction.

Figure 27. Intersection Over Union (IoU)

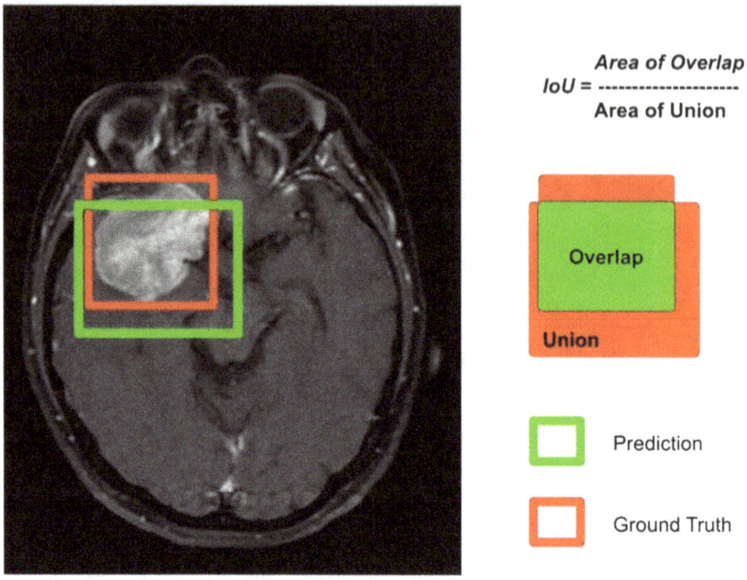

Intersection Over Union (IoU)

Intersection Over Union (IoU) measures the overlap between the ground truth and predicted bounding box. IoU is a ratio of the area of overlap and area of union. IoU is a metric that captures the similarity between ground truth and prediction in terms

Figure 28. Precision-Recall Curve,the formula for AP

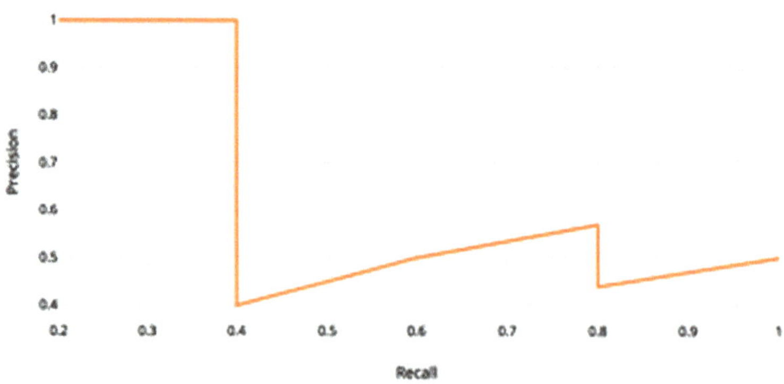

$$\mathbf{AP} = \int_0^1 p(r)dr$$

of boundary box overlap where the value ranges from 0 to 1. In some datasets, there is a threshold (0.5 is widely used) on IoU for classification to define the prediction as false positive or true positive. Figure 26 shows the IoU calculation based on model prediction and ground truth.

Average Precision

Average precision (AP) is the average of all the precision values for recall ranges from 0 to 1. AP is calculated as the area under the precision-recall curve. AP values lie in the range of 0 to 1. Before calculating the AP value for object detection, smoothing is done to reduce zigzag pattern in the precision-recall curve as Figure 27 and Figure 28.

Interpolated AP

PASCAl VOC is a popular dataset for object detection. PASCAL uses an 11-point interpolation method for the AP value calculation. The recall value is divided into 11 points in the range of 0 to 1.0 and at each recall value, the maximum precision is calculated. The interpolated AP is reported as the average of all the AP values. In PASCAL VOC dataset a prediction is considered as a position if the IoU >= 0.5. Figure 29 shows an 11-point interpolation for AP.

Figure 29. Flat Precision-Recall Curve

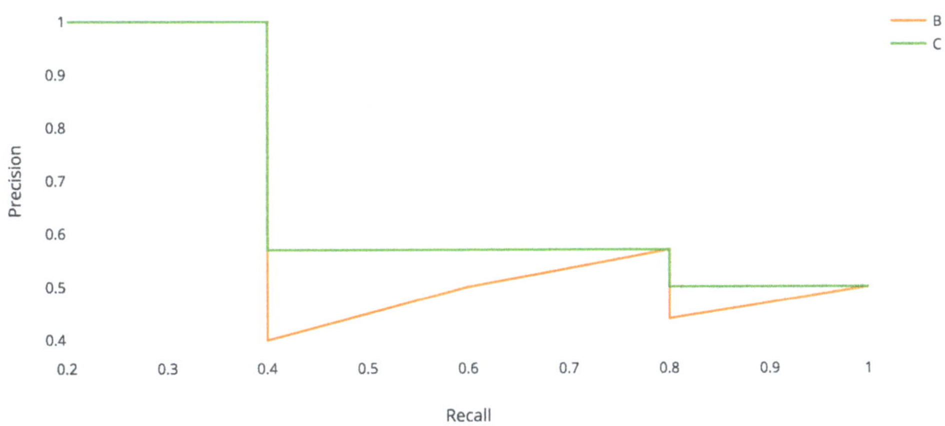

Figure 30. 11-points interpolated precision-recall curve

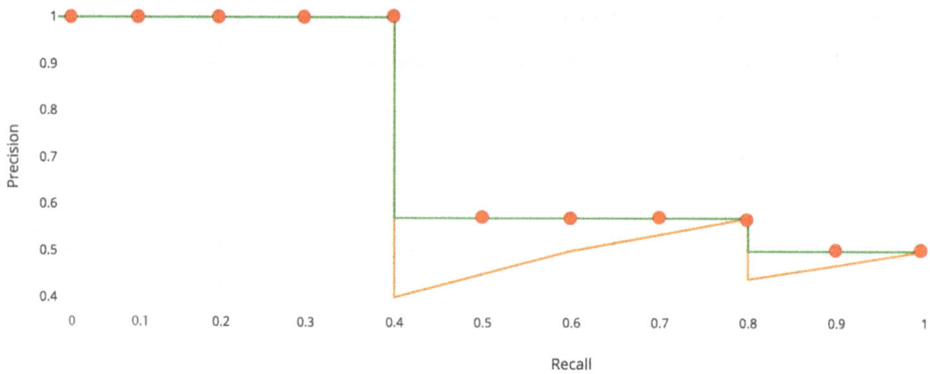

Interpolated AP is an approximation calculation and it losses the ability to find differences of object detection methods which has very low AP.

COCO mAP

Most of the current research on object detection reports the accuracy on the popular COCO dataset. COCO dataset uses Mean Average Precision (mAP) instead of AP. Mean Average Precision is the average of all the AP. COCO uses a 101-points interpolated AP. COCO also uses different IoU threshold for considering a prediction as positive. mAP is the average of 101-points interpolated AP for each of the IoU threshold. In COCO **AP@[0.5:95]** is the average of all the AP for IoU threshold ranging from 0.5 to 0.95 with a step size 0.05.

DATA LABELING AND DATA AUGMENTATION

This section describes different open-source data labelling tools for segmentation and different data augmentation method.

Data Annotation Tools

This section describes different open-source data labelling tools for segmentation and object detection.

VGG Image Annotator

VGG Image Annotator (VIA) is a popular image annotation tool open-sourced by Visual Geometry Group (VGG) at Oxford University. VIA provides key points, bounding boxes and, polygon annotation. Figure 30 shows a sample bounding box and segmentation annotation using VGG image annotator tools.

Computer Vision Annotation Tool (CVAT)

Computer Vision Annotation Tools (CVAT) is another popular image annotation tool that provides semi-automated annotation for instance segmentation. CVAT has a docker image which has provision to use any pre-trained model for the segmentation annotation. There is a popular interactive segmentation model DEXTR which takes 4 extreme points of an object as input and generates instance segmentation mask for that object as output. People normally use DEXTR as a pre-trained model in CVAT annotation tools to accelerate the segmentation annotation process.

Figure 31. VGG Annotation Tools

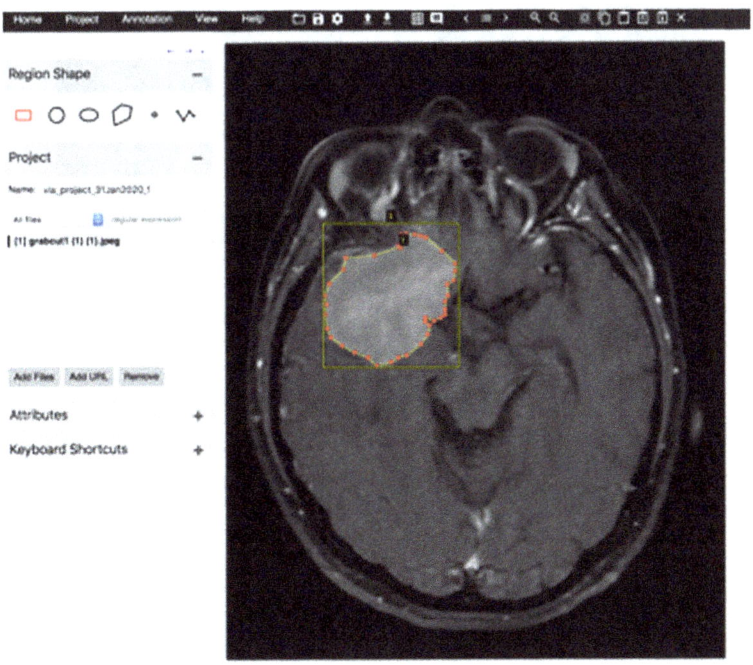

LabelMe - MIT

LabelMe is another popular image annotation tool open-sourced by the image processing group at Massachusetts Institute of Technology (MIT). LabelMe can be used for key points, bounding boxes and, polygon annotation.

DATA AUGMENTATION

Data augmentation is a process of generating new data points without actually collecting more data which increases the diversity in the training dataset. Data augmentation is a very important preprocessing step for training any deep neural network. Image flipping, rotation, cropping, translation, and scale are the most commonly used data augmentation techniques.

Image Processing Based

This section describes each of the image processing based data augmentation techniques to train neural networks.

Figure 32. Example of image flip. Left: original image, middle: h-flip and right: v-flip

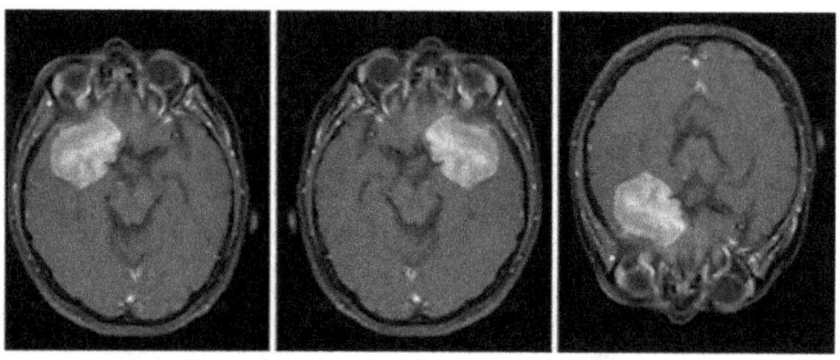

Flip

Flipping is a commonly used data augmentation technique where each image is flipped horizontally or vertically. Figure 31 shows the flip operation on a sample image.

Rotation

The rotation operation in image processing is represented as the following transformation

$$x_2 = \cos(\theta) \times (x_1 - x_0) - \sin(\theta) \times (y_1 - y_0) + x_0 \quad (1)$$

$$y_2 = \sin(\theta) \times (x_1 - x_0) - \cos(\theta) \times (y_1 - y_0) + y_0 \quad (2)$$

In equation (1) and (2) (x_0 , y_0) is the centre of the rotation and θ is the rotation angle. For clockwise rotation, the value θ is positive and negative for otherwise. Rotation is widely used for augmentation for training deep learning model. Most of the deep learning framework have the rotation in their data loader transformer where a random rotation within a range (0° to 45°) is applied to the input image.

Crop

Cropping is a way to select a specific area of an image. Cropping is very popular augmentation technique for training deep learning model. Few deep learning models use random cropping of a specific size from the input image. Some other mode uses fixed-size cropping at the centre and cropping at four corners of the input image. AlexNet (*Krizhevsky, 2012)* uses the centre and four corners cropping of size 227x227 of the input image.

5 Scale

The scale is a geometric transformation which is used to shrink or zoom an image. Subsampling or interpolation is used for scaling. For size reduction subsampling is used where a group of pixels are replaced by one pixel. Inpolating new pixel from neighbouring pixels is used for upscaling an image. There are different method for interpolation. Bilinear, Nearest Neighbour, and Cubic are the most popular interpolation methods for upsampling an image. In most of the deep learning-based methods the input image is resized to a smaller size before training to reduce the computation. In testing, after the model prediction, the output is resized to the original input size to get the actual output.

Figure 33. InstaBoost (a) original image with ground segmentation mask. (b) random InstaBoost, shown multiple appearances of the same object (c) label consistent heatmap (d) one example of the generated image with the mask
(Fang, 2019)

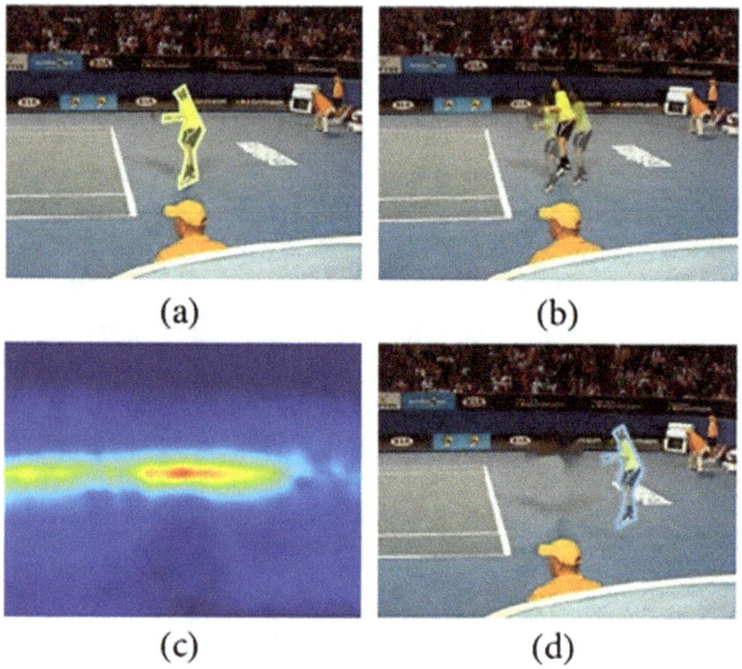

Deep Learning-Based

InstaBoost

InstaBoost *(Fang, 2019)* is a popular deep learning-based method for augmenting detection and segmentation dataset. InstaBoost try to find all possible locations where an object can be placed. It generates a heatmap for all feasible placement of an object and impaint the image by replacing the object location. InstaBoost is a very efficient way to generate more data using the existing object mask and can be integrated with any existing object detection and segmentation pipeline without any bell and whistle for training and inference time. InstaBoost improves the Mask RCNN by 1.7 mAP on COCO dataset and 3.3 mAP on PASCAL VOC dataset. Figure 32 is an example of InstaBoost method.

CONCLUSION

This chapter explains different types of image segmentation and their application in the domain of medical imaging. The chapter mainly highlights the important contribution of deep learning in image segmentation. The authors discuss various state-of-the-art image segmentation techniques, different evaluation metrics and their application in medical imaging. This chapter also highlights popular open-source tools that uses for medical image segmentation data labelling. The chapter ends with implementation details of instance segmentation for medical image.

REFERENCES

Badrinarayanan, V., & Kendall, A. (2017). *Segnet: A deep convolutional encoder-decoder architecture for image segmentation.* ieeexplore.ieee.org

Boykov, Y., Veksler, O., & Zabih, R. (2001). approximate energy minimization via graph cuts. *IEEE Transactions on Pattern Analysis and Machine Intelligence, 23*(11), 1222–1239. doi:10.1109/34.969114

Buckley, Brock, & Oliver.(2009). Interactive segmentation for manipulation in unstructured environments. *ICRA'09: Proceedings of the 2009 IEEE international conference on Robotics and Automation.*

Fang, H. S., Sun, J., Wang, R. M., Gou., Y.L., Li, C., & Lu. (2019). Instaboost: Boosting instance segmentation via probability map guided copy-pasting. ICCV 2019.

He, Gkioxari, Dollár, & Girshick. (2017). *Mask R-CNN International Conference on Computer Vision (ICCV).* Academic Press.

He, K., Zhang, X., Ren, S., & Sun, J. (2016). Deep Residual Learning for Image Recognition. *2016 IEEE Conference on Computer Vision and Pattern Recognition (CVPR)*, 770–778. 10.1109/CVPR.2016.90

Ioffe, S., & Christian, S. (2015). *Batch normalization: Accelerating deep network training by reducing internal covariate shift.* arXiv preprint arXiv:1502.03167

Krizhevsky, Sutskever, & Hinton. (2012). Imagenet classification with deep convolutional neural networks. Advances in Neural Information Processing Systems, 1097-1105.

Krizhevsky, A., Sutskever, I., & Hinton, G. (2012). ImageNet Classification with Deep Convolutional Neural Networks. NIPS 2012: Neural Information Processing Systems.

Lecun, Y., Bottou, L., Bengio, Y., & Haffner, P. (1998). Gradient-based learning applied to document recognition. *Proceedings of the IEEE, 86*(11), 2278–2324. doi:10.1109/5.726791

Levin, A., Lischinski, D., & Weiss, Y. (2008). A closed-form solution to natural image matting. *IEEE Transactions on Pattern Analysis and Machine Intelligence, 30*(2), 228–242. doi:10.1109/TPAMI.2007.1177 PMID:18084055

Li, Z. C., Lang, Y., Chen, J., Liew, J., & Feng. (2019). *Deep reasoning with multi-scale context for salient object detection.* arXiv preprint arXiv:1901.08362

Liao, L. (2019). A Survey of Deep Learning-Based Object Detection. *IEEE Access: Practical Innovations, Open Solutions, 7*, 128837–128868.

Lin, T. Y. P., Dollár, R., Girshick, K., & He. (2017). *Feature pyramid networks for object detection.* openaccess.thecvf.com

Lindeberg, T., & Li, M.-X. (1997). Segmentation and classification of edges using minimum description length approximation and complementary junction cues. *Computer Vision and Image Understanding, 67*(1), 88–98. doi:10.1006/cviu.1996.0510

Liu, S. S., De Mello, J., Gu, G., Zhong, M.H., & Yang. (2017). Learning affinity via spatial propagation networks. Advances in Neural.

Long, J. E., & Shelhamer, T. D. (2015). Fully convolutional networks for semantic segmentation. *Proceedings of the IEEE CVPR 2015.*

Ning, X., Brian, P., Scott, C., Jimei, Y., Thomas, H. (2017). Deep GrabCut for Object Selection. *British Machine Vision Conference (BMVC).*

Ronneberger, O. P., Fischer, T., & Brox. (2015). U-net: Convolutional networks for biomedical image segmentation. In *International Conference on Medical.* Springer.

Simonyan & Zisserman. (2014). *Very deep convolutional networks for large-scale image recognition.* arXiv preprint arXiv:1409.1556

Szegedy, C., Wei, L., Yangqing, J., Pierre, S., Scott, R., Dragomir, A., Dumitru, E., Vincent, V., Andrew, R. (2015). Going deeper with convolutions. *Proceedings of the IEEE conference on computer vision and pattern recognition*, 1-9.

Szegedy, C., Vincent, V., Sergey, I., Jon, S., and Zbigniew, W. (2016). Rethinking the inception architecture for computer vision. *Proceedings of the IEEE conference on computer vision and pattern recognition*, 2818-2826. 10.1109/CVPR.2016.308

Szegedy, C., Sergey, I., Vincent, V., & Alexander, A. A. (2017). Inception-v4, inception-resnet and the impact of residual connections on learning. *Thirty-First AAAI Conference on Artificial Intelligence.*

Xu, N. B., Price, S., & Cohen. (2017). Deep image matting. *Proceedings of the IEEE, CVPR, 2017.* openaccess.thecvf.com

Chapter 3
Relevance of Machine Learning to Cardiovascular Imaging

Sumesh Sasidharan
Imperial College London, UK

M. Yousuf Salmasi
https://orcid.org/0000-0002-4085-1294
Imperial College London, UK

Selene Pirola
https://orcid.org/0000-0003-4368-3940
Imperial College London, UK

Omar A. Jarral
Imperial College London, UK

ABSTRACT

Artificial intelligence (AI) broadly concerns analytical algorithms that iteratively learn from big datasets, allowing computers to find concealed insights. These encompass a range of operations comprising several terms, including machine learning(ML), cognitive learning, deep learning, and reinforcement learning-based methods that can be used to incorporate and comprehend complex biomedical and healthcare data in scenarios where traditional statistical approaches cannot be implemented. For cardiovascular imaging in particular, machine learning guarantees to be a transformative tool that can address many unmet needs for patient-specific management, accurate prediction of disease progression, and the tracking of identifiable biomarkers of disease processes. In this chapter, the authors discuss fundamentals of machine learning algorithms for image analysis in the cardiovascular system by evaluating the need for ML in this field and examining the potential obstacles and challenges of implementation in the context of three common imaging modalities used in cardiovascular medicine.

DOI: 10.4018/978-1-7998-5071-7.ch003

Copyright © 2021, IGI Global. Copying or distributing in print or electronic forms without written permission of IGI Global is prohibited.

INTRODUCTION

The increase in the number of patients with limited clinical and financial resources and the impact of time-consuming manual diagnostic modalities are serious bottlenecks in treatment capacities for healthcare delivery systems. However, recent developments and availability of high-accuracy and high-throughput clinical grade Artificial Intelligence (AI) tools could be part of the sustainable solutions to tackle this crisis in clinical care. Cardiovascular disease remains a leading cause of mortality, despite up to a quarter of deaths being preventable. Accurate diagnosis will support more effective information sharing. Furthermore, it is becoming incumbent for clinicians to provide personalised advice about interventions and disease progression, using improved methods of information sharing and data analytics (Deborah, 2017). The current model of image acquisition, interpretation, and decision-making presents problems with timing, efficiency, missed diagnoses, and false positive diagnoses. The advancement of cardiovascular imaging has come at a significant financial cost, and by facilitating image acquisition, measurement, reporting, and subsequent clinical pathways, artificial intelligence (AI) may reduce cost and improve value. The dynamic characteristics of the cardiovascular system are essential for understanding both its normal physiology and mechanisms of disease. Therefore, the application of ML to cardiovascular imaging lies at the interface of motion analysis, fluid dynamics, electrophysiology, and molecular cardiology.

In practical terms, AI can be interpreted as the ability of a machine, or a device, to make independent decisions based on the data inputted (Russell, 2003). Machine learning (ML) is a technique used to learn rules and identify patterns progressively from large datasets, without being explicitly programmed or without any a priori assumptions. ML takes many forms, but the most relevant to cardiovascular imaging are supervised and unsupervised learning. Supervised learning involves obtaining prior knowledge that is used to train the model, which often consists of human image annotation or objective categorisation. In contrast, unsupervised learning often involves searching for natural clusters in the data that may identify similar groups. Artificial neural networks (ANN) consists of large number of neurons, each having multiple inputs combined into a single output. Deep learning (DL) is a supervised learning method that mimics human cognition in which more internal layers are used than in traditional neural network approaches.

Most published studies have focused on automated segmentation, post-processing and computer-aided diagnosis. This chapter predominantly focuses on research works on machine learning for three modalities that have potential to be useful in the near future on cardiovascular imaging. We aim to provide a non-systematic narrative overview of the early applications and studies of the implementation of ML in cardiac imaging, categorised by the different imaging modalities: echocardiography, computerised-tomography (CT), magnetic resonance imaging (MRI) and nuclear imaging.

EVOLUTION OF MACHINE LEARNING IN CLINICAL IMAGING

Because of the large number of cardiac images that are routinely acquired with a wide range of modalities (Levin, 2019), there has been a surge in research applying deep learning in the cardiac domain (Figure 1). In this chapter, the authors aim to present an introduction to the basic concepts of deep learning and their possibilities, and offer a review of the state-of-the-art of machine learning reported in works on cardiovascular image analysis.

Before the advent of deep learning, a wealth of techniques had been developed to extract clinically relevant information from cardiovascular images. Machine learning algorithms currently in use normally require significant manual adjustment to convert an input image into the desired output (Polonsky, 2010). Although many conventional techniques showed promising results in challenging settings, they were often not robust yet for a routine clinical environment. Many have now been replaced, either in performance or in efficiency, by deep learning-based methods.

Figure 1. A simple illustration of image-based machine learning for cardiovascular imaging.
(Carlos Martin-Isla et al 2020, open-access Creative Commons Attribution License (CC BY))

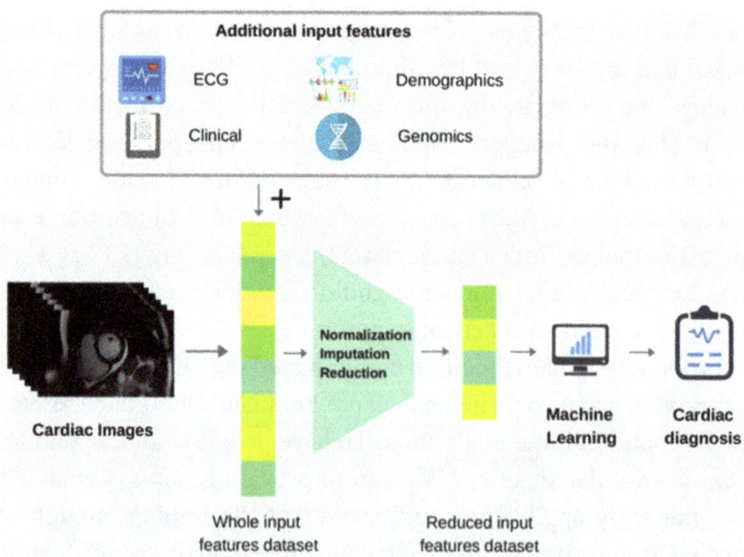

At the heart of all current popular deep learning methods are artificial neural networks (ANNs). The strength of ANNs lies in the fact that by combining many neurons in layers, highly nonlinear relationships between the input and the desired output can be modelled, which is typically needed to obtain accurate predictions. In earlier applications of AI, due to lack of computational power researchers were forced to use networks that were only a few layers deep. Generally, the relationship between a medical image and the desired output is too complex to capture efficiently with such shallow ANNs. However, these issues have been resolved because of the increasing availability of affordable computational power. Currently, researchers can easily build ANNs of tens or even hundreds of layers. This has enabled the direct application of neural networks to medical images without previous feature extraction.

Depending on the task that is being solved (e.g., image classification or enhancement), a specific neural network structure, or architecture (i.e. the number of layers of neurons and how they are connected), is chosen that is optimally suited for that specific task. The most common architecture in image analysis is the convolutional neural network (CNN) where the network architecture can be adapted to perform image segmentation. A second type of neural network architecture used in medical imaging is the recurrent neural network (RNN). RNNs are often used for sequential data, such as electrocardiography, text, or cine-MRI. When deciding on the architecture of a deep neural network, many choices need to be made. Important considerations are the type of network (e.g., ANN, CNN, RNN) Figure 2, the network depth (i.e., the number of layers), or the number of coefficients (i.e., number of nodes in an ANN, number of convolutional filters in a CNN). Over the past decade, the medical imaging field has become dominated by convolutional neural networks (CNNs), the deep learning architecture where the input is typically a matrix of pixel intensities derived from a medical image.

Figure 2. Basic architecture of an ANN and CNN.
(Carlos Martin-Isla et al 2020, open-access Creative Commons Attribution License (CC BY))

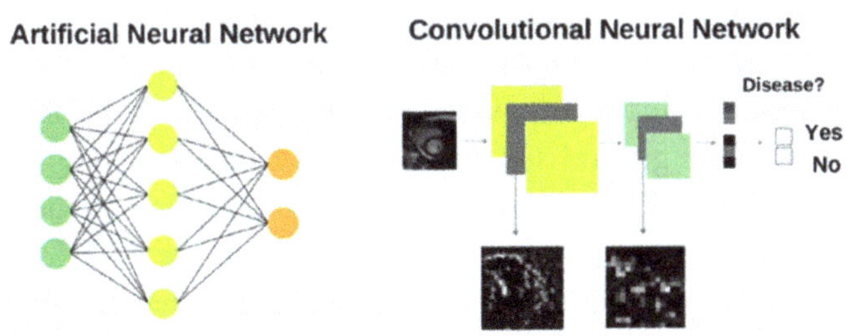

Echocardiography

As an imaging modality, advantageous for its speed, portability and affordability, echocardiography is the most widely used in cardiology (Siegersma, 2019). However, the method of data acquisition is user-dependent and requires intensive training in order to achieve accurate interpretation of the data (Feigenbaum, 1996). To reduce this user dependency, AI allows a more standardised analysis of the echocardiographic images. This has already been demonstrated in its ability to aid in the analysis of echocardiographic images, allowing the automated generation of important measures of cardiac function in real-time, along with automated classification of echocardiographic view.

In the echocardiographic imaging sequence, AI has been applied across various steps. Firstly, in the acquisition of echocardiographic images, automated identification and measurement has been implemented with an ML-based model of the left ventricular wall (Tamborini, 2017). The performance of this algorithm is equivalent to the traditional 3D echocardiographic methods and MRI. However, in pathologies with small ventricular cavities (e.g. congenital disorders), the left ventricular myocardium was not optimally recognised by the algorithm implemented. AI has been applied in the post-processing of echocardiographic images, namely by its classification of standard views, thus enabling a fully automated analysis (Khamish, 2017). Madani et al. demonstrated that in the classification of different views of an image, a deep-learning model can attain matching performance to that of a certified echocardiographer (Madani, 2018). The various parameters of cardiac function have been examined and ascertained with AI-based models trained with data from echocardiography. The published results proved that the determination of left ventricular ejection fraction and longitudinal strain via AI produces similar results as those from expert visual deduction (Knackstedt, 2015).

With the aim for automating ejection fraction measurements, the segmentation of the left and right ventricle is also of interest. The feasibility of using AI models trained with small training sets for the segmentation of the left ventricle has also been demonstrated (Carneiro, 2013). The accuracy of the segmentation is directly dependent on the number of training images used. This is an important characteristic of AI, i.e. increasing the amount of input data will normally improve the performance of the model. In addition, more generalised results can be obtained using a more diverse dataset of images (Carneiri, 2013). A good performance was also demonstrated in the determination of the size and function of the right ventricle (Medvedofsky, 2015). The r-values calculated for the correlation between automated and conventional right ventricular measurements ranged between 0.79 and 0.95. However both end-diastolic and end-systolic volumes were overestimated in the automated analyses. Furthermore, this method was only semi-automated and required manual tracing of the right ventricular wall within one frame (Medvedofsky, 2015). The former mentioned studies also applied post-processing steps, after data acquisition.

Recent developments include introduction of *on-the-fly* echocardiographic analysis into the software of hand-held ultrasound devices. This would enable automated analysis of variables during acquisition. In addition to automation, diagnosis and classification of cardiac pathologies are key features of AI. For example, three different classifiers for the detection of mitral regurgitation has been demonstrated by Moghaddasi and Nourian (2016). Using different input features, the automated identification of mitral regurgitation has been enhanced with AI. The strain rate curves and segmental deformation required for recognition of mitral regurgitation showed an accuracy of 87% (Tabassian, 2017). Another study used texture descriptors derived from discrete wavelet transforms of the ultrasound signal in order to perform analysis of mitral regurgitation yielded an accuracy of 99.5% (Sudarshan, 2015). Narula et al. (2016) used speckle tracking data with three different classifiers to differentiate between a patient's heart and hypertrophic cardiomyopathy. The classifiers demonstrated increased accuracy when combining different echocardiographic features compared to one stand-alone feature. Although clinically these pathologies are similar, the ML models provided the opportunity to distinguish between phenotypes and modify therapy accordingly (Narula, 2016). Similarly, echocardiographic data were also used to differentiate between patients with constrictive pericarditis and restrictive cardiomyopathy. Without AI the differentiation of these structures using four echocardiographic features generates an area under the receiver operating characteristic curve (AUC) of 0.942. A memory classifier trained with features from speckle tracking echocardiography in addition to the four echocardiographic features generated a higher value of AUC (0.962). While similar results were obtained with and without AI, this study demonstrates that implementation of AI for discrimination of these entities is attainable (Sengupta, 2016). The study published by Zhang et al. (2018) segmentation, calculation of numerous clinical parameters and diagnosis of three different cardiac pathologies from around 14000 echocardiograms were performed. Along the imaging pathway, the application of AI was shown to be achievable, e.g. for detection of disease the AUC ranged between 0.85 to 0.93.

Yet another diagnostic domain for the implementation of AI is the characterisation of the phenotype of heart failure with preserved ejection fraction (HFpEF). This management of the disease is restricted by the lack of a true gold standard definition and also due to its heterogeneous profile (Ponikowski, 2016). In a cohort study of 100 subjects including healthy (controls who were hypertensive and breathless) and HFpEF patients, a classifier for the classification of patients with HFpEF had an accuracy of 81% (Tabassian, 2018). The classification was partly determined by ML algorithms based on spatial-temporal rest-exercise features. This study also demonstrated the application of AI in diagnosis and post-processing of imaging data (Tabassian, 2018). A combination of imaging and clinical variables for classification and prediction of outcome in patients with HFpEF was used by Shah et al. (2015). The study showed an AUC between 0.70 and 0.76 during validation. In this study, three different phenotypes with a significant difference in endpoints of cardiovascular hospitalisation or death were generated in an unsupervised phenomapping of HFpEF patients. (Shah, 2015).

In summary, within a short period, AI could be implemented in echocardiography for automated segmentation and analysis of left and right ventricle contours and automated calculation of volumetric parameters, thereby reducing the workload of echocardiographic technicians. In due course, the classification of cardiovascular diseases with AI is likely to be achieved, based exclusively on echocardiographic images, by combining imaging data with clinical variables, supporting clinicians and radiographers. This will also facilitate the generation of improved decision making leading to a better diagnostic and prognostic performance in treatment of different cardiovascular pathologies.

Computed Tomography (CT)

Over the last decade, cardiac CT has improved exponentially, enhancing the accuracy of visualisation of stenosis in the coronary tree, plaque characteristics, coronary calcification and scoring. and more recently the modelling of flow (Nieman, 2015). In the context of image acquisition, the promising opportunities for AI in CT are automated noise reduction, while retaining optimal imaging quality, and the avoidance of invasive coronary angiography for determination of significant stenosis (Budoff, 2008; Wolterink, 2017). Wolterink et al. (2017) developed and validated a method to reduced radiation doses in CT imaging by training a DL model. In the model, low-dose CT images are used to estimate routine-dose CT images. A similar strategy using a convolutional neural network (CNN) was used to determine the calcium score from regular coronary CT angiography (CTA). This eliminated the need for calcium score CT and thereby reduced exposure of the patient to harmful radiation (Wolterink, 2016).

The capability of cardiac CT to perform vessel segmentation and image reconstruction (thus assisting with assessment of coronary stenoses) can be made part of the standard proprietary softwares. Automated segmentation of the left ventricle from coronary CT angiography (CTA)with convolutional neural networks has shown to be a feasible and reliable option (Zreik, 2016). Ascertaining the extent of coronary stenosis from coronary CTA is a clinical area that has been extensively studied. Any significant coronary stenosis is quantified in terms of the fractional flow reserve (FFR) <0.8 determined during invasive angiography. The use of AI generates clear models of local FFR, thereby replacing the need for any invasive measurements in many situations. From coronary CTA, different input features have been derived for modelling: physiological features (Itu, 2016), quantitative plaque measurements (Dey, 2018), features calculated from different spatially connected clusters of heart segmentation (Zreik, 2018), and geometric features of the coronary anatomy (Coenen 2018; Tesche 2017). Also features from CT perfusion are being evaluated for use with AI (Han, 2018). Current methods of non-invasive measurements of FFR using computational fluid dynamics are time consuming and requires expensive processors with high end computational capabilities. The substitution of these methods by AI has been shown to be faster with equally good performance (Itu, 2016; Coenen 2018).

Deep learning algorithms have also been used to segment the blood vessels and create a detailed topology of the lumen and vascular plaques, for use in a computational fluid dynamic (CFD) model investigating lesion-specific ischaemia and evaluating FFR (Taylor, 2017). However, these segmentations are susceptible to image noise, mis-registration, and patient motion that could hinder clinical interpretation. (Tesche, 2017) Recent studies have shown that deep learning algorithms perform equally well as CFD in the prediction of pathology progression (Tesche, 2018).

Another challenge in CT characterisation of coronary disease is that of partial volume effects, leading to an overestimation of the vessel lumen area (Freiman, 2017). Using AI to account for partial volume has led to significant improvements in non-invasive determination of FFR. These modifications may lead to a decrease in the required number of invasive angiograms, reserving such procedures for cases where intervention is required. AI approaches have also been implemented in the automated identification of coronary artery calcium (CAC) in ECG-gated non-contrast-enhanced CT imaging showing an intra-class correlation coefficient of 0.95. This is similar to that of trained personnel (Wolterink, 2015).

In a study to determine the diagnostic value of AI in coronary CTA, Zreik et al. (2019) obtained an accuracy of 0.77 for the detection and characterisation of coronary plaque. From a dataset of 163 patients, an even higher accuracy of 0.80 was obtained in the detection of stenosis and determination of the anatomical significance. Using a more supervised approach with predefined measurements known as radiomics features (Aerts 34; Kolossváry, 2017) identified coronary plaques with a napkin-ring sign (NRS), an independent prognostic marker of major adverse cardiac events (MACE). Data set having a large number of texture features, which were derived from the radiomics set, were used to distinguish between plaques with and without NRS. Another study used texture features derived from calcium score CT as the input in ML models to classify patients with acute or chronic myocardial infarction (MI) and control subjects. The resulting AUC was 0.78, and the model eliminated the need for any MRI scans (Mannil, 2018). However, as an extra non-automated activity, manual segmentation of the coronary plaques and the left ventricular wall was still needed. This poses a limitation for the implementation in the clinical workflow of cardiologists.

Furthermore, automated image analysis, diagnostics and prognostic evaluation have been applied in cardiac CT. Survival analysis was conducted in different patient groups at risk of cardiovascular pathology. ML models exhibited an AUC (0.79) for the classification of all-cause mortality among patients with suspected coronary artery disease (CAD) larger than the individual clinical and coronary CTCA metrics (e.g. Framingham risk score: 0.61, segment stenosis score: 0.64, segment involvement score: 0.64, Duke index: 0.62) (Motwani, 2017). An equivalent prognostic model was established using coronary CTCA features acquired from stenosis. This model predicted a risk score for all-cause death and non-fatal MI during a follow-up after 3 years with an AUC of 0.771. This AUC was greater than for each of the conventional coronary CTCA variables (Rosendael, 2018).

With advances in computing hardware, the iterative image reconstruction algorithms, which were proposed in the initial development stages of CT, have recently seen a revival and have achieved significant reductions in noise leading to lower radiation exposures (Geyer, 2015). Given a ground-truth reconstruction for image processing, CNNs can be used to reconstruct normal-dose CT images from low-dose counterparts. Although this approach has not been applied to gated cardiac CT for de-noising images, it has the potential to significantly reduce doses and for faster reconstruction (Chen, 2017).

Due to the non-invasive, relatively user-independent and faster processing characteristics of CT imaging, a fast growth of ML application in coronary CTCA can be expected. Also, the results of AI-based models are promising for cardiac CT, with added advantage of reduced exposure to radiation, yet preserving spatial resolution for appropriate diagnostic and possibly prognostic decisions. Another benefit of AI in CTCA is the reduced need for invasive angiography, by scaling up the informational value of the diagnostic images. Given the increasing number of studies that incorporate AI in CT, this field is widening and beginning to include other data sources for the analysis. This generates valuable models for personalised treatment in cardiovascular medicine.

Magnetic Resonance Imaging

The field of cardiac MRI allows for imaging of many characteristics of the heart, namely anatomical imaging, flow imaging, perfusion imaging and most importantly myocardial characterisation (Ferreira, 2015). However, given the many aspects that cardiac MRI covers (Fig 3), with regard to AI applications and the technological methods used in MRI, having experienced radiographers with knowledge of the

Figure 3. Cardiovascular magnetic resonance imaging from patient scheduling to image analysis and prognosis
(Tim Leiner 2019 Open Access, https://creativecommons.org/publicdomain/zero/1.0/)

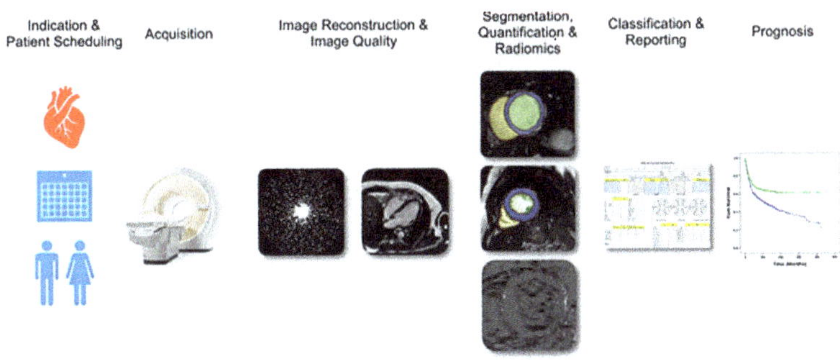

image acquisition and analysis techniques is critical. As a result, the quality of cardiac MR images is not only user dependent, but also scanner and vendor dependent. Automated segmentation of cardiac structures and infarct tissue have been the main topic of interest in cardiac MRI for a long time.

Analysing image data sets from cardiac MRI is time-consuming as it requires contours to be drawn on numerous images to elucidate biventricular volumes and mass (O'Regan, 2020). This introduces subjectivity and inconsistency in a task where precision is key for accurate diagnosis and surveillance. The numbers produced are also unrefined representations of function that are only moderately reproducible and insensitive to the underlying complex disturbances of cardiovascular physiology. Image segmentation, where each voxel is assigned an anatomical label, enables this to be automated. The segmentation labels can be distributed throughout the cardiac cycle for a snapshot of the cardiac chambers in individual images.

Numerous studies have been published on the automated segmentation of cine images (Avendi, 2016; Bratt, 2019; Ngo, 2017; Tan, 2017; Zheng, 2018) and automated calculation of cardiac parameters from MRI data sets (Bai, 2018; Suinesiaputra, 2018). Multiple software programs are also available that can perform automated segmentation based on AI. Karim et al. (2016) tested algorithms for automated segmentation on late gadolinium enhancement imaging. The work showed that AI algorithms provided better accuracy than fixed-model approaches. Beyond the performance metrics, a significant cutting down in time was the remarkably important characteristic of the automated AI-based segmentation. Baessler et al. (2018) used ML models to determine the most salient texture features obtained from cine images, in order to delineate patients with myocardial infarction and control subjects. The use of two texture features in multiple logistic regression analysis produced an AUC of 0.92. Application of this model in a clinical setting avoided the need for gadolinium-enhanced cardiac MRI, thereby expanding the eligible patient data set and in turn reducing costs. Snaauw et al. (2019) presented a novel approach with the possibility of an end-to-end classification of disease pathologies on cardiac MR images, without annotation.

The recent approach has been to apply CNNs to utilize data redundancy in under-sampled MRI through learned representations.(Schlemper, 2018) This has attained a 10-fold acceleration of two-dimensional (2D) cine sequences with real-time reconstruction, even though the performance index in patients with cardiac disease was not ascertained. The idea of moving from a sequential processing of image acquisition, analysis, and interpretation to one that is optimised from end-to-end using ML is also being rigorously undertaken in cardiac MRI. (Rueckert, 2016)

Two studies have reported in detail the performance of ML in predictive modelling based on cardiac MRI data. Principal component analysis was used in one study (Dawes, 2017) to determine the survival rate in patients with pulmonary hypertension. The three-dimensional cardiac motion of the right ventricle was used as the input for the analysis. This method generated an AUC of a time-dependent receiver operating characteristic analysis of 0.73. The inclusion of 3D-MR features in the model along with the clinical, functional and regular MR features derived from right sided heart catheterisation yielded a lower value of 0.6. A second predictive model by Samad et.al (2018) was used to examine the deterioration of left ventricular function in patients with a repaired tetralogy of Fallot. This study (AUC: 0.87) demonstrated that ML models can be useful for planning early intervention in patients at high risk of cardiovascular diseases.

The underlying drawbacks that compromise inter- and intra-patient comparability render the application of diagnostic and prognostic features of AI in MRI data more challenging than other imaging modalities. However as primary steps, the use of AI in cardiac MRI needs to concentrate on automated segmentation and calculation of variables. Software that incorporate these features are indeed emerging. New algorithms are also being developed, optimised and standardised for augmenting the existing approaches. A new deep learning architecture called an auto-encoder is also being used learn compressed representations of cardiac motion that can predict survival of patients. The outcome is a prediction of time-to-event based on learned features of cardiac motion that are clinically interpretable and has been shown to outperform the best available manual parameters (Bello, 2019).

FUTURE RESEARCH DIRECTIONS

In today's healthcare system, AI provides new opportunities for non-invasive cardiac imaging. However, many challenges remain and need to be proactively addressed to keep patients and the public open to the development and introduction of AI solutions. There is a growing potential to improve healthcare systems in terms of quality, equality and cost-effectiveness.

Across the domain of radiology, although automated diagnostic classification has expanded, the application of ML has been far more challenging in cardiovascular disease as both structural and dynamic features need to be captured. The classification of cardiovascular diseases has been enhanced by well-defined, yet arbitrary, haemodynamic or volumetric criteria. Pulmonary hypertension perhaps is one such example as one definition is a resting mean pressure of minimum 25 mmHg in the pulmonary artery. Hypertrophic cardiomyopathy is another where a wall thickness of 15 mm is significant (Elliott, 2014; Galie, 2015). Furthermore, other disease states where conventional imaging struggles to classify adequately may in the future be solved by an effective use of AI. For example, heart failure with preserved ejection fraction (HFpEF) is a very diverse clinical condition with many risk factors. Initial data show that model-based unsupervised clustering can identify homogeneous patient classes with distinct outcomes from multiple variables that include echocardiographic, clinical, and biochemical observations (Shah, 2015). Deep learning architectures have also been implemented to clustering and may provide faster interpretation and grouping of high volume data that could be interesting for image based assignments (Xie, 2016).

Deep learning could also play a major role in directly predicting prognosis from imaging data sets of patients diagnosed with various cardiovascular diseases. To date, this approach has not yet been fully explored, and the applications developed so far have been limited to biomarkers of estimation (e.g., the amount of epicardial fat or the quantity of coronary calcium). These features may in fact aid in the future of AI application, since the accumulation of large amounts of patient and disease-specific data may allow for large association studies and multiscale modelling. . However, such datasets are not widely available and are challenging to gather. This has been the key limitation of published applications of deep learning in cardiovascular imaging.

CONCLUSION

Artificial intelligence approaches have the potential to predict the risk of future cardiac events using the images as inputs and require no human intervention. In MRI, the process starts with cardiac MR images from which time-resolved 3D segmentations of the heart can be created using a type of CNN specialised for this task (Ronneberger, 2015). These can be performed in less than a heartbeat. These examples show the potential of ML algorithms, not just for analysing cardiac image data, but also for providing meaningful outputs leading to development of well-guided disease management strategy.

ML applications has been challenging due to the extra dimension of motion in cardiac imaging but still has the potential in delivering improved predictions, person-specific treatments, and discovery of new therapeutic pathways. Even though the research focus has been to fill the knowledge gaps and address the unmet needs of patients, the distinctive complexities associated with cardiac physiology also demand innovation in the design and implementation of ML architectures. Therefore, a collaborative research endeavour from other time-resolved data domains where ML has been well-established will be the key to the future advancements in this emerging field of research.

Although the inception of deep learning concepts in cardiovascular imaging is having a big impact, from both the perspectives of research and industry, it is important to understand that deep learning is not a solution for-all for critical cardiovascular pathologies. Although algorithms based on deep learning have demonstrated advanced performance in certain medical research assignments, the scope of these works has been quite limited. The rapid digitalization of healthcare presents opportunities to address important medical questions using ML. While traditional statistical methods remain the trade language of medical researchers, ML provides users with novel toolsets for navigating a rapidly evolving diagnosis landscape. Additionally, ML could provide a powerful platform for integration of clinical and imaging datasets, which would be useful for multifactorial and complex cardiovascular diseases.

ACKNOWLEDGMENT

Then authors like to acknowledge the support from Imperial National Institute for Health Research (NIHR) Biomedical Research Centre (BRC).

REFERENCES

Aerts, HJ, Velazquez, ER, & Leijenaar, RT, etal. (2014). Decoding tumour phenotype by non invasive imaging using a quantitative radiomics approach. *Nature Communications*, *5*(4006), 1–8.

Avendi, M. R., Kheradvar, A., & Jafarkhani, H. (2016). A combined deep learning and deformable-model approach to fully automatic segmentation of the left ventricle in cardiac MRI. *Medical Image Analysis*, *30*, 108–119. doi:10.1016/j.media.2016.01.005 PMID:26917105

Baessler, B., Mannil, M., Oebel, S., Maintz, D., Alkadhi, H., & Manka, R. (2018). Subacute and chronic left ventricular myocardial scar: Accuracy of texture analysis on nonenhanced cineMR images. *Radiology*, *286*(1), 103–112. doi:10.1148/radiol.2017170213 PMID:28836886

Bai, W., Sinclair, M., Tarroni, G., Oktay, O., Rajchl, M., Vaillant, G., Lee, A. M., Aung, N., Lukaschuk, E., Sanghvi, M. M., Zemrak, F., Fung, K., Paiva, J. M., Carapella, V., Kim, Y. J., Suzuki, H., Kainz, B., Matthews, P. M., Petersen, S. E., ... Rueckert, D. (2018). Automated cardiovascular magnetic resonance image analysis with fully convolutional networks. *Journal of Cardiovascular Magnetic Resonance*, *20*(65), 1–12. doi:10.118612968-018-0471-x PMID:30217194

Bello, G., Dawes, T. J., Duan, J., Biffi, C., de Marvao, A., Howard, L. S. G. E., Gibbs, J. S. R., Wilkins, M. R., Cook, S. A., Rueckert, D., & O'Regan, D. P. (2019). Deep learning cardiac motion analysis for human survival prediction. *Nat Mach Intell*, *1*(2), 95–104. doi:10.103842256-019-0019-2 PMID:30801055

Bratt, A., Kim, J., Pollie, M., Beecy, A. N., Tehrani, N. H., Codella, N., Perez-Johnston, R., Palumbo, M. C., Alakbarli, J., Colizza, W., Drexler, I. R., Azevedo, C. F., Kim, R. J., Devereux, R. B., & Weinsaft, J. W. (2019). Machine learning derived segmentation of phase velocity encoded cardiovascular magnetic resonance for fully automated aortic flow quantification. *Journal of Cardiovascular Magnetic Resonance*, *21*(1), 1–11. doi:10.118612968-018-0509-0 PMID:30612574

Budoff, M. J., Dowe, D., Jollis, J. G., Gitter, M., Sutherland, J., Halamert, E., Scherer, M., Bellinger, R., Martin, A., Benton, R., Delago, A., & Min, J. K. (2008). Diagnostic performance of 64-multidetector row coronary computed tomographic angiography for evaluation of coronary artery stenosis in individuals without known coronary artery disease. *Journal of the American College of Cardiology*, *52*(21), 1724–1732. doi:10.1016/j.jacc.2008.07.031 PMID:19007693

Carneiro, G., & Nascimento, J. C. (2013). Combining multiple dynamic models and deep learning architectures for tracking the left ventricle endocardium in ultrasound data. *IEEE Transactions on Pattern Analysis and Machine Intelligence*, *35*(11), 2592–2607. doi:10.1109/TPAMI.2013.96 PMID:24051722

Chen, H., Zhang, Y., & Zhang, W. (2017). Low-dose CT via convolutional neural network. *Biomed Opt Express*, *8*(2), 679-94.

Coenen, A., Kim, Y. H., Kruk, M., Tesche, C., De Geer, J., Kurata, A., Lubbers, M. L., Daemen, J., Itu, L., Rapaka, S., Sharma, P., Schwemmer, C., Persson, A., Schoepf, U. J., Kepka, C., Hyun Yang, D., & Nieman, K. (2018). Diagnostic accuracy of a machine-learning approach to coronary computed tomographic angiography-based fractional flow reserve result from the MACHINE Consortium. *Circulation: Cardiovascular Imaging*, *11*(6), 1–11. doi:10.1161/CIRCIMAGING.117.007217 PMID:29914866

Dawes, T. J. W., de Marvao, A., Shi, W., Fletcher, T., Watson, G. M. J., Wharton, J., Rhodes, C. J., Howard, L. S. G. E., Gibbs, J. S. R., Rueckert, D., Cook, S. A., Wilkins, M. R., & O'Regan, D. P. (2017). Machine learning of three-dimensional right ventricular motion enables outcome prediction in pulmonary hypertension: A cardiac MR imaging study. *Radiology*, *283*(2), 381–390. doi:10.1148/radiol.2016161315 PMID:28092203

Deborah Oakley, MRC London Institute of Medical Sciences. (2017). *Putting people at the heart of research.* Available at: https://lms.mrc.ac.uk/putting-people-heartresearch/

Dey, D., Gaur, S., Ovrehus, K. A., Slomka, P. J., Betancur, J., Goeller, M., Hell, M. M., Gransar, H., Berman, D. S., Achenbach, S., Botker, H. E., Jensen, J. M., Lassen, J. F., & Norgaard, B. L. (2018). Integrated prediction of lesion-specific ischaemia from quantitative coronary CT angiography using machine learning: A multicentre study. *European Radiology*, *28*(6), 2655–2664. doi:10.100700330-017-5223-z PMID:29352380

Elliott, P.M., Anastasakis, A., & Borger, M.A. (2014). ESC guidelines on diagnosis and management of hypertrophic cardiomyopathy: the task force for the diagnosis and management of hypertrophic cardiomyopathy of the european society of cardiology (ESC). *Eur Heart J, 35*(39), 2733-79.

Feigenbaum, H. (1996). Evolution of echocardiography. *Circulation*, *93*(7), 1321–1327. doi:10.1161/01.CIR.93.7.1321 PMID:8641018

Ferreira, V. M., Robson, M. D., & Karamitsos, T. D. (2015). Magnetic resonance imaging. In K. Nieman, O. Gaemperli, P. Lancellotti, & S. Plein (Eds.), *Advanced cardiac imaging. Sawston* (pp. 127–169). Woodhead. doi:10.1016/B978-1-78242-282-2.00006-8

Freiman, M., Nickisch, H., Prevrhal, S., Schmitt, H., Vembar, M., Maurovich-Horvat, P., Donnelly, P., & Goshen, L. (2017). Improving CCTA based lesions' hemodynamic significance assessment by accounting for partial volume modeling in automatic coronary lumen segmentation. *Medical Physics*, *44*(3), 1040–1049. doi:10.1002/mp.12121 PMID:28112409

Galie, N., Humbert, M., & Vachiery, J. L. (2015). ESC/ERS guidelines for the diagnosis and treatment of pulmonary hypertension: the joint task force for the diagnosis and treatment of pulmonary hypertension of the European Society of Cardiology (ESC) and the European Respiratory Society (ERS): endorsed by: Association for European Paediatric and Congenital Cardiology (AEPC), International Society for Heart and Lung Transplantation (ISHLT). *Eur Heart J, 37*(1), 67-119.

Geyer, L. L., Schoepf, U. J., & Meinel, F. G. (2015). State of the art: iterative CT reconstruction techniques. *Radiology*, *276*(2), 339-57.

Han, D., Lee, J. H., Rizvi, A., Gransar, H., Baskaran, L., Schulman-Marcus, J., ó Hartaigh, B., Lin, F. Y., & Min, J. K. (2018). Incremental role of resting myocardial computed tomography perfusion for predicting physiologically significant coronary artery disease: A machine learning approach. *Journal of Nuclear Cardiology*, *25*(1), 223–233. doi:10.100712350-017-0834-y PMID:28303473

Itu, L., Rapaka, S., Passerini, T., Georgescu, B., Schwemmer, C., Schoebinger, M., Flohr, T., Sharma, P., & Comaniciu, D. (2016). A machine-learning approach for computation of fractional flow reserve from coronary computed tomography. *Journal of Applied Physiology (Bethesda, Md.)*, *121*(1), 42–52. doi:10.1152/japplphysiol.00752.2015 PMID:27079692

Karim, R., Bhagirath, P., Claus, P., James Housden, R., Chen, Z., Karimaghaloo, Z., Sohn, H.-M., Lara Rodríguez, L., Vera, S., Albà, X., Hennemuth, A., Peitgen, H.-O., Arbel, T., Gonzàlez Ballester, M. A., Frangi, A. F., Götte, M., Razavi, R., Schaeffter, T., & Rhode, K. (2016). Evaluation of state of-the-art segmentation algorithms for left ventricle infarct from late gadolinium enhancement MR images. *Medical Image Analysis*, *30*, 95–107. doi:10.1016/j.media.2016.01.004 PMID:26891066

Khamis, H., Zurakhov, G., Azar, V., Raz, A., Friedman, Z., & Adam, D. (2017). Automatic apical view classification of echocardiograms using a discriminative learningdictionary. *Medical Image Analysis*, *36*, 15–21. doi:10.1016/j.media.2016.10.007 PMID:27816858

Knackstedt, C., Bekkers, S. C. A. M., Schummers, G., Schreckenberg, M., Muraru, D., Badano, L. P., Franke, A., Bavishi, C., Omar, A. M. S., & Sengupta, P. P. (2015). Fully automated versus standard tracking of left ventricular ejection fraction and longitudinal strain: The FAST-EFs Multicenter Study. *Journal of the American College of Cardiology, 66*(13), 1456–1466. doi:10.1016/j.jacc.2015.07.052 PMID:26403342

Kolossváry, M., Karády, J., Szilveszter, B., Kitslaar, P., Hoffmann, U., Merkely, B., & Maurovich-Horvat, P. (2017). Radiomic features are superior to conventional quantitative computed tomographic metrics to identify coronary plaques with napkin- ring sign. *Circulation: Cardiovascular Imaging, 10*(12), 1–9. doi:10.1161/CIRCIMAGING.117.006843 PMID:29233836

Levin, D. C., Parker, L., Halpern, E. J., & Rao, V. M. (2019). Coronary CT angiography: Reversal of earlier utilization trends. *Journal of the American College of Radiology, 16*(2), 147–155. doi:10.1016/j.jacr.2018.07.022 PMID:30158087

Madani, A., Arnaout, R., Mofrad, M., & Arnaout, R. (2018). Fast and accurate view classification of echocardiograms using deep learning. *NPJ Digital Medicine, 1*(6), 1–8. doi:10.103841746-017-0013-1 PMID:30828647

Mannil, M., Von Spiczak, J., Manka, R., & Alkadhi, H. (2018). Texture analysis and machine learning for detecting myocardial infarction in non contrast low-dose computed tomography: Unveiling the invisible. *Investigative Radiology, 53*(6), 338–343. doi:10.1097/RLI.0000000000000448 PMID:29420321

Medvedofsky, D., Addetia, K., Hamilton, J., Leon Jimenez, J., Lang, R. M., & Mor-Avi, V. (2015). Semi-automated echocardiographic quantification of right ventricular size and function. *The International Journal of Cardiovascular Imaging, 31*(6), 1149–1157. doi:10.100710554-015-0672-4 PMID:25948160

Moghaddasi, H., & Nourian, S. (2016). Automatic assessment of mitral regurgitation severity based on extensive textural features on 2D echocardiography videos. *Computers in Biology and Medicine, 73*, 47–55. doi:10.1016/j.compbiomed.2016.03.026 PMID:27082766

Motwani, M., Dey, D., & Berman, D. S. (2017). Machine learning for prediction of all-cause mortality in patients with suspected coronary artery disease: A 5-year multicentre prospective registry analysis. *European Heart Journal, 38*, 500–507. PMID:27252451

Narula, S., Shameer, K., Salem, O. A. M., Dudley, J. T., & Sengupta, P. P. (2016). Machine-learning algorithms to automate morphological and functional assessments in 2D echocardiography. *Journal of the American College of Cardiology, 68*(21), 2287–2295. doi:10.1016/j.jacc.2016.08.062 PMID:27884247

Ngo, T. A., Lu, Z., & Carneiro, G. (2017). Combining deep learning and level set for the automated segmentation of the left ventricle of the heart from cardiac cine magnetic resonance. *Medical Image Analysis*, *35*, 159–171. doi:10.1016/j.media.2016.05.009 PMID:27423113

Nieman, K., Coenen, A., & Dijkshoorn, M. (2015). Computed tomography. In Advanced cardiac imaging. Woodhead. doi:10.1016/B978-1-78242-282-2.00005-6

O'Regan, D. P. (2020). Putting machine learning into motion: Applications in cardiovascular imaging. *Clinical Radiology*, *75*(1), 33–37. doi:10.1016/j.crad.2019.04.008 PMID:31079952

Polonsky, T., McClelland, R., & Jorgensen, N. (2010). Coronary artery calcium score and risk classification for coronary heart disease prediction. *Journal of the American Medical Association*, *303*(16), 1610–1616. doi:10.1001/jama.2010.461 PMID:20424251

Ponikowski, P., Voors, A. A., Anker, S. D., Bueno, H., Cleland, J. G. F., Coats, A. J. S., Falk, V., González-Juanatey, J. R., Harjola, V.-P., Jankowska, E. A., Jessup, M., Linde, C., Nihoyannopoulos, P., Parissis, J. T., Pieske, B., Riley, J. P., Rosano, G. M. C., Ruilope, L. M., Ruschitzka, F., ... van der Meer, P. (2016). The Task Force for the diagnosis and treatment of acute and chronic heart failure of the European Society of Cardiology (ESC). (2016) ESC Guidelines for the diagnosis and treatment of acute and chronic heart failure. *European Heart Journal*, *37*(27), 2129–2200. doi:10.1093/eurheartj/ehw128 PMID:27206819

Ronneberger, O., Fischer, P., & Brox, T. (2015). U-net: convolutional networks for biomedical image segmentation. In Lecture notes in computer science: Vol. 9351. *Medical Image Computing and Computer-Assisted Intervention e MICCAI 2015. MICCAI 2015*. Springer. doi:10.1007/978-3-319-24574-4_28

Rueckert, D. (2016). Engineering, Physical Sciences Research Council. *Smart Heart: next generation cardiovascular healthcare via integrated image acquisition, reconstruction, analysis and learning*. Available at: http://gow.epsrc.ac.uk/NGBOViewGrant.aspx?GrantRef1/4EP/P001009/1

Russell, S., & Norvig, P. (2003). *Artificial Intelligence: A Modern Approach* (2nd ed.). Prentice Hall.

Samad, M. D., Wehner, G. J., Arbabshirani, M. R., Jing, L., Powell, A. J., Geva, T., Haggerty, C. M., & Fornwalt, B. K. (2018). Predicting deterioration of ventricular function in patients with repaired tetralogy of Fallot using machine learning. *European Heart Journal Cardiovascular Imaging*, *19*(7), 730–738. doi:10.1093/ehjci/jey003 PMID:29538684

Schlemper, J., Caballero, J., & Hajnal, J.V. (2018). A deep cascade of convolutional neural networks for dynamic MR image reconstruction. *IEEE Trans Med Imaging*, *37*(2), 491-503.

Sengupta, P. P., Huang, Y. M., Bansal, M., Ashrafi, A., Fisher, M., Shameer, K., Gall, W., & Dudley, J. T. (2016). Cognitive machine-learning algorithm for cardiac imaging; a pilot study for differentiating constrictive pericarditis from restrictive cardiomyopathy. *Circulation: Cardiovascular Imaging*, *9*(6), 1–10. doi:10.1161/CIRCIMAGING.115.004330 PMID:27266599

Shah, S. J., Katz, D. H., Selvaraj, S., Burke, M. A., Yancy, C. W., Gheorghiade, M., Bonow, R. O., Huang, C.-C., & Deo, R. C. (2015). Heart failure phenomapping for novel classification of heart failure with preserved ejection fraction. *Circulation*, *131*(3), 269–279. doi:10.1161/CIRCULATIONAHA.114.010637 PMID:25398313

Shah, S. J., Katz, D. H., Selvaraj, S., Burke, M. A., Yancy, C. W., Gheorghiade, M., Bonow, R. O., Huang, C.-C., & Deo, R. C. (2015). Phenomapping for novel classification of heart failure with preserved ejection fraction. *Circulation*, *131*(3), 269–279. doi:10.1161/CIRCULATIONAHA.114.010637 PMID:25398313

Siegersma, K. R., Leiner, T., Chew, D. P., Appelman, Y., Hofstra, L., & Verjans Neth, J. W. (2019). Artificial intelligence in cardiovascular imaging: State of the art and implications for the imaging cardiologist. *The Hearing Journal*, *27*, 403–413. PMID:31399886

Snaauw, G., Gong, D., & Maicas, G. (2019). End-to-end diagnosis and segmentation learning from cardiac magnetic resonance imaging. *2019 IEEE 16th International Symposium on Biomedical Imaging (ISBI 2019),* 802–5.

Sudarshan, V., Ng, E. Y., & Acharya, U. R. (2015). Computer-aided diagnosis of myocardial infarction using ultrasound images with DWT, GLCM and HOS methods: A comparative study. *Computers in Biology and Medicine*, *62*, 86–93. doi:10.1016/j.compbiomed.2015.03.033 PMID:25912990

Suinesiaputra, A., Sanghvi, M. M., Aung, N., Paiva, J. M., Zemrak, F., Fung, K., Lukaschuk, E., Lee, A. M., Carapella, V., Kim, Y. J., Francis, J., Piechnik, S. K., Neubauer, S., Greiser, A., Jolly, M.-P., Hayes, C., Young, A. A., & Petersen, S. E. (2018). Fully-automated left ventricular mass and volume MRI analysis in the UK Biobank population cohort: Evaluation of initial results. *The International Journal of Cardiovascular Imaging*, *34*(2), 281–291. doi:10.100710554-017-1225-9 PMID:28836039

Tabassian, M., Alessandrini, M., Herbots, L., Mirea, O., Pagourelias, E. D., Jasaityte, R., Engvall, J., De Marchi, L., Masetti, G., & D'hooge, J. (2017). Machine learning of the spatio-temporal characteristics of echocardiographic deformation curves for infarct classification. *The International Journal of Cardiovascular Imaging*, *33*(8), 1159–1167. doi:10.100710554-017-1108-0 PMID:28321681

Tabassian, M., Sunderji, I., Erdei, T., Sanchez-Martinez, S., Degiovanni, A., Marino, P., Fraser, A. G., & D'hooge, J. (2018). Diagnosis of heart failure with preserved ejection fraction: Machine learning of spatiotemporal variations in left ventricular deformation. *Journal of the American Society of Echocardiography*, *31*(12), 1272–1284. doi:10.1016/j.echo.2018.07.013 PMID:30146187

Tamborini, G., Piazzese, C., Lang, R. M., Muratori, M., Chiorino, E., Mapelli, M., Fusini, L., Ali, S. G., Gripari, P., Pontone, G., Andreini, D., & Pepi, M. (2017). Feasibility and Accuracy of automated software for transthoracic three dimensional left ventricular volume and function analysis: Comparisons with two-dimensional echocardiography, three-dimensional transthoracic manual method, and cardiac magnetic resonance imaging. *Journal of the American Society of Echocardiography*, *30*(11), 1049–1058. doi:10.1016/j.echo.2017.06.026 PMID:28916243

Tan, L. K., Liew, Y. M., Lim, E., & McLaughlin, R. A. (2017). Convolutional neural network regression for short-axis left ventricle segmentation in cardiac cine MR sequences. *Medical Image Analysis*, *39*, 78–86. doi:10.1016/j.media.2017.04.002 PMID:28437634

Taylor, C.A., Fonte, T.A., & Min, J.K. (2013). Computational fluid dynamics applied to cardiac computed tomography for noninvasive quantification of fractional flow reserve: scientific basis. *J Am Coll Cardiol*, *61*(22), 2233-41.

Tesche, C., De Cecco, C. N., & Albrecht, M.H. (2017). Coronary CT angiography derived fractional flow reserve. *Radiology*, *285*(1), 17-33.

Tesche, C., De Cecco, C. N., & Baumann, S. (2018). Coronary CT angiography derived fractional flow reserve: machine learning algorithm versus computational fluid dynamics modeling. *Radiology*, *288*(1), 64-72.

Tesche, C., Vliegenthart, R., Duguay, T. M., De Cecco, C. N., Albrecht, M. H., De Santis, D., Langenbach, M. C., Varga-Szemes, A., Jacobs, B. E., Jochheim, D., Baquet, M., Bayer, R. R. II, Litwin, S. E., Hoffmann, E., Steinberg, D. H., & Schoepf, U. J. (2017). Coronary computed tomographic angiography-derived fractional flow reserve for therapeutic decision making. *The American Journal of Cardiology*, *120*(12), 2121–2127. doi:10.1016/j.amjcard.2017.08.034 PMID:29102036 van Rosendael, A. R., Maliakal, G., Kolli, K. K., Beecy, A., Al'Aref, S. J., Dwivedi, A., Singh, G., Panday, M., Kumar, A., Ma, X., Achenbach, S., Al-Mallah, M. H., Andreini, D., Bax, J. J., Berman, D. S., Budoff, M. J., Cademartiri, F., Callister, T. Q., Chang, H.-J., ... Min, J. K. (2018). Maximization of the usage of coronary CTA derived plaque information using a machine learning based algorithm to improve risk stratification; insights from the CONFIRM registry. *Journal of Cardiovascular Computed Tomography*, *12*(3), 204–209. doi:10.1016/j.jcct.2018.04.011 PMID:29753765

Wolterink, J. M., Leiner, T., DeVos, B. D., van Hamersvelt, R. W., Viergever, M. A., & Išgum, I. (2016). Automatic coronary artery calcium scoring in cardiac CT angiography using paired convolutional neural networks. *Medical Image Analysis*, *34*, 123–136. doi:10.1016/j.media.2016.04.004 PMID:27138584

Wolterink, J. M., Leiner, T., Takx, R. A. P., Viergever, M. A., & Išgum, I. (2015). Cardiac CT with ambiguity detection. *IEEE Transactions on Medical Imaging*, *34*(9), 1867–1878. doi:10.1109/TMI.2015.2412651 PMID:25794387

Wolterink, J. M., Leiner, T., Viergever, M. A., & Isgum, I. (2017). Generative adversarial networks for noise reduction in low-dose CT. *IEEE Transactions on Medical Imaging*, *36*(12), 2536–2545. doi:10.1109/TMI.2017.2708987 PMID:28574346

Xie, J., Girshick, R., & Farhadi, A. (2016). Unsupervised deep embedding for clustering analysis. *Proceedings of the 33rd international Conference on international Conference on machine learning*, 48, 478-87.

Zhang, J., Gajjala, S., Agrawal, P., Tison, G. H., Hallock, L. A., Beussink-Nelson, L., Lassen, M. H., Fan, E., Aras, M. A., Jordan, C. R., Fleischmann, K. E., Melisko, M., Qasim, A., Shah, S. J., Bajcsy, R., & Deo, R. C. (2018). Fully automated echocardiogram interpretation in clinical practice. *Circulation*, *138*(16), 1623–1635. doi:10.1161/CIRCULATIONAHA.118.034338 PMID:30354459

Zheng, Q., Delingette, H., Duchateau, N., & Ayache, N. (2018). 3-D consistent and robust segmentation of cardiac images by deep learning with spatial propagation. *IEEE Transactions on Medical Imaging*, *37*(9), 2137–2148. doi:10.1109/TMI.2018.2820742 PMID:29994087

Zreik, M., Leiner, T., & de Vos, B. D. (2016). Automatic segmentation of the left ventricle in cardiac CT angiography using convolutional neural networks. *IEEE 13th International Symposium on Biomedical Imaging (ISBI)*, 40–43. 10.1109/ISBI.2016.7493206

Zreik, M., Lessmann, N., vanHamersvelt, R. W., Wolterink, J. M., Voskuil, M., Viergever, M. A., Leiner, T., & Išgum, I. (2018). Deep learning analysis of the myocardium in coronary CT angiography for identification of patients with functionally significant coronary artery stenosis. *Medical Image Analysis*, *44*, 72–85. doi:10.1016/j.media.2017.11.008 PMID:29197253

Zreik, M., van Hamersvelt, R. W., Wolterink, J. M., Leiner, T., Viergever, M. A., & Isgum, I. (2019). A Recurrent CNN for Automatic Detection and Classification of Coronary Artery Plaque and Stenosis in Coronary CT Angiography. *IEEE Transactions on Medical Imaging*, *7*(38), 1588–1598. doi:10.1109/TMI.2018.2883807 PMID:30507498

Chapter 4
A CONVblock for Convolutional Neural Networks

Hmidi Alaeddine
https://orcid.org/0000-0002-2417-3972
Laboratory of Electronics and Microelectronics, Faculty of Sciences of Monastir, Monastir University, Tunisia

Malek Jihene
Higher Institute of Applied Sciences and Technology of Sousse, Sousse University, Tunisia & Laboratory of Electronics and Microelectronics, Faculty of Sciences of Monastir, Monastir University, Tunisia

ABSTRACT

The reduction in the size of convolution filters has been shown to be effective in image classification models. They make it possible to reduce the calculation and the number of parameters used in the operations of the convolution layer while increasing the efficiency of the representation. The authors present a deep architecture for classification with improved performance. The main objective of this architecture is to improve the main performances of the network thanks to a new design based on CONVblock. The proposal is evaluated on a classification database: CIFAR-10 and MNIST. The experimental results demonstrate the effectiveness of the proposed method. This architecture offers an error of 1.4% on CIFAR-10 and 0.055% on MNIST.

INTRODUCTION

In recent years, Convolutional Neural Networks (CNN) is a well-known deep learning architecture. It has achieved very good performance on various issues, such as visual recognition and detection. In 1959, Hubel and Wiesel (D. H. Hubel, 1968) discovered

DOI: 10.4018/978-1-7998-5071-7.ch004

Copyright © 2021, IGI Global. Copying or distributing in print or electronic forms without written permission of IGI Global is prohibited.

that animal visual cortex cells were responsible for detecting light in the receiving fields. Inspired by this discovery, in 1980, Fukushima proposed the neocognitron (K. Fukushima, 1982), which could be considered as the first work that deserves to be depth. After 10 years, Yann leCun et al. (B. B. Le Cun, 1989) proposed a network of artificial neurons multilayer capable of classifying the handwritten digits. This network is called LeNet-5. The LeNet-5 integrates several layers (Convolution, Pooling, Fully connected) and can be trained with the back propagation algorithm (Hecht-Nielsen, 1988). Since 2006, many methods have been proposed to overcome the difficulties encountered in the formation of deep CNN (X.-X. Niu, 2012),(O. Russakovsky, 2015), (K. Simonyan, 2015), (C. Szegedy, 2015). Since AlexNet's (Alex Krizhevsky, 2012) success in 2012, several enhancements have been made to CNN's convolution layers. However, various proposals have been made to this layer to improve its representational capacity. Convolution using filters whose weights are automatically learned during training extract different characteristics. There is a wide variety of filters that can be chosen for convolution. The purpose of the convolution layer is to learn the representations of the input features. Convolution techniques are proposed for convolution management in the other two directions (height and width), as well as arithmetic convolution . A 1×1 convolution is described as a solution of treatment with depth in convolution. The advantages of this type of convolution are the reduction of dimensionality for efficient calculations, pooling of functionalities and also include the use of new non-linearity such as ReLU after convolution. This convolution layer is equivalent to the parametric grouping operation between channels that is followed by ReLU (V. Nair, 2010) . The convolution of size 1×1 has been proposed in Network in Network (NiN) (M. Lin, 2014). It was then heavily exploited in the Google Inception architecture (C. Szegedy, 2015). Szegedy et al. (C. Szegedy, 2015), which can be considered as a logical outcome of NIN (M. Lin, 2014), introduce the Inception module. They use variable filter sizes to capture different visual models of different sizes. The Inception module integrates layers of convolution that are placed before the convolutions of sizes 3×3 and 5×5 for reducing the depth and width of CNN. This solution has reduced the parameters of this network (C. Szegedy, 2015) up to 5 million, which is much lower than AlexNet (Alex Krizhevsky, 2012) (60 million) and ZFNet (M. D. Zeiler, 2014) (75 million). In Deep Learning, several architectures, CNN (Convolutional Neural Network), take their name from the convolutional layer. Diluted CNN (F. Yu, 2016) is a CNN proposal that introduces an additional hyper-parameter into the suitable layer. This extra hyper-parameter l (dilation rate) indicates how much we want to expand the kernel. CNN dilated performed interesting performances in different tasks such as speech synthesis (Aaron van den Oord, 2016) and synthesis and speech recognition (T. Sercu, 2016). The technique of diluted convolution has been introduced in (F. Yu, 2016) and (L.-C. Chen, 2015). The dilated convolutions "inflate" the size of the network's reception field and allow it to cover more suitable information, thanks to insertion by inserting spaces between the elements of the kernels (there are usually 1-1 spaces inserted between the elements of the kernel). The mechanism of weight sharing in CNNs can play an important role in reducing the number of parameters. Tiled CNN (J. Ngiam, 2010) is a CNN variation of tiles and multi-feature maps to learn invariant rotation and scale characteristics. Their experiments conducted by (J. Ngiam, 2010). In (Z. Wang, 2015), Wang et al. found that Tiled CNN generates higher results than traditional CNN (. Zheng, 2014) for small time series databases. For many network architectures, it is desired to perform transformations going in the opposite direction to a normal convolution, It can be seen as the backward step of a traditional convolution. It is also known as de-convolution (M. D. Zeiler, 2014), (M. D. Zeiler D. K., 2010), (M. D. Zeiler G. W., 2011), (J. Long, 2017) and fractional convolution (F. Visin, 2015). De-convolution combines a single activation with several output activations. Unlike the normal convolution that links several input activations to a single activation, the de-convolution has been widely used for visualization (M. D. Zeiler G. W., 2011), recognition (C. Cao, 2015), (J. Zhang, 2016), (Y. Zhang, 2016) semantic segmentation (H. Noh, 2015), and localization (B. Zhou, 2016).

The reduction in the size of convolution filters has demonstrated their effectiveness in image classification models, both to obtain better models than before what was possible for a given number of parameters and to significantly reduce the number of parameters to be executed at a given level. In this work, convolutional networks based on CONVblock are proposed and implemented. We introduce a new architecture that allows a significant reduction of the number of parameters and the amount of computation required and to obtain advanced results in terms of classification accuracy.

The rest of his papers are organized like this, we will first briefly describe the background in Section II. The third section describes the proposed architecture. Subsequently, the experimental results are provided in Section IV. We then conclude in section V on the basis of the experimental results.

CONVblock

The principle of "CONVblock" is to divide a kernel into two smaller kernels. In our case, we divide a kernel 3×3 into a kernel 3×1 and 1×3 . We note that there is no relation between convolution weights 3×3 and convolution weights 3×1 and 1×3 as in separable spatial convolution. Typically, the size convolution kernel 3×3 convolve directly with the incoming image. In CONVblock, the convolution kernel of 3×1 convolutes first with the incoming image. Then, the 1×3 kernel is applied to the resulting image of the first convolution.

Figure 1. CONVblock VS Normal Convolution.

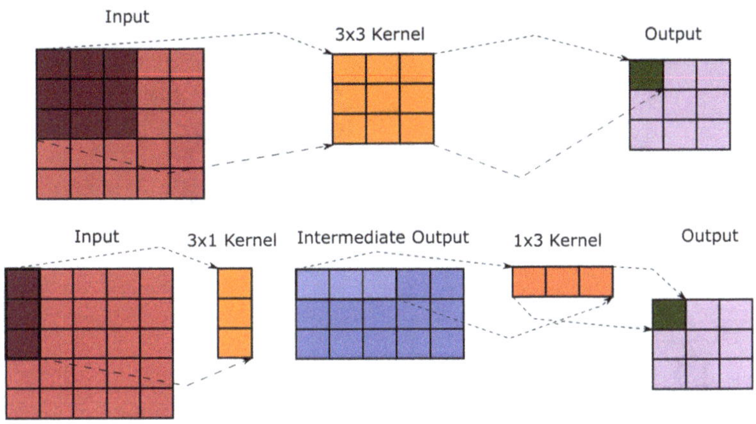

Figure 1 shows these two convolution techniques. Calculating a 2D convolution using two separate linear convolutions may allow more efficient convolution calculations than using more expensive explicit CPU techniques. In addition, this technique can reduce costs while maintaining quality, especially for large convolution kernels. The main problem is that not all cores can be split into two smaller kernel. A convolution of size 3×3 requires 9 parameters. On the other hand, CONVblock requires only 6 parameters by performing the same operations. In addition, a number of convolution matrix multiplications are consumed in the CONVblock. Instead of doing a 3×3 convolution with 9 multiplications, we use two convolutions with 3 multiplications for each convolution (3×2 = 6 in total) for bit to get the same effect. The reduction in the number of multiplications leads to a reduction in computational complexity and an increase in network speed. For each convolution layer inside the block we use 32 different kernels. The selection of the numbers of the CONVblock (NB) is ensured by this formula:

$$NB = \frac{SP_0}{2} - 1$$

The size of the resulting images after each CONVblock is calculated by the following formula:

$$SP_0 - \left(2 \times N_{NB}\right) \times \left(SP_0 - \left(2 \times N_{NB}\right)\right)$$

Figure 2. The architecture of the proposed model.

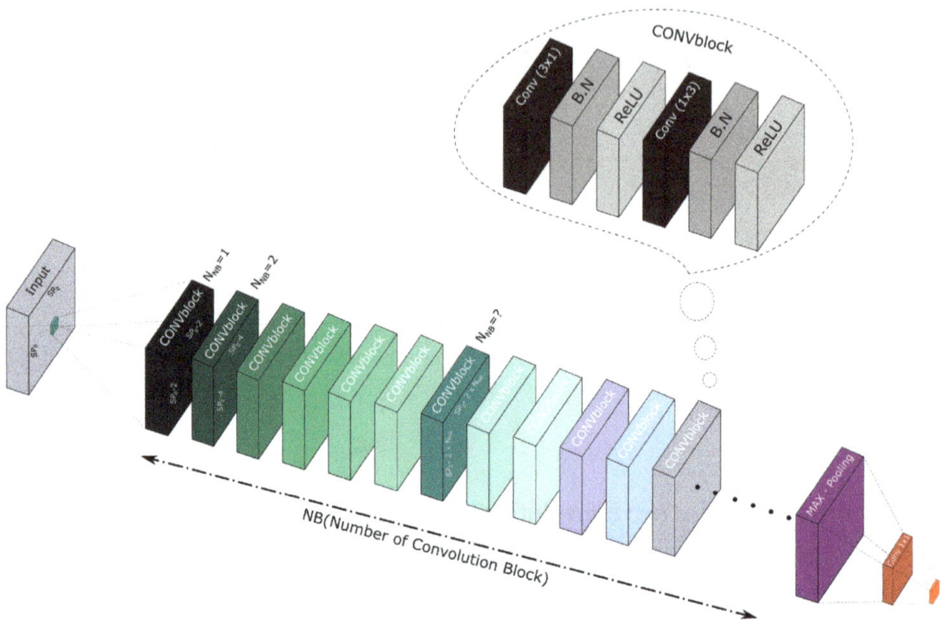

Knowing that SP_0 denotes the initial size of the image of the database and N_{NB} is the number of local convolution block.

Each block integrates two convolution layers of size 3×1 and 1×3. A Batch normalization and Relu layer follow these two convolutional layers. Generally, CONVblock uses parameters equivalent to 6144.

The Proposed Architecture

It was widely known that the smaller the size of the filter, the better the accuracy would be. Likewise for the increase of the numbers of the channels. This is what we can see from the comparison between Alexnet (Alex Krizhevsky, 2012) and ZFnet (M. D. Zeiler, 2014).

Although the increase of the number of the kernels leads to the increase of the precision, the reduction of the sizes of the filters is more favorable because it leads to the increase of the precision while also ensuring a decrease in the numbers of the parameters. For this in our case we made the decision to use the CONVblock with 3×1 and 1×3 size convolution filters instead of using the 3×3 size filters as in most of the proposed architectures [(K. Simonyan, 2015), (Komodakis., 2016), (Saining Xie, 2016), (I. J. Goodfellow, 2013). The use of the 3×1 and 1×3 size filters leads to a reduction in the size of the image, which helps us to avoid the use of several pooling layers and especially leads to increased numbers of ReLU activation functions used in architectures. We propose a new architecture with NB CONVblock localized after a convolutional layer with 32 kernels for a 3×3 size filter with an "S = 1" and "P = 1". This type of filter was used to increase the feature maps from the incoming RGB image while keeping the same image size. Figure 2 illustrates our proposed architecture.

A single layer of pooling is located after the NB_{neme} CONVblock. This layer is of type average pooling layer of size 2×2 and a stride equivalent to 1 and padding equal to 0. A convolution layer 1×1 was used to ensure the adaptation with the number of the class of the database. This layer is located after the average-pooling layer and before the Softmax layer. Note that the CIFAR-10 database includes 10 classes. In CNNs, there really is no "Fully Connected layers". There are only convolutional layer with kernels of size 1×1 MatConvNet (A. Vedaldi and K. Lenc, 2015) does exactly this: the vlnnconv function implements both convolutional layers and fully connected layers.

Table 1 describes the different parameters of our architecture and the number of parameters and the data memory size used for each layer (CIFAR-10).

The Table 2 describes the different parameters of our architecture and the number of parameters and the data memory size used for each layer. For CIFAR-10, our architecture consumes a data memory equivalent to 537.520 MB. For parameter memory, our architecture consumes nearly 384KB. Note that each convolution and batch normalization layer consumes respectively 12 KB and 512B (parameter memory). For MNIST, the data memory is nearly à 362 MB.

Experimental Results

CNN model initially incorporates random parameters (weight, bias) that produce no significant results before learning. The parameters must be modified during the formation of the CNN model performed on a database. There are two possible approaches to forming a CNN model: supervised learning and unsupervised learning. A CNN model is fed with batch training images. Usually, batches of 128 images or 256 images are the most used. It is recalled that the duration of formation of a CNN model on a complete set of training images is called an epoch. A CNN model can converge after training over several periods, depending on the complexity of the task and the structure of the model. CNN models use a loss function that defines the difference between the model output and the input label. The loss function is calculated for each image and is accumulated for the training batch. After processing a batch of images, the accumulated loss is used in the optimization algorithms to update the parameters in the model. Optimization algorithms are used to minimize the error calculated as a loss. By updating parameters and minimizing errors,

Table 1. The number of parameters and the data memory size used for each layer (CIFAR-10).

N	type	patch size	Stride	Pad	output Data size		Kernel	Data mem Mégabit(MB)
0	INPUT	-	-	-	32	32	3	2
1	Conv	3x3	1	1	32	32		16
2	Batch.Norm	n/a	n/a	n/a	32	32		16
3	ReLU	n/a	n/a	n/a	32	32		16
4	Conv	3x1	1	0	30	32		15
5	Batch.Norm	n/a	n/a	n/a	30	32		15
6	ReLU	n/a	n/a	n/a	30	32		15
7	Conv	1x3	1	0	30	30		14,0625
8	Batch.Norm	n/a	n/a	n/a	30	30		14,0625
9	ReLU	n/a	n/a	n/a	30	30		14,0625
10	Conv	3x1	1	0	28	30		13,125
11	Batch.Norm	n/a	n/a	n/a	28	30		13,125
12	ReLU	n/a	n/a	n/a	28	30		13,125
13	Conv	1x3	1	0	28	28		12,25
14	Batch.Norm	n/a	n/a	n/a	28	28		12,25
15	ReLU	n/a	n/a	n/a	28	28		12,25
16	Conv	3x1	1	0	26	28		11,375
17	Batch.Norm	n/a	n/a	n/a	26	28		11,375
18	ReLU	n/a	n/a	n/a	26	28		11,375
19	Conv	1x3	1	0	26	26		10,5625
20	Batch.Norm	n/a	n/a	n/a	26	26		10,5625
21	ReLU	n/a	n/a	n/a	26	26		10,5625
22	Conv	3x1	1	0	24	26		9,75
23	Batch.Norm	n/a	n/a	n/a	24	26	32	9,75
24	ReLU	n/a	n/a	n/a	24	26		9,75
25	Conv	1x3	1	0	24	24		9
26	Batch.Norm	n/a	n/a	n/a	24	24		9
27	ReLU	n/a	n/a	n/a	24	24		9
28	Conv	3x1	1	0	22	24		8,25
29	Batch.Norm	n/a	n/a	n/a	22	24		8,25
30	ReLU	n/a	n/a	n/a	22	24		8,25
31	Conv	1x3	1	0	22	22		7,5625
32	Batch.Norm	n/a	n/a	n/a	22	22		7,5625
33	ReLU	n/a	n/a	n/a	22	22		7,5625
34	Conv	3x1	1	0	20	22		6,875
34	Batch.Norm	n/a	n/a	n/a	20	22		6,875
35	ReLU	n/a	n/a	n/a	20	22		6,875
36	Conv	1x3	1	0	20	20		6,25
37	Batch.Norm	n/a	n/a	n/a	20	20		6,25
38	ReLU	n/a	n/a	n/a	20	20		6,25
39	Conv	3x1	1	0	18	20		5,625
40	Batch.Norm	n/a	n/a	n/a	18	20		5,625
41	ReLU	n/a	n/a	n/a	18	20		5,625
42	Conv	1x3	1	0	18	18		5,0625
43	Batch.Norm	n/a	n/a	n/a	18	18		5,0625
44	ReLU	n/a	n/a	n/a	18	18		5,0625
45	Conv	3x1	1	0	16	18		4,5
46	Batch.Norm	n/a	n/a	n/a	16	18		4,5
47	ReLU	n/a	n/a	n/a	16	18		4,5

N	type	patch size	Stride	Pad	output Data size		Kernel	Data mem Mégabit(MB)
48	Conv	1x3	1	0	16	16		4
49	Batch.Norm	n/a	n/a	n/a	16	16		4
50	ReLU	n/a	n/a	n/a	16	16		4
51	Conv	3x1	1	0	14	16		3,5
52	Batch.Norm	n/a	n/a	n/a	14	16		3,5
53	ReLU	n/a	n/a	n/a	14	16		3,5
54	Conv	1x3	1	0	14	14		3,0625
55	Batch.Norm	n/a	n/a	n/a	14	14		3,0625
56	ReLU	n/a	n/a	n/a	14	14		3,0625
57	Conv	3x1	1	0	12	14		2,625
58	Batch.Norm	n/a	n/a	n/a	12	14		2,625
59	ReLU	n/a	n/a	n/a	12	14		2,625
60	Conv	1x3	1	0	12	12		2,25
61	Batch.Norm	n/a	n/a	n/a	12	12		2,25
62	ReLU	n/a	n/a	n/a	12	12		2,25
63	Conv	3x1	1	0	10	12		1,875
64	Batch.Norm	n/a	n/a	n/a	10	12		1,875
65	ReLU	n/a	n/a	n/a	10	12		1,875
66	Conv	1x3	1	0	10	10		1,5625
67	Batch.Norm	n/a	n/a	n/a	10	10		1,5625
68	ReLU	n/a	n/a	n/a	10	10		1,5625
69	Conv	3x1	1	0	8	10		1,25
70	Batch.Norm	n/a	n/a	n/a	8	10		1,25
71	ReLU	n/a	n/a	n/a	8	10		1,25
72	Conv	1x3	1	0	8	8	32	1
73	Batch.Norm	n/a	n/a	n/a	8	8		1
74	ReLU	n/a	n/a	n/a	8	8		1
75	Conv	3x1	1	0	6	8		0,75
76	Batch.Norm	n/a	n/a	n/a	6	8		0,75
77	ReLU	n/a	n/a	n/a	6	8		0,75
78	Conv	1x3	1	0	6	6		0,5625
79	Batch.Norm	n/a	n/a	n/a	6	6		0,5625
80	ReLU	n/a	n/a	n/a	6	6		0,5625
81	Conv	3x1	1	0	4	6		0,375
82	Batch.Norm	n/a	n/a	n/a	4	6		0,375
83	ReLU	n/a	n/a	n/a	4	6		0,375
84	Conv	1x3	1	0	4	4		0,25
85	Batch.Norm	n/a	n/a	n/a	4	4		0,25
86	ReLU	n/a	n/a	n/a	4	4		0,25
87	Conv	3x1	1	0	2	4		0,125
88	Batch.Norm	n/a	n/a	n/a	2	4		0,125
89	ReLU	n/a	n/a	n/a	2	4		0,125
90	Conv	1x3	1	0	2	2		0,0625
91	Batch.Norm	n/a	n/a	n/a	2	2		0,0625
92	ReLU	n/a	n/a	n/a	2	2		0,0625
93	Max.pool	3x1	1	0	1	1		0,015625
94	Conv 1x1	1x1	1	0	1	1	10	0,00488281
95	Softmax	n/a	n/a	n/a	1	1	1	3,8147E-06

CNN models learn features and dependencies to produce correct outputs. Several optimization algorithms are used, namely the Adaptive Moment Estimation (ADAM), the Stochastic Descending Gradient (SGD), the Nesterov Accelerated Gradient (NAG), and so on. The learning and execution of CNN models is usually done on graphics processing units (GPUs) because they can use massive parallelism for floating-point number calculations. Processors, such as Tensor Processing Units (TPUs), FPGAs, and ASICs, can provide alternatives to GPUs.

Table 2. The number of parameters and the data memory size used for each layer (MNIST).

	N	type	patch size	Stride	Pad	output Data size		Kernel	Data mem Mégabit(MB)
	0	INPUT	-	-	-	28	28	1	1,53125
	1	Conv	3x3	1	1	28	28		12,25
	2	Batch.Norm	n/a	n/a	n/a	28	28		12,25
	3	ReLU	n/a	n/a	n/a	28	28		12,25
CONVblock - 1	4	Conv	3x1	1	0	26	28		11,375
	5	Batch.Norm	n/a	n/a	n/a	26	28		11,375
	6	ReLU	n/a	n/a	n/a	26	28		11,375
	7	Conv	1x3	1	0	26	26		10,5625
	8	Batch.Norm	n/a	n/a	n/a	26	26		10,5625
	9	ReLU	n/a	n/a	n/a	26	26		10,5625
	10	Conv	3x1	1	0	24	26		9,75
	11	Batch.Norm	n/a	n/a	n/a	24	26		9,75
	12	ReLU	n/a	n/a	n/a	24	26		9,75
	13	Conv	1x3	1	0	24	24		9
	14	Batch.Norm	n/a	n/a	n/a	24	24		9
	15	ReLU	n/a	n/a	n/a	24	24		9
CONVblock - 2	16	Conv	3x1	1	0	22	24		8,25
	17	Batch.Norm	n/a	n/a	n/a	22	24		8,25
	18	ReLU	n/a	n/a	n/a	22	24		8,25
	19	Conv	1x3	1	0	22	22		7,5625
	20	Batch.Norm	n/a	n/a	n/a	22	22	32	7,5625
	21	ReLU	n/a	n/a	n/a	22	22		7,5625
	22	Conv	3x1	1	0	20	22		6,875
	23	Batch.Norm	n/a	n/a	n/a	20	22		6,875
	24	ReLU	n/a	n/a	n/a	20	22		6,875
	25	Conv	1x3	1	0	20	20		6,25
	26	Batch.Norm	n/a	n/a	n/a	20	20		6,25
	27	ReLU	n/a	n/a	n/a	20	20		6,25
	28	Conv	3x1	1	0	18	20		5,625
	29	Batch.Norm	n/a	n/a	n/a	18	20		5,625
	30	ReLU	n/a	n/a	n/a	18	20		5,625
	31	Conv	1x3	1	0	18	18		5,0625
	32	Batch.Norm	n/a	n/a	n/a	18	18		5,0625
	33	ReLU	n/a	n/a	n/a	18	18		5,0625
	34	Conv	3x1	1	0	16	18		4,5
	34	Batch.Norm	n/a	n/a	n/a	16	18		4,5
	35	ReLU	n/a	n/a	n/a	16	18		4,5
	36	Conv	1x3	1	0	16	16		4
	37	Batch.Norm	n/a	n/a	n/a	16	16		4
	38	ReLU	n/a	n/a	n/a	16	16		4
	39	Conv	3x1	1	0	14	16		3,5
	40	Batch.Norm	n/a	n/a	n/a	14	16		3,5
	41	ReLU	n/a	n/a	n/a	14	16		3,5

N	type	patch size	Stride	Pad	output Data size		Kernel	Data mem Mégabit(MB)
42	Conv	1x3	1	0	14	14		3,0625
43	Batch.Norm	n/a	n/a	n/a	14	14		3,0625
44	ReLU	n/a	n/a	n/a	14	14		3,0625
45	Conv	3x1	1	0	12	14		2,625
46	Batch.Norm	n/a	n/a	n/a	12	14		2,625
47	ReLU	n/a	n/a	n/a	12	14		2,625
48	Conv	1x3	1	0	12	12		2,25
49	Batch.Norm	n/a	n/a	n/a	12	12		2,25
50	ReLU	n/a	n/a	n/a	12	12		2,25
51	Conv	3x1	1	0	10	12		1,875
52	Batch.Norm	n/a	n/a	n/a	10	12		1,875
53	ReLU	n/a	n/a	n/a	10	12		1,875
54	Conv	1x3	1	0	10	10		1,5625
55	Batch.Norm	n/a	n/a	n/a	10	10		1,5625
56	ReLU	n/a	n/a	n/a	10	10		1,5625
57	Conv	3x1	1	0	8	10		1,25
58	Batch.Norm	n/a	n/a	n/a	8	10		1,25
59	ReLU	n/a	n/a	n/a	8	10	32	1,25
60	Conv	1x3	1	0	8	8		1
61	Batch.Norm	n/a	n/a	n/a	8	8		1
62	ReLU	n/a	n/a	n/a	8	8		1
63	Conv	3x1	1	0	6	8		0,75
64	Batch.Norm	n/a	n/a	n/a	6	8		0,75
65	ReLU	n/a	n/a	n/a	6	8		0,75
66	Conv	1x3	1	0	6	6		0,5625
67	Batch.Norm	n/a	n/a	n/a	6	6		0,5625
68	ReLU	n/a	n/a	n/a	6	6		0,5625
69	Conv	3x1	1	0	4	6		0,375
70	Batch.Norm	n/a	n/a	n/a	4	6		0,375
71	ReLU	n/a	n/a	n/a	4	6		0,375
72	Conv	1x3	1	0	4	4		0,25
73	Batch.Norm	n/a	n/a	n/a	4	4		0,25
74	ReLU	n/a	n/a	n/a	4	4		0,25
75	Conv	3x1	1	0	2	4		0,125
76	Batch.Norm	n/a	n/a	n/a	2	4		0,125
77	ReLU	n/a	n/a	n/a	2	4		0,125
78	Conv	1x3	1	0	2	2		0,0625
79	Batch.Norm	n/a	n/a	n/a	2	2		0,0625
80	ReLU	n/a	n/a	n/a	2	2		0,0625
81	Max.pool	3x1	1	0	1	1		0,015625
82	Conv 1x1	1x1	1	0	1	1	10	0,00488281
83	Softmax	n/a	n/a	n/a	1	1	1	3,8147E-06

MatConvNet

MatConvNet (A. Vedaldi and K. Lenc, 2015) is an implementation on the MATLAB environment with a VLFeat open source library for computer vision applications and image understanding. It is described as a Matlab Toolbox used for implementation and rapid prototyping of CNN architectures (Convolutional Neural Networks) using only the MATLAB code. In addition, it presents CNN's various building blocks in a simple and flexible way such as convolution with filter banks, pooling, activation function and classification and other blocks that allow to form complex models on from different datasets such as CIFAR, MNIST and ImageNet ILSVRC. MatConvNet can be easily extended; it offers the ability to make efficient calculations on CPU and GPU.

Figure 3. The first convolutional layer.

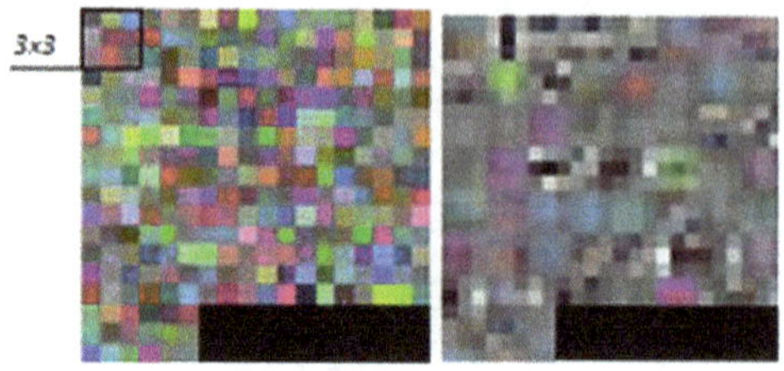

Implementation Details

We initialized the weights of our architecture with a Gaussian distribution and for the learning; we used stochastic gradient descent (often-abbreviated SGD) with a Momentum equivalent to 0.9. Our model is trained during more than 90 epoches for CIFAR-10 and more than 45 for MNIST.The network is formed using mini-batch of size equivalent to 128. The learning rate is initialized to 0.001 and it reduces by a scale of 10 in the 80 and 90 epochs knowing that we have trained our architecture for more of 90 epochs for a batch size equivalent to 128 on CIFAR-10 and MNIST for the same batch sizes where we get a 0.14% test error on CIFAR- 10 and 0.055% for MNIST. All the experiments are performed in the Matlab (R2018a). Our approach is driven on MatConvnet Toolbox (A. Vedaldi and K. Lenc, 2015) on CPU - Intel Xeon Processor E5-2620 v4. This framework (A. Vedaldi and K. Lenc, 2015) provides features for creating layers for CNN models: model building; execution inferences without back propagation. Unfortunately, these frameworks do not offer solutions that can be implemented directly on an FPGA like the other frameworks.

Visualization

The figure 3 shows the 32-convolution kernel 3×3 of the first CONV layer of our architecture before (a) and after (b) the learning phase. Visualization of the first convolutional layer is usually more preferable than other layers since it is applied directly to the raw pixel data of the 32×32 input images.

Evaluation

During training, the performance of a CNN-based model can be measured by accuracy and loss function. Usually, the performance is performed on a validation set, a set containing images that were not used during the training to update the settings. We evaluate our configurations on a set of reference data: CIFAR-10, MNIST. The CIFAR-10 consists of 60,000 images grouped into 10 image classes (6000 images

Figure 4. Objective, Top-1 and Top-5 test error (%) of our model on the CIFAR-10 dataset.

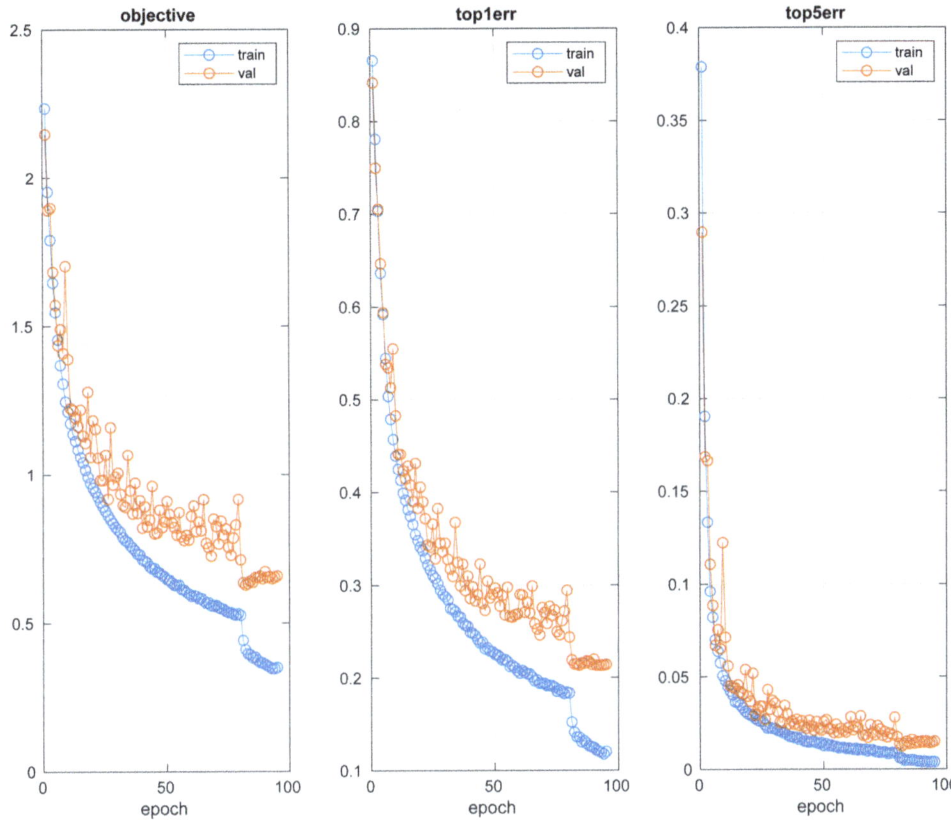

in each class). These 60,000 images are separated between 50,000 total training images and 10,000 test images.

Figure 4 shows the curve of the formation, test and loss of our architecture on CIFAR-10.

The MNIST represents a modification of an original database called "NSIT" that integrates binary images of handwritten digits. It was built from the NIST database and consists of different hand-written numbers ranging from 0 to 9, this dataset contains 28×28 size images divided between 60,000 training images and 10,000 images in total. Figure 5 shows the curve of the formation, test and loss of our architecture on MNIST.

In terms of precision, our architecture reaches an error of 1.4% (Top5error) with 32 convolution layer on Cifar-10 where we can notice that the CONVblock and the reduction of the size of the convolution filters represents one of the best solution for the increase in performance with the decrease in the number of parameters,

Figure 5. Objective, Top-1 and Top-5 test error (%) of our model on the MNIST dataset.

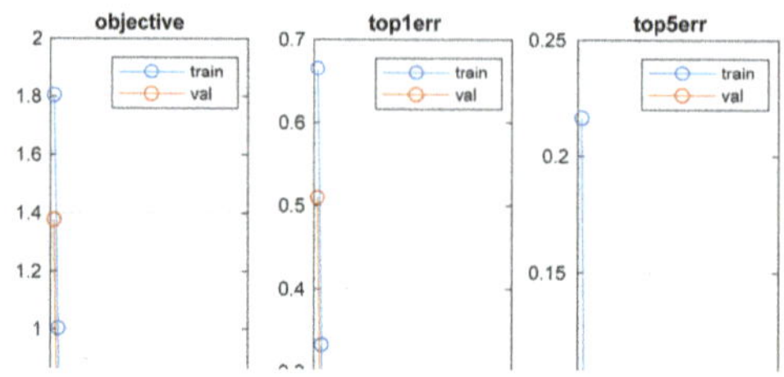

memory data and memory parameters. This is what we can see from comparisons with ResNET (Komodakis., 2016) which is the closest architecture where our results exceed the results of (Komodakis., 2016) in terms of the parameters and more precisely with a number of layers lower than that of (Komodakis., 2016) (32 instead of 101). Moreover, it exceeds the other architecture (Saining Xie, 2016), (I. J. Goodfellow, 2013) even that it is based on the width more than the depth like the architecture (O. Russakovsky, 2015) (K. Simonyan, 2015).

A comparison between our work and the architectures already accomplished is shown in Table 3. The results of our work are presented with the size of the mini batch 128. Our results were obtained by calculating the average of three executions.

CONCLUSION

We propose a new CNN for image classification. This architecture achieves new results for CIFAR-10 and MNIST. This architecture consists of NB convolution blocks (CONVblock). A spatial Average pooling layer that subsamples the input

Table 3. The number of parameters and the data memory size used for each layer (MNIST)

REF	CIFAR-10(%)	MNIST (%)
(I. J. Goodfellow, 2013)	9,38%	0,9%
(M. Lin, 2014)	8,81%	0,47%
(C.-Y. Lee, 2015)	8,22%	0,32%
(He X. Zhang, 2015)	6,43%	-
(Komodakis., 2016)	3,89%	-
(Saining Xie, 2016)	3,58%	-
Our (CONVbloc)	1,4%	0,055%

image by a factor of two follows the last block. As a rule, the Batch Normalization layer is applied after all the convolutional layers to the last convolutional layer of size 1×3, which ensures the same operation of the FC layer. This architecture facilitates both real-time implementation and embedded on a System-on-Chip.

REFERENCES

Aaron van den Oord, S. D. (2016). *WaveNet: A Generative Model for Raw Audio.* arXiv:1609.03499 [cs.SD]

Alex Krizhevsky, I. S. (2012). *Imagenet classification with deep convolutional.* Academic Press.

Cao, C. X. L. (2015). Look and think twice: Capturingtop-down visual attention with feedback convolutional neural networks. *Proceedings of the International Conference on Computer Vision (ICCV),* 2956–2964.

Chen, L.-C., G. P. (2015). Semantic image segmentation with deep convolutional netsand fully connected crfs. *Proceedings of the International Conference on Learning Representations (ICLR).*

Fukushima, K. S. M. (1982). Neocognitron: A self-organizing neural network model for a mechanism of visual pattern recognition. Competition and cooperation in neural nets, 267–285.

Goodfellow, I. J., D. W.-F. (2013). Maxout networks. *Proceedings of the 30th International Conference on Machine Learning (ICML 2013)*, 28, 1319– 1327.

He, X., & Zhang, S. R. (2015). *Deep residual learning for image recognition.* ArXiv preprint arXiv:1512.03385

Hecht-Nielsen, R. (1988). Theory of the backpropagation neural network. *Neural Networks, 1*, 445–448. doi:10.1016/0893-6080(88)90469-8

Hubel, D. H., & Wiesel, T. N. (1968). Receptive fields and functional architecture of monkey striate cortex. *The Journal of Physiology, 195*(1), 215–243. doi:10.1113/jphysiol.1968.sp008455 PMID:4966457

Komodakis, S. Z. (2016). Wide residual networks. *BMVC.*

Le Cun, B. B., J. S. (1989). Handwritten digit recognition with a back-propagation network. *Proceedings of the Advances in Neural Information Processing Systems (NIPS)*, 396–404.

Lee, C.-Y., S. X. (2015). Deeply supervised nets. *Proceedings of AISTATS.*

Lin, M., Q. C. (2014). Network in network. *International Conference on Learning Representations.*

Long, J., E. S. (2017). Fully convolutional networks for semantic segmentation. *IEEE Transactions on Pattern Analysis and Machine Intelligence*, 640–651. PMID:27244717

Nair, V., G. E. (2010). Rectified linear units improve restricted boltzmann machines. *Proceedings of the International Con-ference on Machine Learning (ICML)*, 807–814.

Ngiam, J., Z. C. (2010). Tiled convolutional neural networks. *Proceedings of the Advancesin Neural Information Processing Systems (NIPS)*, 1279–1287.

Niu, X.-X., & Suen, C. Y. (2012). A novel hybrid cnn–svm classifier for recognizing handwritten digits. *Pattern Recognition*, *45*(4), 1318–1325. doi:10.1016/j.patcog.2011.09.021

Noh, H., S. H. (2015). Learning deconvolution network for semantic segmentation. *Proceedings of the InternationalConference on Computer Vision (ICCV)*, 1520–1528.

Russakovsky, J. D. (2015). Magenetlarge scale visual recognition challenge. *International Journal of Conflict and Violence*, 211-252.

Sercu, V. G. (2016). Dense prediction on sequences with time-dilated convolutions for speech recognition. *Proceedings of the Advances in Neural Information Processing Systems (NIPS) Workshops.*

Simonyan, K., A. Z. (2015). Very deep convolutional networks for large-scale image recognition. *Proceedings of the International Conference on Learning Representations (ICLR).*

Szegedy, C., W. L. (2015). Going deeper with convolutions. *Proceedings of the IEEE Conference on Computer Vision and Pattern Recognition (CVPR)*, 1-9.

Vedaldi, A., & Lenc, K. (2015). MatConvNet - Convolutional Neural Networks for MATLAB. *Proc. of the ACM Int. Conf. on Multimedia.*

Visin, F., K. K. (2015). A recurrent neural network for object segmentation. *Proceedings of the IEEE Conference on Computer Vision and Pattern Recognition (CVPR) Workshops.*

Wang, Z. T. O. (2015). Encoding time series as images for visual inspection and classification using tiled convolutional neural networks. *Proceedings of the Association for the Advancement of Artificial Intelligence (AAAI) Workshops.*

Xie, S. (2016). R. G. Aggregated Residual Transformations for Deep Neural Networks. Academic Press.

Yu, F., V. K. (2016). Multi-scale context aggregation by dilated convolutions. *Proceedings of the International Conference onLearning Representations (ICLR).*

Zeiler, M. D., D. K. (2010). Deconvolutional networks. *Proceedings of the IEEE Conference onComputer Vision and Pattern Recognition (CVPR)*, 2528-2535.

Zeiler, M. D., G. W. (2011). Adaptive deconvolutional networks for mid and high level feature learning. *Proceedings of the International Conference on Computer Vision (ICCV)*, 2018–2025. 10.1109/ICCV.2011.6126474

Zeiler, M. D., R. F. (2014). Visualizing and understanding convolutional networks. *Proceedings of the European Conference onComputer Vision (ECCV)*, 818–833.

Zhang, J., Z. L. (2016). Top-down neural attention by excitation backprop. *Proceedings of theEuropean Conference on Computer Vision (ECCV)*, 543-559.

Zhang, Y. E. K. (2016). Augmenting supervised neural networks with unsupervised objectives for large-scaleimage classification. *Proceedings of the International Conference on Machine Learning (ICML)*, 612-621.

Zheng, Q. L. (2014). Time series classification using multi-channels deep convolutional neural networks. *Proceedings ofthe International Conference on Web-Age Information Management (WAIM)*, 298–310. 10.1007/978-3-319-08010-9_33

Zhou, B. A. K. (2016). Learning deep features for discriminative localization. *Proceedings of the IEEE Conference on Computer Vision and Pattern Recognition (CVPR)*, 2921–2929.

KEY TERMS AND DEFINITIONS

BN: Batch normalization layer.
L x C: The filter size.
MD: Memory data.
N_{NB}: Number of local convolution block.
NB: Number of convolution block.
P: Padding.
S: Stride.
SP: Size picture.
SP_0: Size of picture of dataset.

Chapter 5
Machine Learning for Prediction of Lung Cancer

Nikita Banerjee
College of Engineering and Technology, Rourkela, India

Subhalaxmi Das
College of Engineering and Technology, Bhubaneswar, India

ABSTRACT

This work is focused on lung cancer prediction using machine learning technique. Lung cancer is one of the widespread diseases due to the growth of irregular cell in both the lungs as a result of which this irregular cell starts growing into tumour, and this tumour can be cancerous as well as non-cancerous. In the traditional approach CT scan images has been used based on the report image segmentation has been done to remove the noise so that a clear picture can be generated to detect the location of tumor. Once the location is known then classification or clustering approach can be used to predict the stage of cancer. Previously supervised machine learning algorithm has been used to predict lung cancer. In this work a prediction model is proposed that is based on the median filter, watershed segmentation, and then feature extraction has done like texture and region. And on the extracted feature classification technique was applied for prediction of cancer.

INTRODUCTION

Cell division is one of important part of a life, every time an old cell dies and gets replaced with new one in controlled fashion. But when there is abnormal growth of cell occur it lead to cancer, and a mask of abnormal cell is called tumor. At the same

DOI: 10.4018/978-1-7998-5071-7.ch005

Copyright © 2021, IGI Global. Copying or distributing in print or electronic forms without written permission of IGI Global is prohibited.

time every tumor are not cancerous, a tumor has been divided into two categories one is benign which is also called as non-cancerous tumor that means it does not spread to other part of the body and other one is malignant or the cancerous tumor which spread through the blood vessel to other part of the body. There is various type of cancer like leukemia, lymphoma, carcinoma, sarcoma, and melanoma. Out of all this type carcinoma is one the common type of cancer; Carcinomas are cancers that occur in epithelial tissues in the body. They comprise 80% to 90% of all cancers. Most breast, lung, colon, skin, and prostate cancers are carcinomas. This class includes the two most common skin cancers, basal cell carcinoma and squamous cell carcinoma. Also in this class is the glandular cancer adenocarcinoma (Stoppler, n.d).

Among the carcinoma cancer lung cancer has become one of the root cause of death from a survey done by national cancer institute it has been estimated as 23.5% of death from all other cancer. The main cause of lung cancer is smoking and other causes are second hand smoking, explore to radon gas, asbestos fiber etc. Basically lung cancers are of two type's small cell lung cancer and non small cell lung cancer, and this can be distinguished based on the tumor size. A small cell lung cancer occur to those who smoke it has spread to other part of the body very rapidly whereas non small cell lung cancer is the most common type of lung cancer which can be further divided into other type based on the cancer cell found the tumor. Symptoms of lung cancer are cough that produce blood, shortness of breath, unexpected weight loss, change in the appearance of finger, persistent cough etc (Cancer treatment center of America 2020). Diagnosis of lung cancer at early stage is very crucial so that based on the diagnoses report stage of cancer can be detected and based on that treatment can be given at early stage, the diagnosis process include Computed tomography, X-Ray of chest, Magnetic Resonance Imaging, Blood test etc.

In prediction of cancer CT scan report is basically used. But CT scan report is full of noise which cannot be seen by human eye for that reason various digital image processing plays a important role to get a noise free image. Digital image processing is the process where the analysis and manipulation of image is used to extract some useful information from the image. Digital image processing involve various step like image pre-processing where we can enhance the image using histogram equalization, spatial filter etc. Then image restoration can be done where various kind of noise like salt and pepper noise, Gaussian noise etc are applied and filter like median filter, mean filter can be applied on the pre-processed image. After that color conversions is applied only if the image is colored image then convert it to gray level.

Image segmentation is a process which divides the image into several segment based on the pixel, once the image segmentation is over the feature extraction can be applied. Feature extraction is a type of dimensionality reduction where a set of raw data is reduced to more manageable group image data for extracting the feature like region and texture .After extracting the feature different machine learning technique is used to classify the image.

Machine learning is a subset of Artificial Intelligence the main difference between artificial intelligence and machine learning is that artificial intelligence allows the computer to think like human where as machine learning is a process where system learns from its past experience. In machine learning a set of data is trained using different machine learning methods which is called as training dataset. Once the training is complete then the machine is feed with new dataset which is called testing data set. Now machine can predict the object based on its training data. Machine learning is categorized into three categories supervised, unsupervised and reinforcement learning. This work is focused on supervised learning. Supervised learning is a learning in which machine learn or train the dataset which are already marked with correct answer (labeled data) after which machine is feed with testing dataset on that supervised approach is used to provide correct result. Supervised learning is classified into two categories Classification where the output variables are categorical (or discrete) and Regression where the output variables are continuous (or numerical) .Some traditional algorithms used in machine learning are Decision Tree, K Nearest Neighbor and Logistic Regression.

RELATED WORK

Since many year various research is going on for prediction of lung cancer at early stage like D.Palani et al., has proposed a new Internet of Thing (IoT) based predictive modeling by using fuzzy cluster based augmentation and classification for predicting the lung cancer disease through continuous monitoring. Fuzzy C-Mean clustering algorithm is used to group the transition region feature extracted from segmented image. Otsu threshold has been applied for segmentation. Morphological thinning operation has been used for enhancing segmentation and morphological cleaning operation has been applied for image filling and to get a good edge image of lung. After pre-processing a incremental model has been used, in incremental model association rule mining has applied to extract rule and on that decision tree is applied then at last convolutional neural network has been used for decision making (Palani et al.,2019). H. Yang et al., has proposed a model were he has used clinical data and pathological data, the pathologic staging is based on pathological report which describe the size and to detect whether the tumor has spread or not, and the clinical report consist of previous history of patient, number of smoking per year etc, as the pathological data take longer time so the study was more focus on clinical dataset. On clinical data decision tree was applied and on pathological data pre-processing was applied and then separately two dataset are generated and on both the dataset association rule mining was applied and based on association rule mining support and confidence are calculated but at the same time based on the clinical data one cannot decide whether the person has cancer or not (Yang et al., 2015).

Jadhav et al., has proposed a automated system to detect cancer at early stage, on the image dataset first pre-processing was applied and then on the pre-processed image artificial neural network was applied for training the dataset and on the trained dataset genetic algorithm was applied for feature extraction on the extracted feature back propagation algorithm was applied to remove the error from the image and finally it was classified as cancerous or non cancerous, author has not only classified the tumor but also provided the stage of cancer based on the tumor size (D'Cruz et al. 2016).

Pradeep K R et al., has proposed a model using various machine learning algorithm where in first phase data has been collected from various doctors who are undergoing treatment and data has been collected from The north central cancer group on both the data preprocessing has applied then feature has been extracted. Features are selected based on pathological report and surgery. Then training and testing of these features are made by applying machine learning algorithms like Support vector machine, decision tree under decision tree only C4.5 was only applied, Naïve Bayes. At the end comparison was made based on accuracy, Area Under the Curve (AUC), Receiver Operating Characteristic (ROC) (Pradeep et al.,2018)

Fenwa et al., has proposed a classification model classification of cancer using artificial neural network and support vector machine. In image pre-processing stage first the image was classified into gray image after image conversation feature were extracted based on textures, then on the extracted feature selection was applied using forward selection feature selection is usually used to select the best feature out of all the selected feature and then machine learning algorithm was applied to compare the performance of the ANN and SVM classifiers on acquired online cancer datasets. The performance of both classifiers is evaluated using different measuring parameters namely; accuracy, sensitivity, specificity, true positive, true negative, false positive and false negative (Fenwa et al.,2016).

CANCER DETECTION STAGES

From the related work it can be seen that there are various way for detection of cancer but detection with correct process is very much important. From the related work it can be seen that some of the authors were using clinical data whereas some of them were using pathological data. And it can be seen that pathological data is giving more accurate result as compare to clinical data.

Pathological data mostly comprises of Computed Tomography (CT scan), chest X-Ray, blood test, MRI etc, based on this pathological dataset detection of cancer is shown in figure 1

Figure 1. Stage for detection of cancer.

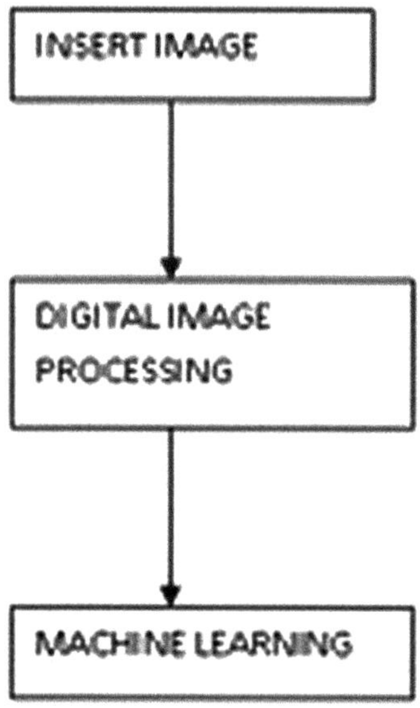

DATASET

Image dataset are mostly used for cancer detection and the image data can be taken from

- **TCIA:** TCIA (The Cancer Imaging Archive) is a service which consists of images of cancer and is accessible for public download. The data are organized as "collections"; typically patients' imaging related by a common disease (e.g. lung cancer), image modality or type (MRI, CT, digital histopathology, etc) or research focus. DICOM is the primary file format used by TCIA for radiology imaging. Supporting data related to the images such as patient outcomes, treatment details, genomics and expert analyses are also provided when available (The cancer imaging archive 2020).
- **LIDC:** The lung image database consortium image collection (LIDC-IDRI) is a part of the cancer imaging archive, basically lidc consist of diagnostic and lung cancer screening thoracic computed tomography (CT) scans with

marked-up annotated lesions. This dataset are accessible to all researchers. I was initiated by National cancer institute and further it was advanced by the foundation for the National institute of health. It consist of 1018 cases and image images in CT scan format and each image is associated with XML file which consist the record of the patient and the nodules are categorized into three categories (“nodule > or =3 mm,” “nodule <3 mm,” and “non-nodule > or =3 mm”) (The cancer imaging archive 2020).

Digital Image Processing

Digital image processing is the method of manipulating and performs some activity for generating some valuable data from the image. The basic step or the first step is image pre-processing where we increase the brightness of the image by using various technique like histogram process, log transformation, etc once the image is brightened we perform image restoration where on the enhanced image we adding some noise like Gaussian noise, salt and pepper noise and based on the noise individual noise we add filter to remove the noise filter like mean filter, median filter etc, noise is added in image to get more clear picture. After noise is removed color conversion is adapted to convert the image from red, green, blue (RGB) to grey level or from RGB to HSV (hue, saturation, value).Then we apply image segmentation the work of image segmentation is to segment the image into constituent parts, there are various techniques for image segmentation like edge detection, point detection, region based detection etc. Image segmentation is very important in digital image processing because it keeps only that part which is needed. After image segmentation is executed it is proceed by feature extraction so feature extraction can be defined as the process by which we can reduce the dimensionality by which a set of the raw data is reduced to more manageable group for process there are various process of feature extraction like based on region, based on texture etc once the feature are extracted we can classify the data using machine learning technique.

Machine Learning

Machine learning is a part of artificial intelligence where the machine tries to answer question whether machine can learn or not. The main difference between artificial intelligence and machine learning is that in artificial intelligence the computer is made to think like human being or it can be defined as artificial intelligence is a decision maker on the other hand machine learning simple take the concept of artificial intelligence and make the system learn from its past experience. Generally artificial intelligence think about the rate of success of the task rather than concentrating on the accuracy whereas machine learning is more focused on accuracy rather the success of the event. Hence machine learning can be defined as a set of methods that focuses on the automatic representation of the input data and generalization of the learned patterns for use on future unseen data (Tong et al.,2020). Or in general term machine learning can be described as it automatically learn different pattern from a given data set and predict the output for the unknown dataset.

At first machine is trained with a set of sampled data which is also called as training data using a specific machine learning algorithm once the machine is trained then the machine is feed with unknown samples with is called as testing dataset set based on the trained data or the past experience machine can predict the result about the unknown sample. Machine learning has been broadly classified into three categories that are supervised, unsupervised and reinforcement learning again each of these categories has been sub divided into other different categories that is supervised learning has been divided into classification and regression, unsupervised learning has been classified into clustering and association rule mining and each of this sub categories consist of some algorithm which has been shown in block diagram in figure 2.

- Supervised learning is a process where we first a random dataset set is trained with a target value then based on the training new set of data is feed and that new set of data is tested based on the training data set to check whether the training data set is generating the desire output or not. Then the supervised learning has been classified into two categories one is classification and other one is regression. Some of the classification algorithms are decision tree, K nearest neighbor, Naïve bayes, neural network etc and regression algorithm are linear regression, non linear regression, logistic regression etc.
- In unsupervised learning the machine has to learn from its past experience, it is also known as self organized learning technique here the correct answered is not assigned so machine has to learn itself unless and until it gets similar pattern. Once it starts getting the similar pattern it starts divining it into groups or start generating the rules. Again unsupervised learning has been divided into two types clustering and association rule mining. Some of the unsupervised learning are K means, DBSCAN, K medians etc.
- Reinforcement learning is about taking action to maximize the reward in a particular environment like supervised learning reinforcement learning is not marked with correct values but the reinforcement agent knows what action is to be taken in absences of training dataset.

Figure 2. Machine learning architecture

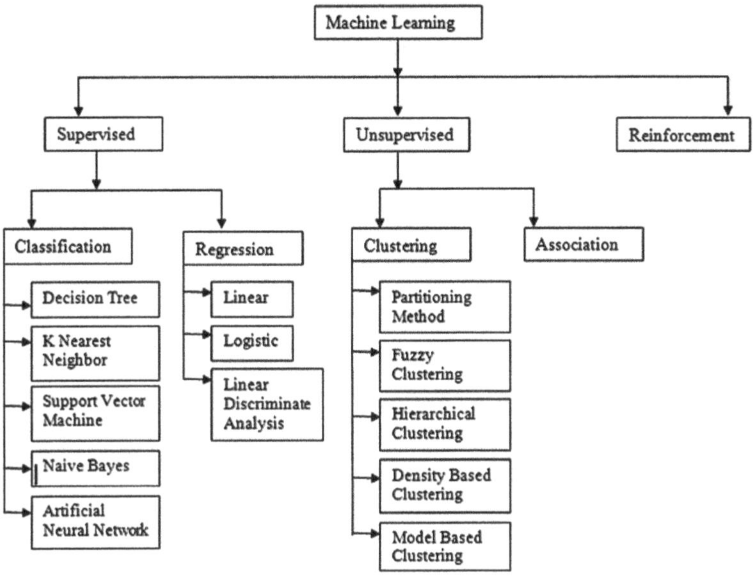

Classification

Classification is a supervised machine learning algorithm where the machine which is used to predict when the output variable are categorical. Some of the classification algorithms are

Decision Tree

A decision tree is a tree like structure or a flowchart which is used for taking decision. In a decision tree, each internal node represents a "test" on an attribute, each branch represents the outcome of the test, and each leaf node represents a decision after computing all attributes. Each root-to-leaf path shows the decision-making process. An example of decision tree has show in figure 3 where decision tree has been used for classification of Lung .Decision tree learning by splitting the training dataset into subset recursive based by testing different attribute present on the dataset. Basically a class label is always given based on that class label it predict the rest by testing each of the attribute. First entropy of the class label is calculated based on probability of occurrence (P) and probability of not occurrence (N) and the formula for calculating entropy is

Figure 3. Decision Tree

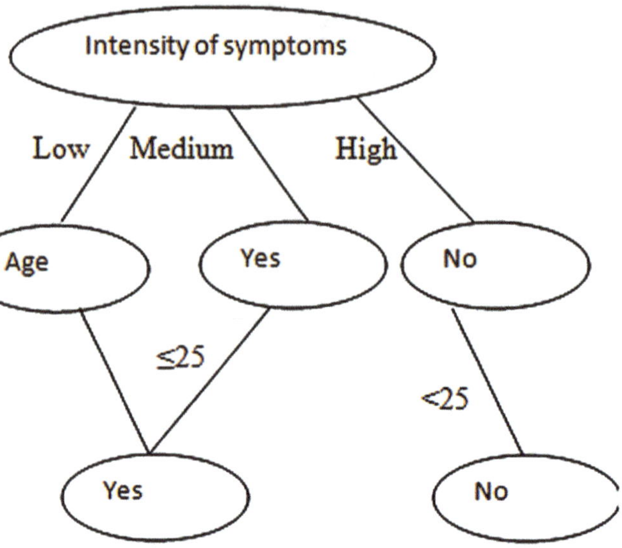

$$\text{Entropy (class)} = \frac{-P}{P+N}\log_2\left(\frac{P}{P+N}\right) - \frac{N}{P+N}\log_2\left(\frac{N}{P+N}\right)$$

The concept entropy was borrowed from thermodynamics Extended the thermodynamic entropy concept, (Shannon et al.,1948) introduced statistical entropy in 1948 to measure the randomness in statistics and the amount of information of a transmitted message in information theory. Entropy of class is always taken as the root node. Once the root node is decided next step is to calculate entropy of each attribute.

Based on the entropy of the class entropy of each attribute is calculated and the formula for calculating entropy of each attribute is

$$I(P_i, N_i) = \frac{-P}{P+N}\log_2\left(\frac{P}{P+N}\right) - \frac{N}{P+N}\log_2\left(\frac{N}{P+N}\right)$$

$$\text{Entropy (attribute)} = \frac{\sum P_{i+N_i}}{P+N}\left(I(P_i, N_i)\right)$$

Once the entropy of attribute is calculate then information gain is measured and the formula for information gain is:

Information gain = Entropy (class) – Entropy (attribute)

Once all the information gain is measured, then the next node is decide by taking the highest information gain as it is said to be recursive process it will continue till it reach the target variable or the prediction stage.

K- Nearest Neighbor

The K-Nearest Neighbor algorithm (KNN) is a non-parametric method used for classification. The input consists of the K closest training examples in the feature space. KNN is a type of instance-based learning. In KNN Classification, the output is a class membership. Classification is done by a majority vote of neighbors. If K = 1, then the class is single nearest neighbor (Bhuvaneswari et al.,2015).

Nearest neighbor classification is based on learning by comparison that by distinguishing given test dataset with the training dataset which are similar in pattern. The training data set are described by the k attributes and each k attributes represent a point in a k dimensional space. In this way all the training dataset are stored in a k dimensional pattern space when given unknown dataset or test dataset, a space of n training data that is closest to the test data, these k training data are the K nearest neighbor of the test data.

Closeness is measured in tern of a distance metric such as Euclidean distance, Minkowski distance, and Manhattan distance etc

Minkowski Distance

Minkowski distance is a metric in normed vector space. A Normed vector space is a vector space on which a norm is defined. Suppose X is a vector space then a norm on X is a real valued function $||x||$which satisfies below conditions –

- **Zero Vector-** Zero vector will have zero length.
- **Scalar Factor-** The direction of vector doesn't change when you multiply it with a positive number though its length will be changed.
- **Triangle Inequality-** If distance is a norm then the calculated distance between two points will always be a straight line (Sharma 2019)

$$\left(\sum_{i=1}^{n} \left| Xi - Yi \right| \hat{}\ p \right)^{1/p}$$

Manhattan Distance

We use Manhattan Distance if we need to calculate the distance between two data points in a grid like path. As mentioned above, we use Minkowski distance formula to find Manhattan distance by setting ***p's*** value as ***1*** (Sharma 2019)

$$D = \sum_{i=1}^{n} \left| Xi - Yi \right|$$

Euclidean Distance

Euclidean distance is one of the most used distances metric. It is calculated using Minkowski Distance formula by setting ***p's*** value to ***2***. This will update the distance 'd' formula as below (Sharma 2019)

$$D\left(X,Y\right) = sqroot\left(\left(\sum_{i=1}^{n} \left| Xi - Yi \right| \right) \hat{} \, 2 \right)$$

Naïve Bayes

Naïve bayes classification is a probability model which comes under supervised learning classification algorithm. It can predict the class membership probability that means probably of a data belong to that particular class or not.

Formula for calculation naïve bayes is

$$P\left(A \mid B\right) \frac{P\left(B \mid A\right) P\left(A\right)}{P\left(B\right)}$$

Where A is evidence and B is the event P(A) is the prior of A, P(B|A) is posteriori

Support Vector Machine

Support vector machine is a supervised learning algorithm; it is a classification as well as regression technique. It predict the model based on its arrangement that is if the arrangement of the dataset are in linear manner then it can be plot in 2 dimensional space and can be separated using a hyperplane but at the same time it the arrangement of the dataset are in non linear form it use kernel function to predict the model and plot it in 3 dimensional space. A diagram of SVM has been shown in figure 4.

Figure 4. Support vector Machine

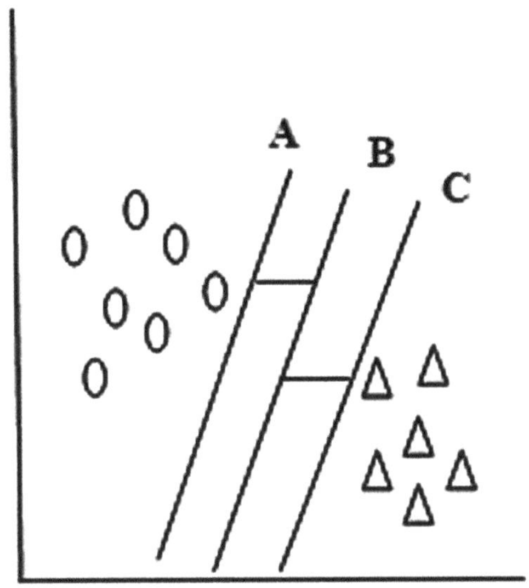

Artificial Neural Network

Artificial neural network was inspired from biological neural network. Like in human brain the neuron is the basic computational unit, neuron receives signal from dendrites and then it product output through axon. In the sample the artificial neural network consist of three layers that is input layer, hidden layer and output layer. Each input layer receives signal and pass it to the hidden layer hidden layer consist of weight and activation function and after the evaluation of the activation the result of hidden layer is forwarded to output layer. And output layer final gives the prediction.

Some common artificial neural network algorithm is multilayer feed forward network, back propagation algorithm, Convolution neural network.

Regression

A regression problem is when the output variable is a real or continuous value. Regression model tries to fit data with the best hyper plane which goes through the point. The benefit of regression is that it shows relationship between dependent and independent variable that is training and testing data, it shows the strength of impact between different dependent and independent variable. Regression analysis allows comparing the effect of variable measured in different parameter.

One of the commonly used regression algorithm is logistic regression. Logistic regression is used to measure the probability of occurrence of event that is the event can be either successful or failure. Logistic regression is basically used when there is binary a binary condition that is the class label or the dependent variable can be either true or false, up or down, 0 or 1 etc in nature. The value of depended variable ranges from 0 to 1 and can be represented in equation that is

$$Odd = {}^{p}\!\big/_{1-p}$$

$$Ln\left(odd\right) = \ln\left({}^{p}\!\big/_{1-p}\right)$$

$$Logit(p) = \ln\left({}^{p}\!\big/_{1-p}\right)$$

Above p is the probability of presence of the characteristic of interest, and logit is used in the equation because the working is in the form of binomial distribution (dependent variable) and prediction will made by selecting a link function which is best suited for that function.

1. **Logistic regression:** Logistic regression is basically used for classification problem and one of its advantages is that it does not require any linear relationship as it can handle any type of relationship. The reason behind this is that it uses a non linear log transformation to predict odd ratio and it is not necessary that the independent variable has to be correlated with each other.
2. **Linear regression:** Linear regression is most widely used regression technique for prediction of a class. In this technique the class label are continuous and all other attributes can be either continuous or discrete by using a regression line which is also known as best fit straight line

It can be calculated by the formula

$Y = B_0 + B_1 * x + e$

Here "e" is the error rate

3. 3. **Linear Discriminate Analysis:** Linear discriminate analysis is used to avoid the drawback of logistic regression as logistic regression is limited only for two class classification problem. When there are more than two classes that time linear discriminate analysis is preferred for classification. LDA can be solved by statistical properties that is mean, variance, covariance and Gaussian mean.

$$Mean(k) = \frac{1}{N} * \sum_{i=1}^{n} X\ of\ i$$

Clustering

Clustering is a method of grouping the data into classes of similar object that is partitioning the data and arranging it in similar group. Clustering is a unsupervised machine learning technique because here machine learn from its past experience. Some of the clustering algorithm is K means, K medians, DBSCAN etc

1. **K Means:** The K means algorithm take dataset K and partitions a set of m object into k cluster so that the resulting intra cluster similarity is high but the inter cluster similarity is low.

K mean cluster can be solved by first selecting the k object randomly from a given dataset then find the next element which is closer to that k valve the more closer will form one group and the far one will form another cluster then find the mean of the first cluster form and again find the closest element to that next mean. This process iterate until the similar type of cluster start forming. K means clustering is a type of partitioning clustering.

2. **Hierarchical Clustering:** A hierarchical clustering method work by grouping data object into a tree of cluster. The demerit of hierarchical clustering is that it become difficult to adjust the performance once a merge or split decision has been executed. As it cannot backtrack so it always better to decide first before

splitting or merging the tree. There are two type of hierarchical clustering one is agglomerative another is divisive.

3. **Density Based Method:** A density based clustering method is based on connected region with sufficiently high density. One of its famous techniques is DBSCAN.

DBSCAN begins with an arbitrary starting data point that has not been visited. It starts visiting the node within its neighbor. If the distance is nearer to its neighbor then it start forming the cluster once it has visited the node it mark the visited node. Once it is done with the current cluster. It starts the process again with the unvisited node and it continues till it form cluster of the entire node present.

Association

Association rule mining is a used for solving the pattern that is appear in the dataset frequently.

Association rule mining is a popular and well known method for discovering interesting relation between variable in large database. Some important term of association rule mining are support, confidence, lift and conviction.

Suppose there are two attribute A and B so support can be calculated by:

$$Support = \frac{Number\ of\ transaction\ in\ which\ A\ apper}{total\ number\ of\ transation}$$

$$Confidence\left(A \rightarrow B\right) = \frac{Support\left(A\,UB\right)}{Support\left(A\right)}$$

$$Lift = \frac{Support\left(A\,UB\right)}{Support\left(A\right)Support\left(B\right)}$$

METHODOLOGY

The aim of this work is to predict whether the tumor is grown to cancer or not by taking a CT scan image and further it is compared with different classification techniques. In the existing model the use of image enhancement, classification and feature extraction technique were limited. Here two types of feature extraction techniques are used, one is texture based and another is region description. In texture based the gray level Co-occurrence Matrix is used to extract feature based on color, contrast of the image and in region based feature like area and perimeter are extracted. After feature extraction different classification technique is applied individually to known which classification method is giving more accuracy.

Figure 5 shows the proposed novel framework.

Figure 5. Proposed framework

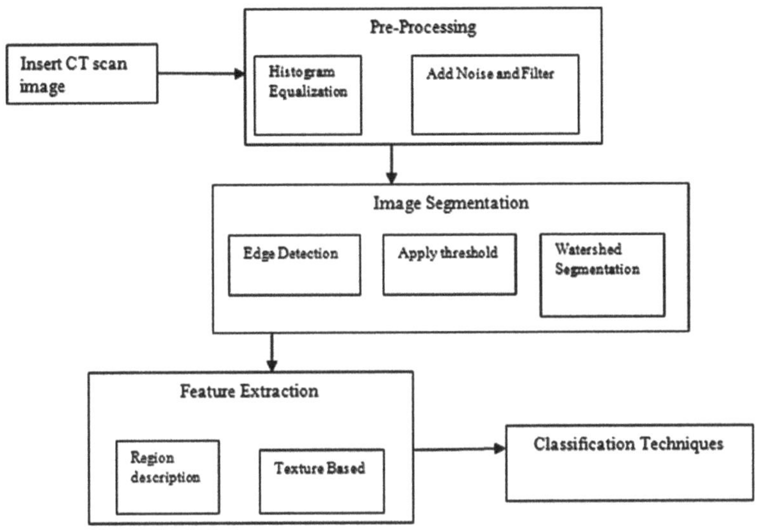

The different stages of these models are as follows:

- **Pre-processing module:** The original image is enhanced and filter are added in the image to get a clear and noise free image as we know that the original image is full of noise and the image is not clear. So for getting a clear image pre-processing step is carried out. In Pre- processing block first histogram equalization is applied to get clear and enhanced image. Then on enhanced image some noise are added, noise which is added is salt and pepper noise for removing the noise that is the noise which was already present in the image and the extra noise which was added latter on median filter has been used. And for salt and pepper noise the best filter is median filter other all filters can be applied but the maximum might not be removed and pre-Processing is the crucial stage because if the image is not pre-processed properly then there is a chance of getting less accuracy. The pre- processing image is shown in figure 6

Figure 6. Pre-processed image (a) original image (b) gray image (c) gray histogram graph (d) histogram equalization (e) histogram

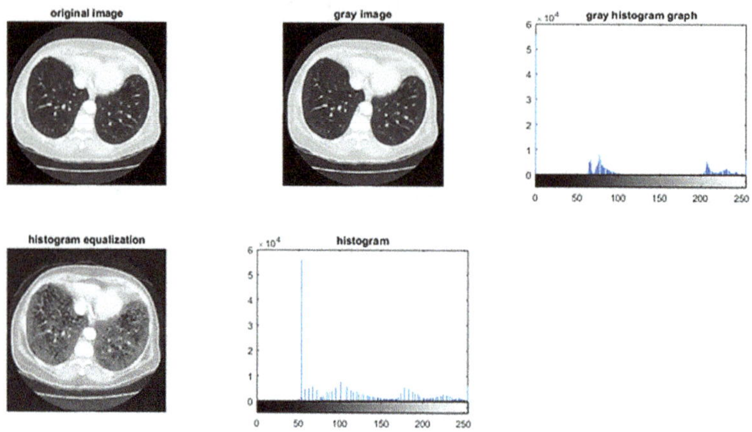

- **Segmentation module:** Image segmentation is a method of partitioning the image into various parts. After pre-processing the image on the pre-processed image segmentation is applied to acquire the information from the image. For image segmentation first we have applied edge detection technique through edge detection we can segment the boundary of the image for edge detection sobel operator has been used, sobel edge detector compute the gradient by using the discrete differences between row and columns of there neighbor. On that operator threshold has been applied that is Otsu threshold if the intensity value which is less than threshold is removed and the intensity value which is higher than or equal to threshold will consider for further segmentation after getting the segmented image by applying threshold we will apply watershed segmentation on the output image. There are various ways to segment using watershed segmentation here we have used watershed segmentation using gradient. The gradient magnitude is used to preprocess the gray scale image that is it has high pixel value along the object edge and low pixel value in another left region. And through this we can get the segmented image by which we can extract features. Segmented image is shown in figure 7

Figure 7. Segmented Image

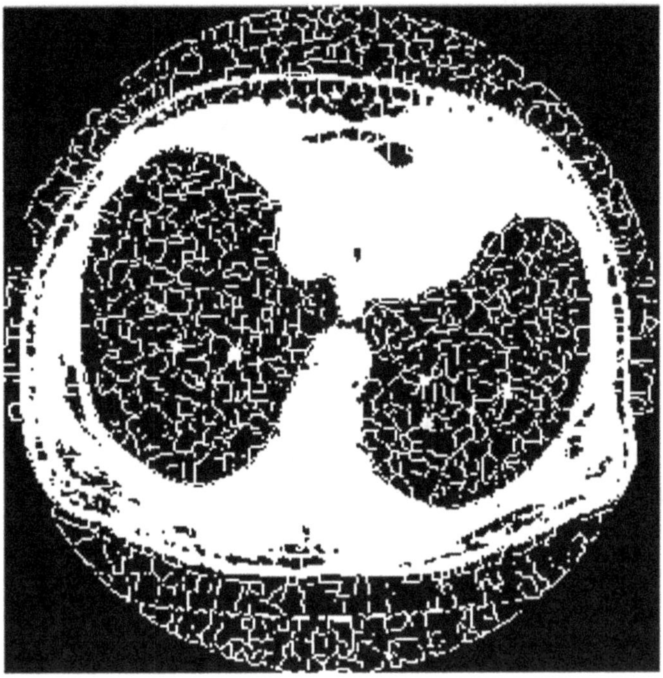

- **Feature extraction module:** It is used to reduce the dimension of the image using texture and region based feature. On the region based feature extracted are area(The number of pixel in the image), perimeter(if there are N numbers of element then that N element vector consist of distance around the boarder of each of the N region in the image), centroid (The center of the region on the image), Bounding Box (it is used to define the smallest rectangle consist of region), Euler Number (it is used to find the difference between number of object in the mage and number of holes on that image), Equiv Diameter (it is used to find the diameter of the circle with the same area as the region), Extent (The proportion of the pixel in the bounding box that is also present in the region). On the basis of texture features that are extracted are contrast (it returns a measure of intensity brightness between the pixel and its neighbors. Correlation (it gives a measure that how well pixels are correlated to its neighbor over the entire image). Energy (it gives the sum of squared element in the co occurrence matrix). Homogeneity (it gives a value that measures the closeness of the distribution of element in the co occurrence matrix to the diagonal of co occurrence matrix).

- **Classification module:** Machine learning classification technique will be used like Logistic Regression, decision tree, and K-Nearest Neighbor to classify whether the tumor is cancerous or not. Based on the classification performance is evaluated and comparison is made based on accuracy, precision, recall and F1 score to predict which algorithm is giving the best output.

PERFORMANCE MATRIX

Confusion Matrix

A confusion matrix is a detail study of prediction result on a classification problem. The number of correct and incorrect predictions are summarized with count values and broken down by each class. This is the key to the confusion matrix (https://machinelearningmastery.com/confusion-matrix-machine-learning/).

Table 1. Confusion Matrix

	Prediction(yes)	Prediction (no)
Actual (yes)	True Positive	False Negative
Actual(no)	False Positive	True Negative

- **True Positive:** When we want to predict yes and the actual value is also yes it is called true positive
- **True Negative:** When we want to predict no and the actual value is also no is called true negative
- **False Positive:** When we want to predict yes and actual value is no is called false positive
- **False Negative:** When we want to predict no and actual value is yes is called false negative
- **Precision:** The precision for a class is the number of true positives (i.e. the number of items correctly labeled as belonging to the positive class) divided by the total number of elements labeled as belonging to the positive class (i.e. the sum of true positives and false positives, which are items incorrectly labeled as belonging to the class) (Precision 2020).

$$Precision = \frac{True\,positive}{True\,positive + False\,Positive}$$

- **Recall:** Recall for a class is defined as the number of true positives divided by the total number of elements that actually belong to the positive class (i.e. the sum of true positives and false negatives, which are items which were not labeled as belonging to the positive class but should have been) (Precision 2020).

$$Recall = \frac{True\,positive}{True\,positive + False\,Negative}$$

- **F1 Score:** A measure that combines precision and recall is the harmonic mean of precision and recall, the traditional F-measure or balanced F-score. This measure is approximately the average of the two when they are close, and is more generally the harmonic mean, which, for the case of two numbers, coincides with the square of the geometric mean divided by the arithmetic mean. There are several reasons that the F-score can be criticized in particular circumstances due to its bias as an evaluation metric (Precision 2020).

$$F1\,Score = 2 * \frac{1}{\frac{1}{Precision} + \frac{1}{Recall}}$$

- **Accuracy**: Classification Accuracy is what we usually mean, when we use the term accuracy. It is the ratio of number of correct predictions to the total number of input samples. It works well only if there are equal number of samples belonging to each class.

$$Accuracy = \frac{Number\,of\,correct\,prediction\,made}{Total\,Number\,of\,prediction\,made}$$

RESULT AND DISCUSSION

For the experiment image data was used which was collected from LIDC, and after the feature extraction some of the machine learning supervised algorithm were used like logistic regression, Decision Tree, and K-nearest neighbor. The image dataset consist of 1018 cases out of which 20 cases have been considered for the evaluation of the proposed model. Out of 20 images 15 images has been trained and rest 5 images has been used for testing. After training and testing the data set performance metrics was evaluated to check which algorithm is giving more accuracy. Comparison of accuracy, Recall, Precision and F1 score has been shown in bar chart in figure 8

Figure 8. Region based classification

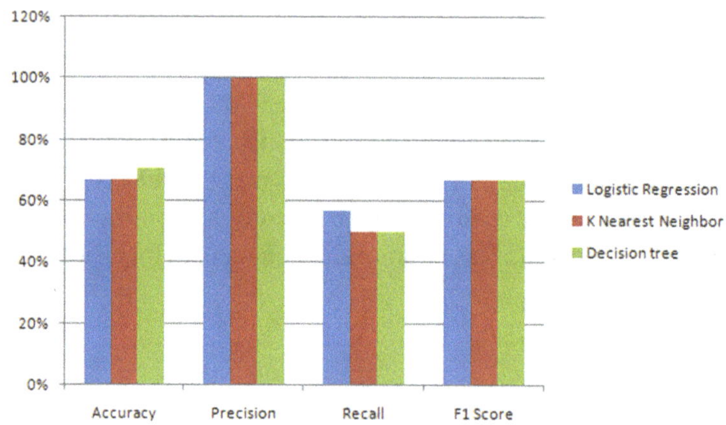

Figure 9. Texture based classification

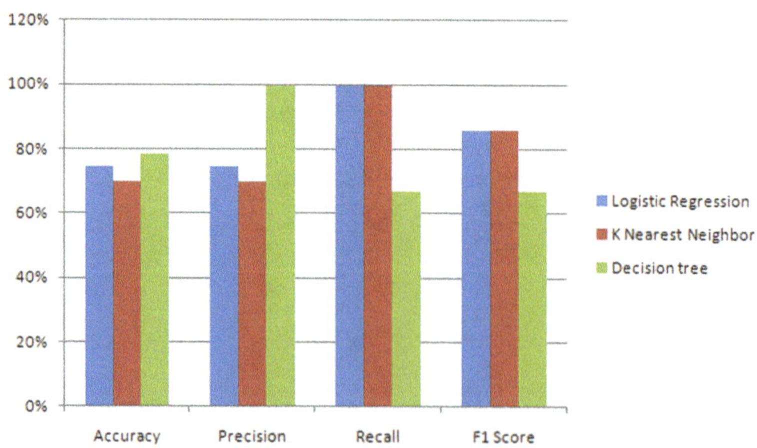

and figure 9. Tool which has been used for pre- processing was Matlab (R2017a) and for classification google colab was used.

Table 2. Performance of region based feature extraction

	Accuracy	Precision	Recall	F1 Score
Logistic Regression	67%	100%	57%	67%
K Nearest Neighbor	67%	100%	50%	67%
Decision Tree	71%	100%	50%	67%

Table 3. Performance of texture based feature extraction

	Accuracy	Precision	Recall	F1 Score
Logistic Regression	75%	75%	100%	86%
K Nearest Neighbor	70%	70%	100%	86%
Decision Tree	79%	100%	67%	80%

TOOLS

There are several tools available for machine learning and digital image processing. Before going to tools some of the common programming languages that are used for machine learning are Python, R, C++, Java, JavaScript, C# etc, and for digital image processing programming language are matlab, openCV etc. As said a good programming language can result a better result in the same way it is important to decide which tool is to be used for that particular scenario. The most common tools used for machine leaning are:

1. **Keras:** keras is a high level neural network API written in python. It allow easy and fast computation, it is used for executing the algorithm of deep neural network like CNN and RNN. Beside this it can run smoothly on CPU and GPU. It put the user experience very properly, provides simple and consistent API and reduces the number of user action required. New classes or function can be added simply. Modules described in python code are easier to debug and allow extensibility. A model is understood as sequence or graph of standalone that can be plugged together with few very restrictions (Keras Documentation, n.d.)

2. **Pandas:** Panda is a python package that provides fast, flexible and suggestive data structure design to make working with structured data and time series data very easily. Panda are well suited for different kind of data like tabular data with heterogeneous column, ordered or unordered time series data. Pandas are well known for handling the missing data, Column can be inserted or deleted from dataframe, flexible reshape and pivoting datasets. Panda is well known data analytics and data manipulation tool (PyPI- Pandas 2020).
3. **NumPy:** NumPy is the fundamental package for scientific computing with Python. It also contains N-Dimensional array object, well defined functions. It can integrate C, C++ and forton code (NumPy 2020).
4. **Scikit-Learn:** It gives simple and efficient tools for predictive data analytics and provide accessibility to everybody, and reusable in various contexts. It is an open source tool. Scikit-Learn provide a friendly API. Its main features include classification, regression, clustering, dimensionality reduction, model selection, and preprocessing (Scikit Learn 2020)
5. **Matplotlib:** Matplotlib is a Python 2D plotting library which produces publication quality figures in a variety of hardcopy formats and interactive environments across platforms. Matplotlib can be used in Python scripts, the Python and IPython shells, the Jupyter notebook, web application servers, and four graphical user interface toolkits. Through matplotlib you can create bar chart, scatter plots, histogram etc (Matplotlib n.d).
6. **TensorFlow:** Tensorflow is a python package. TensorFlow is an open source platform for machine learning. It has a comprehensive, flexible ecosystem of tools, libraries and community resources that lets researchers push the state-of-the-art in Machine learning and developers easily build and deploy ML applications. TensorFlow offers many levels of abstraction so you can choose the best one according to your requirement. Build and train models by using the high-level Keras API, which makes getting started with TensorFlow and machine learning easy. If you need more flexibility, eager execution allows for immediate iteration and intuitive debugging. For large ML training tasks, use the Distribution Strategy API for distributed training on different hardware configurations without changing the model definition (TensorFlow n.d.).
7. **Google Colab:** Colaboratory is a free Jupyter notebook environment where you can write python code and it requires no setup and runs entirely in the cloud. With Colaboratory you can write and execute code, save and share your analyses, and access powerful computing resources, all for free from your browser (https://colab.research.google.com/notebooks/welcome.ipynb#scrollTo=xitplqMNk_Hc).

CONCLUSION

As the dataset which was taken for classification was a Dicom image and data set was taken from LIDC. LIDC consist of 1018 cases. The main difficulty which is faced is the Dicom was not able to run neither in python nor in matlab environment.

Based on the literature survey, the given proposed model provides precision and recall. From the proposed model it can be seen that texture based feature extraction is giving more accuracy as compare to region based and in both the cases decision tree is giving better accuracy. If both the feature is compared separately then in region based feature extraction precision was improved and decision tree was giving more accuracy as compared to logistic regression and K Nearest neighbor. And in texture based feature extraction recall and F1 score was improved and decision tree was giving more accuracy as compared to logistic regression and K Nearest neighbor.

In future other machine learning classification algorithm along with other technique can be applied to generate more accuracy, precision, F1 score. And other than machine learning deep learning can be applied for the prediction of cancer as deep learning work more appropriately with image and the probability of generating proper result is more in deep learning as compare to machine learning.

REFERENCES

Bhuvaneswari, P., & Therese, A. B. (2015). Detection of cancer in lung with k-nn classification using genetic algorithm. *Procedia Materials Science*, *10*, 433–440. doi:10.1016/j.mspro.2015.06.077

Cancer treatment center of America. (2020). *About lung cancer.* Retrieved from https://www.cancercenter.com/cancer-types/lung-cancer/symptoms

Colaboratory. (n.d.). Retrieved from https://colab.research.google.com/notebooks/welcome.ipynb#scrollTo=xitplqMNk_Hc

D'Cruz, J., Jadhav, A., Dighe, A., Chavan, V., & Chaudhari, J. (2016). Detection of lung cancer using backpropagation neural networks and genetic algorithm. *Computer Technology and Application*, *6*(5), 823–827.

Fenwa, O. D., Ajala, F. A., & Adigun, A. (2016). Classification of cancer of the lungs using SVM and ANN. *International Journal of Computers and Technology*, *15*(1), 6418–6426. doi:10.24297/ijct.v15i1.1715

Jason Brownlee. (2016). *Machine learning Mastery.* Retrieved 18 November 2016, from https://machinelearningmastery.com/confusion-matrix-machine-learning/

Keras Documentation. (n.d.). *Keras-The Python Deep Learning Library.* Retrieved from https://keras.io/

LIDC. (n.d.). Retrieved from https://wiki.cancerimagingarchive.net/display/Public/LIDC-IDRI

Matplotlib. (n.d.). *Matplotlibcontents.* Retrieved from https://matplotlib.org/

National Cancer Institute. (2019). *Lung and bronchus cancer.* Retrieved from https://seer.cancer.gov/statfacts/html/lungb.html

NumPy. (2020). *NumPy.* Retrieved from https://numpy.org/

Palani, D., & Venkatalakshmi, K. (2019). An IoT based predictive modelling for predicting lung cancer using fuzzy cluster based segmentation and classification. *Journal of Medical Systems, 43*(2), 21. doi:10.100710916-018-1139-7 PMID:30564924

Pradeep, K. R., & Naveen, N. C. (2018). Lung cancer survivability prediction based on performance using classification techniques of support vector machines, C4. 5 and Naive Bayes algorithms for healthcare analytics. *Procedia Computer Science, 132*, 412–420. doi:10.1016/j.procs.2018.05.162

Precision. (2020). Retrieved May 18, 2020 from https://en.wikipedia.org/wiki/Precision_and_recall

PyPI- Pandas. (2020). *Pandas 1.0.1.* Retrieved May 18,2020 from https://pypi.org/project/pandas/

Scikit Learn. (2020). *Scikit-Learn Machine learning in python.* Retrieved from https://scikit-learn.org/stable/

Shannon, C. E. (1948). A mathematical theory of communication. *The Bell System Technical Journal, 27*(3), 379–423. doi:10.1002/j.1538-7305.1948.tb01338.x

Stöppler & Marks. (n.d.). *Lung cancer article.* Retrieved from https://www.medicinenet.com/lung_cancer/article.htm

TensorFlow. (n.d.). *TensorFlow About.* Retrieved from https://www.tensorflow.org/about/

The cancer imaging archive. (2020). Retrieved from https://www.cancerimagingarchive.net/about-the-cancer-imaging-archive-tcia/

Tong, W. (2020). Machine learning for spatiotemporal big data in air pollution. In *Spatiotemporal Analysis of Air Pollution and Its Application in Public Health* (pp. 107–134). Elsevier. doi:10.1016/B978-0-12-815822-7.00005-4

Toward Data Science Natasha Sharma. (2019). *Importance of distance Metrics in Machine learning modeling.* Retrieved 13 January, 2019 from https://towardsdatascience.com/importance-of-distance-metrics-in-machine-learning-modelling-e51395ffe60d

Yang, H., & Chen, Y. P. P. (2015). Data mining in lung cancer pathologic staging diagnosis: Correlation between clinical and pathology information. *Expert Systems with Applications*, *42*(15-16), 6168–6176. doi:10.1016/j.eswa.2015.03.019

Chapter 6
A Survey on Prematurity Detection of Diabetic Retinopathy Based on Fundus Images Using Deep Learning Techniques

Amiya Kumar Dash
KIIT University, India

Puspanjali Mohapatra
International Institute of Information Technology, Bhubaneswar, India

ABSTRACT

Diabetic retinopathy (DR) is a disease related to eye correlated with long-standing diabetes. It is a leading cause of blindness among working adults. Detection of this condition in the early stage is critical for good prognosis. Present day detection of DR normally requires digital fundus image or images generated using optical coherence tomography (OCT). As OCT are high-priced, diagnosis of DR using fundus image will benefit for the patient and the ophthalmologists. Manual inspection of morphological changes in blood vessels, microaneurysms, exudates, hemorrhages, and macula are time consuming and tedious tasks. So, designing a computer-aided system helps in analyzing the morphological changes and identifying the DR. This chapter reviews the applications of machine learning and deep learning algorithms for detection of nonproliferative diabetic retinopathy by analyzing fundus images.

DOI: 10.4018/978-1-7998-5071-7.ch006

Copyright © 2021, IGI Global. Copying or distributing in print or electronic forms without written permission of IGI Global is prohibited.

INTRODUCTION

Medical image analysis is an active area of research in present days which attracts scientists and physicians from different domain. This area entails the examination of digital images to provide computational tools as a way to help the quantification and visualization of interesting pathology and anatomical structures. This field has brought off significant improvement over past few years. Physicians have advanced diagnostic tools to evaluate their patients in order to plan different forms of management and monitor the progress more efficiently than before.

Diabetic is a very common diseases Now-a-days. It is identified as a widespread epidemic that has progressive effect on every country across the globe irrespective of any age group. A survey was conducted by 'International Diabetes Federation', where they have generated a report showing that approximately 415 million people were suffering from diabetes worldwide and this number has increased in the past 30 years, especially in Asia. Of them, around one-thirds are diagnosed with diabetic retinopathy (DR), a chronic disease which can cause impaired vision and also complete vision loss in many cases. ***Diabetic Retinopathy*(DR*)*** is a major source of visual impairment among grown-ups and the older segment of the populace. It is connected with type 1 and type 2 diabetes. The reason for this is increase in glucose levels in veins in the retinal region, leading little spillages of blood, blood proteins, serum and blood fats. Detection of DR in the early stage prevents its progress.

Diagnosis of DR based on the examination of retinal images. Clinically, DR is categorized into different types. (1) ***Non-proliferative Diabetic Retinopathy (NPDR)*** is the first stage of this taxonomy. At this phase, fats and other deposits create microaneurysms which are spots on the walls of veins in the retina. At the point when the smaller scale aneurysms outpouch and spill, there is inflammation in the macula and in the nerve fibers. Blood Vessels might be obtruded and macula stops to work appropriately because of absence of oxygen, and obscuring the vision of the patient all the while. (2) ***Proliferative Diabetic Retinopathy (PDR)*** is the second phase. This happens when many blood vessels close and afterward the retina attempts to **make restitution** that by producing fresh blood vessels. This procedure is called neovascularization. However, these unusual vessels don't supply the proper quantity of blood to the retina. Another conceivable outcome is a harm to the optic nerve bringing about glaucoma. Figure 1 shows the images of NPDR and PDR (Li et al.,2014) with different levels.

There are many ways to get the imaging and hence diagnosis of Diabetic Retinopathy. In the recent past, a fluorescein test during angiography was the most common method of imaging the eye. In this method a fluorescein is visible in the arteries, which is absorbed in the tissue and lastly go back through the veins. A video clip is generated for the entire procedure as output. Diabetic Retinopathy screening detects spill of blood and alternative parts, offering confirmation to the headway of the sickness.

OCT is a present day method to carry out Diabetic Retinopathy screening. In this, the ophthalmologist offers an exact angiography image without being it invasive for the patient. There is no injection of substance. This wipe out many side-effects. Another strategy utilizes ultrasound to identify Diabetic Retinopathy side effects. B-scan ultrasonography additionally empowers the screening of veins in the retinal region.

An algorithmic way to automatically diagnose and evaluate Diabetic Retinopathy has to perform many tasks like finding the blood spills, identifying the development of new vessels, which show the presence of micro aneurysm. These tasks are done by checking every pixel precisely. This is a time taking process when executed by a human. This justify the need of an automated technique for detection of microaneurysm. Microaneurysm are localized capillary dilatations which are usually saccular, that is, round in shape.

Figure 1. ¬

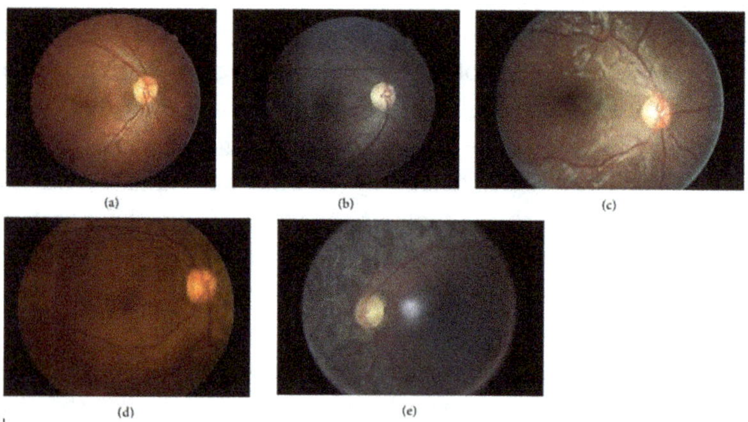

Early detection of this disease is very difficult as it requires skilled clinical facilities and of a lot of manual labour. Symptoms are limited and this often prevents a timely and appropriate treatment. For this reason, various scientists are trying various automated methods for early detection of Diabetic Retinopathy. With the development of various methods and technology, this work has become successful to a great extent.

Literature Review

Identification of DR from fundus image basically involved image segmentation and identification of DR. Major goal of image segmentation is to locate the retinal vessel. The valid data about vessels precise location and thickness plays a vital role for determining the patient is DR or not. As the fundus images contain many other substances so, vessel tracking is a complex task. Numerous vessel segmentation techniques have been suggested by many authors. Those techniques can be divided broadly into five types such as Morphological processing, Matched filtering, Vascular tracking, Deformation model and Machine learning.

Review on Image Segmentation

Morphological Processing

Here we analyze the binary image for segmentation and identification of target object. Linear and circular elements of the blood vessels are selected by isolating the desired structure rather than the background image. A mathematical approach based on morphology which separate vessels from all possible undesirable patterns are given by Zana and Klein (2001). Based on Zana and Kleinapproach Ayala (2005) build a model using fuzzy set. Miri and Mahloojifar (2010) have analyzed the fundus image using curvelet transformation and morphological reconstruction. It results the enhancement in boundaries of the image and determines the vascular ridge. Karthika and Marimuthu (2014) have combined above methods of multi-structural elements for segmentation and identification of vessels with strongly connected component analysis (SCCA) .

Matched Filtering

Chaudhuri and Chatterjee (1989) applied Gaussian filters for vessel tracking by considering that vessels are darker than the background. He has designed a two dimensional Gaussian filter. It has the capability to detect the vessels in twelve directions. An improved methodology has developed by Hoover et al., 2000 which considers the regional characteristics of vessels to identify blood vessels in retinal images. Zhang et al.,2009 has used local bilateral thresholding on vessels cross section for match filtering.

Vascular Tracking Method

In the year 1993, Liu and Sun (1993) have derived a tracking system which extracts the vascular from X-ray angiograms. This method needs an initial point and the direction of the vessel as an input. The author uses an "extrapolation-update" method to estimate the local vessel trajectories. After tracking the vessel fragment, it is being removed from the image. The above process is repeated till the vascular tree has been extracted. The drawbacks of this technique are, firstly, the user has to specify the starting point inside the vessel and secondly, it is also not suitable for three-dimensional extraction. A generalized threshold method is given by Jiang et al. (Jiang and Mojon,2003). It is based on the concept of multithreshold detection. Zhang et al., 2009 has used local bilateral thresholding for enhancement matching filtering scheme by applying local vessel cross section (pp.528-534). For the extraction of tiny vessels, Li et al., 2012 has proposed a multi-scale production of the matched filter.

Methods of Deformation Models

In 1988 Kass introduced this model. This model (Kass et al.,1988)has the ability to produce smooth surfaces and curves. Deformation models are categorized into two types: parametric deformation model and geometric deformation model . Espona (2007) has implemented parametric deformation model on fundus image and upgrade an improved method with morphological segmentation. Al-Diri and Hunte proposed a deformation model named as ribbon of twins (ROT) to calculate the vessel width. However parametric deformation model has several disadvantage because the output of segmentation depends on the initial contour and difficulties arise in segmenting complex objects.

It has been found that as compared to parametric deformation model geometric deformation model can well solve the problems. Zhang (2009) used nonlinear orthogonal projection scheme. It captures the characteristics of retinal image and obtains an adaptive local thresholding algorithm which can be implemented for blood vessel segmentation. Zhao (2014) have suggested a model which is a region-based active contour model which has level set implementation and a region growing attribute.

Machine Learning

These are the algorithms that train the computers to learn achieve goals automatically from the given data sets by building discriminative and generative models. Machine Learning can be broadly classified into Supervised learning and Unsupervised learning. A supervised classification with 2-dimensonal Gabor wavelet was proposed by Cesar and Jelinek. Feature vector is used to represents each pixel. It consists of grey scale feature along with the responses of distinct sizes of two-dimensional Gabor wavelet (Cesar and Jelinek,2016).Marin (2011) has proposed a scheme that uses neural network. It has one input layer in the beginning, three hidden layers in the intermediate level and one output layer at the end. In this technique, he has trained the network with the help of seven dimensional feature vector of each pixel.Another technique proposed by Shanmugam and Banu to create seven dimensional feature vector which is based on grey scale features. Retinal vessels are detected by using extreme learning machine (ELM) (Shanmugam and Banu, January,2013). Wang et al., 2015 proposed a hierarchical retinal vascular segmentation. In this scheme author used iterative clustering. It is useful to achieve super-pixel segmentation and random selection of pixel to represent the entire super-pixel. This method is easy and one of the efficient means of feature extraction.

Review on Diabetic Retinopathy Detection

Machine learning algorithms can be used to extract retinal vessels before detecting DR. It results high accuracy in comparison to other techniques. This is time consuming to create the marked ground-truth for retinal vessels. An alternative model can be used to train the computer. It learns automatically and distinguishs different level of DR from fundus image directly without performing vessel segmentation. Ege et al., 2000 developed a statistical classifier, including Bayseian, Mahalanobis distance and K-nearest neighbor classifier for automatic identification of DR. Silberman (2010) proposed an automatic analysis of DR system and record an equal error rate of 87%. Karegowda (2011) used a back-propagation neural network algorithm to find exudates in the retinal images where features were decided by decision tree and genetic algorithms with correlation-based feature selection. In their experiment they reported an accuracy of 98.45%. Kavitha and Duraiswamy used color histogram thresholding to classify hard and soft exudates. This experiment resulted 99.07%, 89% and 99% of accuracy, sensitivity and specificity respectively (Kavitha and Duraiswamy,2011,pp.493-504). In the year of 2014, Calleja et al. used local binary patterns (LBP) for feature selection and for classification they have used support vector machine (SVM), random forest (RF) and Artificial Neural Network (ANN). They used a dataset that contains 71 images and they achieved 97.46% accuracy with RF (Calleja et al.,2014).

OUTLINE OF DEEP LEARNING METHODS

Over the past years ophthalmic imaging has developed rapidly but recently researcher started applying deep learning algorithm for analysis of retinal images. Most of the works applied convolutional Neural Network (CNN) for analysis of color fundus image. Recent research addresses a wide variety of applications such as image quality assessment, diagnosis of eye diseases, segmentation of anatomical structures, segmentation and detection of retinal abnormalities. Kaggle has organized a competition in 2015 on the topic diabetic retinopathy detection. The dataset had 35,000 color fundus images as the training sample and to test the severity of the disease 53,000 test images were provided. Total 661 teams participated in the competition and all of them have applied deep learning technique to detect the presence of diabetic retinopathy.

Neural networks are the basis of most deep learning techniques. The word "neural" refers to the adjective form of neurons and "networks" refers to the graph like structures. So artificial neural network is a computation system that is inspired by the neural connection of our nervous system. A Neural Network consists of neurons which has a few activation function '*a*', fixed weights (*W*) and a set of biases (*B*). This activation function can be characterized as the linear combination of parameters *(W, B)* and the input (X) to the neurons, followed by a piece wise transfer function which is non-linear in nature.

$$a = \sigma\left(W^{T}X + b\right) \tag{1}$$

Standard transfer functions for neural networks are hyperbolic tangent function and sigmoid function. A traditional well known neural network is multi-layered perceptron (MLP) having a few layers of these transformations:

$$F\left(X,W,B\right) = \sigma\left(W^{L}\sigma\left(w^{L-1}\,.........\,\sigma\left(w^{0}X + b^{0}\right) + b^{L-1}\right) + b^{L}\right) \tag{2}$$

Here,

w^{n} : two dimensional matrix which consists of rows as w_{k}
k: activation in the output sequence
n: number of current layer,
L: final layer

Layers present between the input and output are called as hidden layers. A neural network model having more than one hidden layers is called as a deep neural network.

Generally, final layer's activation functions of the network are plotted to a distribution over classes $p\left(y \mid x;\Theta\right)$. It is done through a softmax function.

$$p\left(y \mid x;\Theta\right) = soft\max\left(x;\Theta\right) = \frac{\left(e^{w_i^L}\right)^T x + b_i^L}{\sum_{K=1}^{K}\left(e^{w_i^L}\right)^T x + b_i^L} \tag{3}$$

Where, w_i^L : Weight vector of the output node associated with class *i*.

In earlier days, Deep Neural Networks were very difficult to be trained by the machine to achieve an efficient result. After 2006, it gains the popularity as Bengio et al. and Hinton et al. have proved that training a deep neural network unsupervised manner layer wise, followed by a supervised fine tuning of the network have performed good. Stack auto encoder(SAE) and deep belief networks(DBN) are the two popular network trained on the above method. Even so, these methods have complex working principles and require a momentous work to produce an adequate result.

Convolutional Neural Networks(CNNS)

CNN is different than MLP in two ways. The existing network executes convolution operation on images by sharing the weights in the network. Hence, for a given object, present at separate location in an image, model does not require to learn other different detectors. This makes the network equivalent to translations of the input. The network also tries to lessen the number of parameters that need to be learned.

In CNN, set of *m* kernels are taken at each layer. Input in the form of image is convoluted with the kernels. Let's assume *w* as the kernel set i.e. $w = \left\{w_1, w_2, \ldots. w_m\right\}$ .A added bias set $B = \left\{b_1, b_2 \ldots\ldots\ldots b_m\right\}$ is taken for creating a new feature map $\boldsymbol{X}_{m}$. A nonlinear transformation is applied to these newly generated features element wise and it is iterated for every convolutional layer l:

$$X_m^l = \sigma\left(W_m^{l-1} * X^{l-1} + b_k^{l-1}\right) \tag{4}$$

Use of pooling layers is another way to differentiate between CNNs and MLPs. In CNN, neighborhood pixel values are summed using a permutation of a uniform function which can enhance the receptive field of subsequent convolutional layers. At the end of this method, fully connected layers are added. Here weights are not shared further. Figure 2 shows the architecture of CNN model [42]. Close to this in MLPs, a distribution is generated over each class by applying the activation in the final layer. Here also a softmax function is used for the purpose. The existing network is trained using maximum likelihood.

Figure 2. Convolutional neural network architecture with two hidden layers
Blue represents input node, red represents hidden layers, green represents output node.

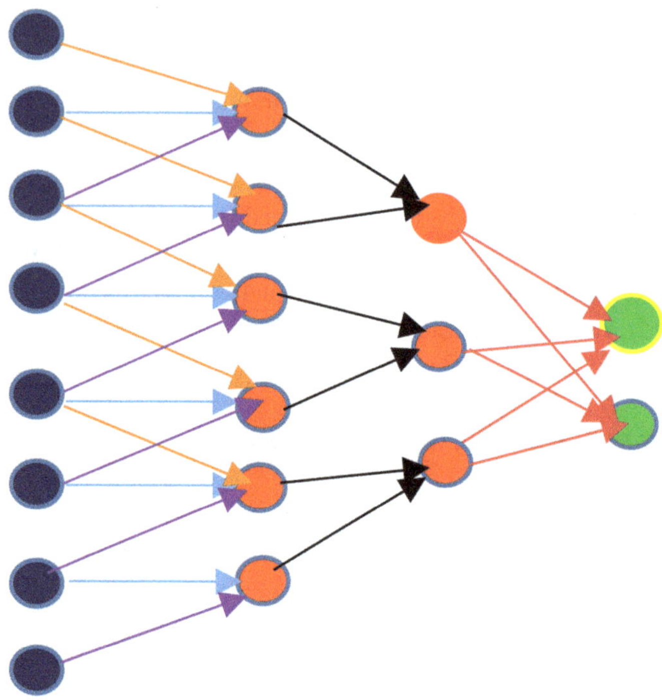

Given the fact and conditions of CNN in the analysis of clinical or medical, the most well-known architectures that are broadly used are LeNet and AlexNet proposed by LeCun et al., 1998 and Krizhevsky et al., 2012 respectively. The essences of these two models are very much similar. Both the networks are relatively shallow, consisting of 2 and 5 convolution layers respectively. These networks implemented in such a way that near to the input it uses kernels with wide receptive fields in layers and small size kernel near to the output. Alexnet employed rectified linear units as activation function as opposed to the hyperbolic tangent function, that is the most common choice in CNN.

The research on novel architecture on deep learning models took off after 2012. Researchers now give preference to far deeper models and rather deploying a one-layer kernel with large receptive fields, deeper model uses smaller kernels with less number of parameters.

The deeper networks are explored by Simonyan and Zisserman in 2014. They have used a small kernel of fixed size at every layer. In 2014, a 19-layer model VGG19 or OxfordNet has won the ImageNet challenge.

A more complex model has been developed on the top of these networks to increase the efficiency of the training method and to decrease the parameters number. A 22-layer network model has been introduced by szegedy et al. (2014) [25] named *GoogLeNet*. He et al. (2015) proposed *ResNet* which won the ImageNet contest in 2015 and consist of so called ResNet blocks.

Present studies say that all researchers use Inception v3 (Gulshan et al., 2016; Esteva et al., 2017; Liu et al., 2017) which is a version of GoogleNet but still AlexNet or other simple models such as VGG are still popular for medical data.

Discussion

In this survey we reviewed 41 research articles of medical image analysis using deep learning. Out of these 41 articles 16 articles applied deep learning methods for diabetic retinopathy detection and majority of the papers were published on 2016 or January 2017. From the survey it has been observed that for medical imaging end-to-end trained CNN have become the preferred method for interpretation clinical image. Sometimes these CNNs are combined with traditional machine learning methods or image analysis techniques for better interpretation of medical images. Table 1 shows the detail application of deep learning methods on diabetic retinopathy detection.

CONCLUSION

After reviewing so many papers it is evident that, use of end-to-end CNN followed by traditional machine learning techniques or image analysis techniques gives better result and a large group of researchers applied these techniques as a standard practice. From the study it has been found that expert knowledge about the task to be solved plays a greater role for increasing the performance of the model. We have seen that, in challenges like CAMELYON16 and Kaggles Diabetic retinopathy detection, most of the researchers apply same architecture but gets different performance by applying data preprocessing and augmentation outside the network. Hence from the survey we can conclude that application of deep learning on medical image analysis gives better performance as compared to other traditional image analysis techniques and serves as the current standard practice.

Table 1. Overview of usage of deep learning techniques for analysis of retinal image

Reference	Application	Methods
Quality Assessment and Segmentation of Anatomical Structures of Color Fundus Image		
Mahapatra et al. year 2016	Retinal image quality assessment (IQA)	Unsupervised saliency maps fused with supervised CNN for classification of the Image quality.
Fu et al. Year-2016b	Segmentation of retinal vessel	A fully connected CNN combined with fully connected CRF to design a framework for long range pixel segmentation
Fu et al. Year-2016a	Segmentation of retinal vessel	Redeveloped his approach (sFu et al. 2016b) using RNN instead of CRF
Maninis et al. Year-2016	Retinal vessel and optic disc segmentation.	For each segmentation task VGG-19 network model is expanded with specialized layers.
Wu et al. Year-2016	Segmentation of retinal vessel	CNN followed by mapping Principal component analysis solution of the last layer features map to the full segmentation
Zilly et al. Year-2017	Optic cup and disc segmentation of retinal image	Ensemble learning based CNN with several layers of sequentially learned filters using boosting.
Diseases and Abnormalities Detection of Color Fundus Image		
Chen et al. Year-2016b	Detection of Glaucoma	A simple CNN with six learned six learned layers (4 convolutional and 2 fully connected) are used. And to boost the performance of glaucoma diagnosis dropout and data augmentation strategies are used.
Abramoff et al. Year-2016	Detection of diabetic retinopathy	Used end-to-end convolutional neural network on public dataset.
Burlina et al. (2016)	Detection of degenerated macular due to age	For extraction of the features they overfeat the pretrained network
Van Grinsven et al. Year-2016	Detection of Hemorrhage	Dynamically trained CNN using perceptive data sampling to perform hard negative mining.
Gulshan et al. Year-2016	Detection of diabetic retinopathy	Used inception network for detection of DR. Performance of the model was verified by a group of ophthalmologists.
Prentasic & Loncaric Year-2016	Detection of hard exudate	Output of traditional classifier combined with end-to-end CNN for detection of exudates.
Worall et al.(2016)	Prematurity detection of retinopathy	Used GoogleNet followed by feature map visualization to highlight disease.
Other Method for Medical Imaging		
Gao et al. Year-2015	Classification of cataract in slit lamp image	A set of recursive neural networks are applied after using CNN techniques for extracting high order features.
Schlegl et al. Year-2015	Segmentation of fluid in OCT	Clinical reports are analyzed using CNN combined with semantic descriptors
Prentasic et al. Year-2015	Segmentation of retinal vessel in OCT angiography	Used simple convolutional neural network for segmentation of capillary networks.

REFERENCES

Abràmoff, M. D., Lou, Y., Erginay, A., Clarida, W., Amelon, R., Folk, J. C., & Niemeijer, M. (2016). Improved automated detection of diabetic retinopathy on a publicly available dataset through integration of deep learning. *Investigative Ophthalmology & Visual Science*, *57*(13), 5200–5206. doi:10.1167/iovs.16-19964 PMID:27701631

Ayala, G., León, T., & Zapater, V. (2005). Different averages of a fuzzy set with an application to vessel segmentation. *IEEE Transactions on Fuzzy Systems*, *13*(3), 384–393. doi:10.1109/TFUZZ.2004.839667

Burlina, P., Freund, D. E., Joshi, N., Wolfson, Y., & Bressler, N. M. (2016, April). Detection of age-related macular degeneration via deep learning. In *2016 IEEE 13th International Symposium on Biomedical Imaging (ISBI)* (pp. 184-188). IEEE. 10.1109/ISBI.2016.7493240

Cesar, R. M., Jr., & Jelinek, H. F. (2003). Segmentation of retinal fundus vasculature in nonmydriatic camera images using wavelets. In J. S. Suri & S. Laxminarayan (Eds.), Angiography and Plaque Imaging: Advanced Segmentation Techniques (pp. 193–224). Academic Press.

Chaudhuri, S., Chatterjee, S., Katz, N., Nelson, M., & Goldbaum, M. (1989). Detection of blood vessels in retinal images using two-dimensional matched filters. *IEEE Transactions on Medical Imaging*, *8*(3), 263–269. doi:10.1109/42.34715 PMID:18230524

Chen, X., Xu, Y., Wong, D. W. K., Wong, T. Y., & Liu, J. (2015, August). Glaucoma detection based on deep convolutional neural network. In *2015 37th annual international conference of the IEEE engineering in medicine and biology society (EMBC)* (pp. 715-718). IEEE. 10.1109/EMBC.2015.7318462

De la Calleja, J., Tecuapetla, L., Medina, M. A., Bárcenas, E., & Nájera, A. B. U. (2014, September). LBP and machine learning for diabetic retinopathy detection. In *International Conference on Intelligent Data Engineering and Automated Learning* (pp. 110-117). Springer. 10.1007/978-3-319-10840-7_14

Ege, B. M., Hejlesen, O. K., Larsen, O. V., Møller, K., Jennings, B., Kerr, D., & Cavan, D. A. (2000). Screening for diabetic retinopathy using computer based image analysis and statistical classification. *Computer Methods and Programs in Biomedicine*, *62*(3), 165–175. doi:10.1016/S0169-2607(00)00065-1 PMID:10837904

Espona, L., Carreira, M. J., Ortega, M., & Penedo, M. G. (2007, June). A snake for retinal vessel segmentation. In *Iberian Conference on Pattern Recognition and Image Analysis* (pp. 178-185). Springer. 10.1007/978-3-540-72849-8_23

Fu, H., Xu, Y., Lin, S., Wong, D. W. K., & Liu, J. (2016, October). Deepvessel: Retinal vessel segmentation via deep learning and conditional random field. In *International conference on medical image computing and computer-assisted intervention* (pp. 132-139). Springer. 10.1007/978-3-319-46723-8_16

Fu, H., Xu, Y., Wong, D. W. K., & Liu, J. (2016, April). Retinal vessel segmentation via deep learning network and fully-connected conditional random fields. In *2016 IEEE 13th international symposium on biomedical imaging (ISBI)* (pp. 698-701). IEEE. 10.1109/ISBI.2016.7493362

Gao, X., Lin, S., & Wong, T. Y. (2015). Automatic feature learning to grade nuclear cataracts based on deep learning. *IEEE Transactions on Biomedical Engineering*, *62*(11), 2693–2701. doi:10.1109/TBME.2015.2444389 PMID:26080373

Gulshan, V., Peng, L., Coram, M., Stumpe, M. C., Wu, D., Narayanaswamy, A., ... Kim, R. (2016). Development and validation of a deep learning algorithm for detection of diabetic retinopathy in retinal fundus photographs. *Journal of the American Medical Association*, *316*(22), 2402–2410. doi:10.1001/jama.2016.17216 PMID:27898976

Hoover, A. D., Kouznetsova, V., & Goldbaum, M. (2000). Locating blood vessels in retinal images by piecewise threshold probing of a matched filter response. *IEEE Transactions on Medical Imaging*, *19*(3), 203–210. doi:10.1109/42.845178 PMID:10875704

Jiang, X., & Mojon, D. (2003). Adaptive local thresholding by verification-based multithreshold probing with application to vessel detection in retinal images. *IEEE Transactions on Pattern Analysis and Machine Intelligence*, *25*(1), 131–137. doi:10.1109/TPAMI.2003.1159954

Karegowda, A. G., Nasiha, A., Jayaram, M. A., & Manjunath, A. S. (2011). Exudates detection in retinal images using back propagation neural network. *International Journal of Computers and Applications*, *25*(3), 25–31. doi:10.5120/3011-4062

Karthika, D., & Marimuthu, A. (2014, February). Retinal image analysis using contourlet transform and multistructure elements morphology by reconstruction. In *2014 World Congress on Computing and Communication Technologies* (pp. 54-59). IEEE. 10.1109/WCCCT.2014.15

Kass, M., Witkin, A., & Terzopoulos, D. (1988). Snakes: Active contour models. *International Journal of Computer Vision, 1*(4), 321–331. doi:10.1007/BF00133570

Kavitha, S., & Duraiswamy, K. (2011). Automatic detection of hard and soft exudates in fundus images using color histogram thresholding. *European Journal of Scientific Research, 48*(3), 493–504.

Li, Q., You, J., & Zhang, D. (2012). Vessel segmentation and width estimation in retinal images using multiscale production of matched filter responses. *Expert Systems with Applications, 39*(9), 7600–7610. doi:10.1016/j.eswa.2011.12.046

Li, Y. H., Yeh, N. N., Chen, S. J., & Chung, Y. C. (2019). Computer-assisted diagnosis for diabetic retinopathy based on fundus images using deep convolutional neural network. *Mobile Information Systems, 2019.*

Litjens, G., Kooi, T., Bejnordi, B. E., Setio, A. A. A., Ciompi, F., Ghafoorian, M., van der Laak, J. A. W. M., van Ginneken, B., & Sánchez, C. I. (2017). A survey on deep learning in medical image analysis. *Medical Image Analysis, 42*, 60–88. doi:10.1016/j.media.2017.07.005 PMID:28778026

Liu, I., & Sun, Y. (1993). Recursive tracking of vascular networks in angiograms based on the detection-deletion scheme. *IEEE Transactions on Medical Imaging, 12*(2), 334–341. doi:10.1109/42.232264 PMID:18218423

Mahapatra, D., Roy, P. K., Sedai, S., & Garnavi, R. (2016, October). Retinal image quality classification using saliency maps and CNNs. In *International Workshop on Machine Learning in Medical Imaging* (pp. 172-179). Springer. 10.1007/978-3-319-47157-0_21

Maninis, K. K., Pont-Tuset, J., Arbeláez, P., & Van Gool, L. (2016, October). Deep retinal image understanding. In *International conference on medical image computing and computer-assisted intervention* (pp. 140-148). Springer.

Marín, D., Aquino, A., Gegúndez-Arias, M. E., & Bravo, J. M. (2010). A new supervised method for blood vessel segmentation in retinal images by using gray-level and moment invariants-based features. *IEEE Transactions on Medical Imaging, 30*(1), 146–158. doi:10.1109/TMI.2010.2064333 PMID:20699207

Miri, M. S., & Mahloojifar, A. (2010). Retinal image analysis using curvelet transform and multistructure elements morphology by reconstruction. *IEEE Transactions on Biomedical Engineering, 58*(5), 1183–1192. doi:10.1109/TBME.2010.2097599 PMID:21147592

Prentašić, P., & Lončarić, S. (2016). Detection of exudates in fundus photographs using deep neural networks and anatomical landmark detection fusion. *Computer Methods and Programs in Biomedicine, 137*, 281–292. doi:10.1016/j.cmpb.2016.09.018 PMID:28110732

Prentašić, P., & Lončarić, S. (2016). Detection of exudates in fundus photographs using deep neural networks and anatomical landmark detection fusion. *Computer Methods and Programs in Biomedicine, 137*, 281–292. doi:10.1016/j.cmpb.2016.09.018 PMID:28110732

Schlegl, T., Waldstein, S. M., Vogl, W.-D., Schmidt-Erfurth, U., & Langs, G. (2015). Predicting semantic descriptions from medical images with convolutional neural networks. *Lecture Notes in Computer Science, 9123*, 437–448. 10.1007/978-3-319-19992-4_34

Shanmugam, V., & Banu, R. D. W. (2013, January). Retinal blood vessel segmentation using an extreme learning machine approach. In 2013 IEEE Point-of-Care Healthcare Technologies (PHT) (pp. 318-321). IEEE. doi:10.1109/PHT.2013.6461349

Silberman, N., Ahrlich, K., Fergus, R., & Subramanian, L. (2010, March). Case for automated detection of diabetic retinopathy. *2010 AAAI Spring Symposium Series.*

Szegedy, C., Liu, W., Jia, Y., Sermanet, P., Reed, S., Anguelov, D., . . . Rabinovich, A. (2014). *Going deeper with convolutions.* arxiv:1409.4842.

Tachibana, R., Näppi, J. J., Hironaka, T., Kim, S. H., & Yoshida, H. (2016). Deep learning for electronic cleansing in dual- energy ct colonography. *Proceedings of the SPIE Medical Imaging, 9785.*

Van Grinsven, M. J., van Ginneken, B., Hoyng, C. B., Theelen, T., & Sánchez, C. I. (2016). Fast convolutional neural network training using selective data sampling: Application to hemorrhage detection in color fundus images. *IEEE Transactions on Medical Imaging, 35*(5), 1273–1284. doi:10.1109/TMI.2016.2526689 PMID:26886969

Wang, S., Yin, Y., Cao, G., Wei, B., Zheng, Y., & Yang, G. (2015). Hierarchical retinal blood vessel segmentation based on feature and ensemble learning. *Neurocomputing, 149*, 708–717. doi:10.1016/j.neucom.2014.07.059

Worrall, D. E., Wilson, C. M., & Brostow, G. J. (2016). Automated retinopathy of prematurity case detection with convolutional neural networks. In *Deep Learning and Data Labeling for Medical Applications* (pp. 68–76). Springer. doi:10.1007/978-3-319-46976-8_8

Wu, A., Xu, Z., Gao, M., Buty, M., & Mollura, D. J. (2016, April). Deep vessel tracking: A generalized probabilistic approach via deep learning. In *2016 IEEE 13th International Symposium on Biomedical Imaging (ISBI)* (pp. 1363-1367). IEEE. 10.1109/ISBI.2016.7493520

Zana, F., & Klein, J. C. (2001). Segmentation of vessel-like patterns using mathematical morphology and curvature evaluation. *IEEE Transactions on Image Processing*, *10*(7), 1010–1019. doi:10.1109/83.931095 PMID:18249674

Zhang, L., Li, Q., You, J., & Zhang, D. (2009). A modified matched filter with double-sided thresholding for screening proliferative diabetic retinopathy. *IEEE Transactions on Information Technology in Biomedicine*, *13*(4), 528–534. doi:10.1109/TITB.2008.2007201 PMID:19389699

Zhang, L., Li, Q., You, J., & Zhang, D. (2009). A modified matched filter with double-sided thresholding for screening proliferative diabetic retinopathy. *IEEE Transactions on Information Technology in Biomedicine*, *13*(4), 528–534. doi:10.1109/TITB.2008.2007201 PMID:19389699

Zhang, Y., Hsu, W., & Lee, M. L. (2009). Detection of retinal blood vessels based on nonlinear projections. *Journal of Signal Processing Systems for Signal, Image, and Video Technology*, *55*(1-3), 103–112. doi:10.100711265-008-0179-5

Zhao, Y. Q., Wang, X. H., Wang, X. F., & Shih, F. Y. (2014). Retinal vessels segmentation based on level set and region growing. *Pattern Recognition*, *47*(7), 2437–2446. doi:10.1016/j.patcog.2014.01.006

Zilly, J., Buhmann, J. M., & Mahapatra, D. (2017). Glaucoma detection using entropy sampling and ensemble learning for automatic optic cup and disc segmentation. *Computerized Medical Imaging and Graphics*, *55*, 28–41. doi:10.1016/j.compmedimag.2016.07.012 PMID:27590198

Chapter 7
Deep Learning Applications in Medical Imaging:
Introduction to Deep Learning-Based Intelligent Systems for Medical Applications

Janani Viswanathan
Sri Ramakrishna Engineering College, India

N. Saranya
Sri Ramakrishna Engineering College, India

Abinaya Inbamani
Sri Ramakrishna Engineering College, India

ABSTRACT

Deep learning (DL) and artificial intelligence (AI) are emerging tools in the healthcare sector for medical diagnostics. This chapter elaborates on general reasons for the popularity of computational techniques such as deep learning and machine learning (ML) applications in the medical image processing domain. The initial part of this chapter focuses on reviewing the fundamental concepts of DL algorithms, competence with machine learning, need in healthcare, applications, and challenges in medical image processing. Doing so allows understanding the reasons for the construction of all of them and offers a different view on various domains in the medical sector. The tools and technology required for DL, selection, implementation, optimization, and testing are discussed with respect to an application of cancer detection. Thus, this chapter gives an overall vision of deep learning concepts related to biomedical research.

DOI: 10.4018/978-1-7998-5071-7.ch007

Copyright © 2021, IGI Global. Copying or distributing in print or electronic forms without written permission of IGI Global is prohibited.

INTRODUCTION

Deep learning (DL) and artificial intelligence (AI) is becoming an emerging tool in the healthcare sector for medical diagnostics. This chapter elaborates on general reasons for the popularity of computational techniques such as deep learning, Machine learning (ML) applications in the medical image processing domain. The emergence of exploratory and confirmatory DL based decision making is the need for the most developed and developing countries. This fertile field of research is now the area of interest for multidisciplinary people such as computer science, biomedical, biochemistry, bioinformatics etc... However, the practical applications of DL in clinical diagnosis techniques are relatively small, with many challenges added to it. The initial part of this chapter focuses on reviewing the fundamental concepts of the neural network's algorithms. The ML versus DL algorithm is elaborated in brief. The major players in healthcare industries with AI support are also been discussed. The performance and assessment of different architectures for deep neural networks are discussed using the open-source software. Doing so allows us to understand the reasons for the construction of intelligent architectures like multilayer, feedforward, recurrent algorithms. All of them serve a different purpose and offer a different view on various domains in the medical sector. The tools and technology required for DL, selection, Implementation, optimization, testing are discussed with respect to an application of cancer detection. Thus this chapter giver overall vision of deep learning concepts related to biomedical research.

In today's vision, observably medical image processing is one of the thirst areas which have been largely intervening domain progressing back again with DL. The impact of the DL algorithms and models in healthcare domain has narrowed down its way for data mining, analysis and has also attracted attention in the area of medical image analysis. At present, DL is been employed to involve the classification problems in medical image segmentation, recognition, and brain function studies. The images mainly include ultrasound, X-rays, computed tomography (CT), nuclear magnetic resonance (MRI), digital blood vessel silhouette (DSA), and positron emission tomography (PET). In the field of medical image analysis, the main research directions are image segmentation, image registration, and information fusion, time-series image analysis, and content-based image retrieval. Hence, it is important to select methods of significance and describe them in high detail which is served in this chapter.

Added on, how to effectively perform medical image analysis is a major problem in the field of disease diagnosis, and further diagnostic methods in pieces of literature are also discussed in this chapter. At this stage, DL could be viewed as a black box requiring knowledge of its internal workings, and hence presents some crucial technical challenges that need further methodological development techniques which are critically reviewed. By looking toward the contribution of DL in today's era, researchers are thinking that by the next 20 years, DL will serve for full automation for all kind of cyclic works. The deployment of DL models gives great benefits in healthcare.

Figure 1. Schematic representation of Network models and its applications

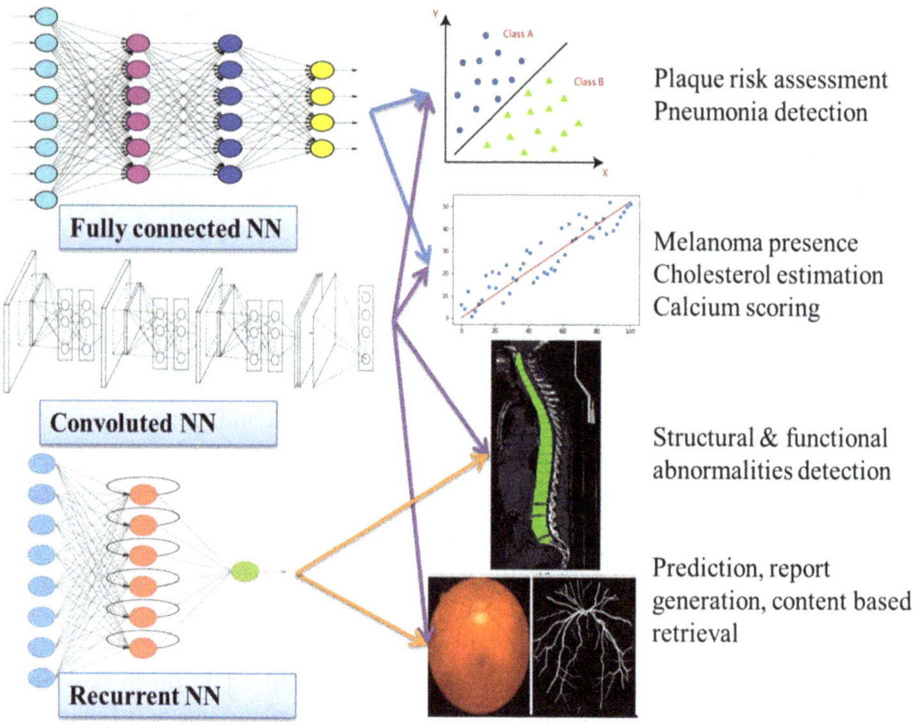

As an overall summary, first, the chapter has initially placed the basic requirements of the DL algorithm over machine learning architectures, followed by the understanding of all architectures along with its own significance. The chapter had also accelerated towards the implementation environments for validating the algorithm performance. In the final section, applications of biomedical imaging analysis using DL for various imaging modalities are presented as state-of-art for the readers. Therefore, several researchers are highly concentrating on DL, based on the efficient solution that mainly encourages using these techniques on biomedical imagining.

By evaluating ML or DL, with respect to effects on the real world, a human will soon be replaced in almost all medical-related applications. However, we are focusing on the solution but there also several challenges that reduce the growth of medical data which is the impression on the other coin. This crucial part is now addressed by any means. One of the greatest challenges are the unavailability of such a structured or unstructured dataset. Generally, Deep Learning methods provides positive feedback but if we are considering healthcare data for analysis it is also a challenging task for DL methods because healthcare data required higher sensitive values.

Nowadays, the healthcare system plays a vital role in a person's wellbeing. It helps to develop the community with good physical and mental health. It is all about maintenance or improvement of health via the prevention, diagnosis, treatment, recovery or cure of disease [Krivhezsky 2012]. A good health care system throughout the country boosts its economy across all the fields.

Need of Intelligent Systems

Artificial Intelligence (AI), Machine Learning (ML) and Deep Learning (DL) is used in all kind of industries which rule out mundane work and helps in intelligent decision making. Analyzing medical data such as summary reports, different scan reports, graph data, and disease diagnosis should be done in a faster way. World Economic Forum Annual Meeting 2020 report states that

- By 2030, AI will access multiple sources of data to reveal patterns in disease and aid treatment and care.
- Healthcare systems will be able to predict an individual's risk of certain diseases and suggest preventative measures.
- AI will help to reduce waiting times for patients and improve efficiency in hospitals and health systems.

In 2030, Health care systems are able to deliver truly proactive, predictive healthcare (De Bruijne, 2016). AI, ML, DL gain their attention in health care due to accurate analysis of clinical data. These techniques help to take preventive measures or corrective actions at the earliest. Clinical data includes data collected from patients during clinical trials or treatments. Data are collected in different forms (Summers, 2003). It includes

- Narrative- Recording by clinician
- Numeric Measurements- Values obtained as a result of measuring blood pressure, temperature, etc…
- Recorded Signals – ECG, EEG, EKG, etc…
- Coded data – Selection from controlled terminology environment

- Text data – Electronic Health Report (EHR or any information in text form
- Images – Scan reports from X-ray radiography, Magnetic Resonance Imaging (MRI), medical ultrasonography or ultrasound, Computed Tomography (CT), and nuclear medicine functional imaging techniques like Positron Emission Tomography (PET).

Medical imaging is a part of the health care system which involves creating images of different parts of the human body for disease identification and its treatment. Even though medical imaging is one of the complex forms of image representation it contains more information about the patients. In recent days, many kinds of research have revolutionized medical imaging and diagnostic.

Fundamentals of Artificial Intelligence

Artificial intelligence (AI) refers to the imitation of human intelligence in machines where it is programmed to think like humans and mimic their actions (Langley, 2011). With the huge clinical data availability, AI can able to outperform humans in disease diagnosis and spotting malignant tumors. AI in healthcare is used to emulate human cognition in the analysis of complicated medical records. AI is not a single technique it is a collection of many others like machine learning, deep learning, Natural Language Processing (NLP), Robotic Process Automation (RPA), etc...

Figure 2. Relationship between AI, ML and DL

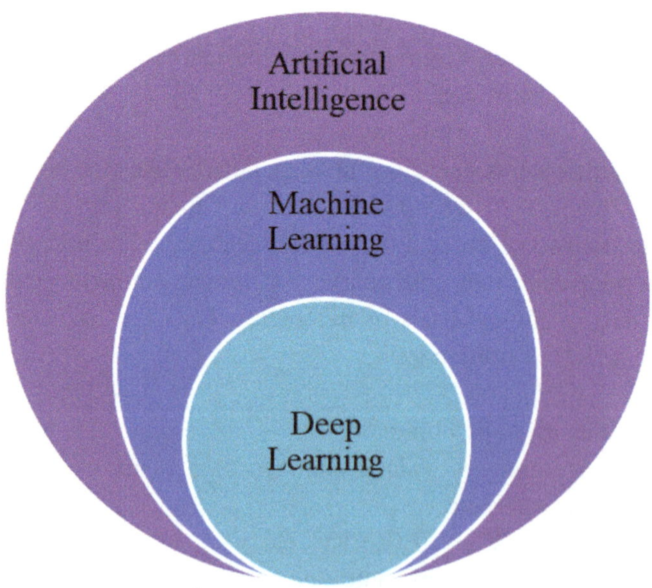

Types of AI

AI is divided into two broad categories based on its capability and functionality.

Based on Capabilities

Narrow AI

It is also called week AI. It is trained to outperform only for specific tasks. Build to work on a highly focused set of tasks like chess-playing algorithm, Alexa, Siri, etc.

Figure 3. Categories of AI

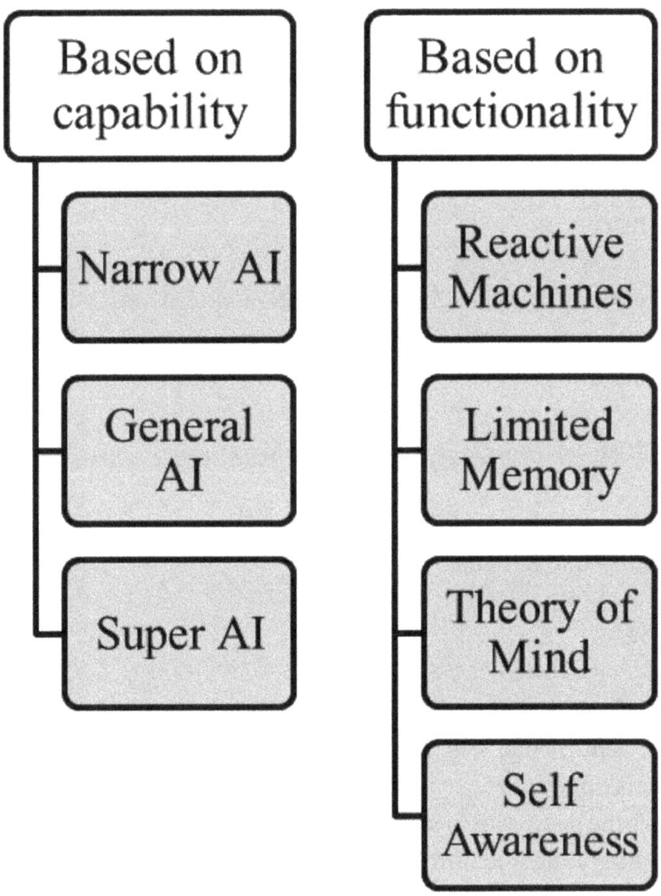

Broad AI

It is also called strong AI. It is trained to perform any intellectual task with efficiency like a human in a smarter way. A system with general AI is still under research.

Super AI

It aims to build an intelligent system which outperforms human intelligence. Some of the key characteristics include ability to think, reason, and solve the make judgment on its own. It is still a hypothetical concept in the field of AI.

Based on Functionality

Reactive AI

It is a reactive form of AI. These systems do not store past memories or experiences for future actions. IBM's Deep Mind, Google's Alpha Go are some of the examples of reactive AI.

Limited Memory

Unlike reactive AI systems, a limited AI system stores only a limited amount of memory for a short period for intelligent decision making. Self-driving cars are one of the examples.

Theory of Mind

It aims to build a system which can understand human emotions, beliefs and able to interact socially like humans.

Self-Awareness

It is the future of AI. Machines will be intelligent on their own and have their own consciousness, sentiments, and self-awareness. It does not exist in reality but a hypothetical concept.

Narrow AI is the most widely used form to do single tasks more precisely. AI used in medical imaging for the identification of diseases or anomalies from the scanned images. It helps in predicting Amyotrophic Lateral Sclerosis (ALS), Alzheimer's, cardiovascular disease, tumour diagnosis, etc…

Fundaments of Deep Learning and Machine Learning:

Machine Learning had become important in day to day life, making an individual's life easier by developing decision-making intelligent systems, recommendation systems, searching (ALEXA),etc. Basically these use training examples to explore hidden patterns, construct models, and then make predictions on the new database (testing phase). There are several MLAs used for classification. These simple architecture of ANN consists of an input layer, an output layer, and hidden layers with processing units. These processing units take input as training examples and learn features that are used to predict different classes with appropriate choosing of activation functions and parameters called weight. The network thus results in a descent response to noisy or incomplete input because of its distributed associative memory Conventional machine-learning techniques were limited in their ability to process natural data in their raw form.

If we construct ML systems, then we require domain expertise and careful engineering to develop feature extractors, which convert raw data in to feature vectors that we can use as input to the neural network whereas perceptron and other NN requires features as input whereas DNNs extract features automatically with multiple hidden layers. DL is a subfield of ML. In DL feature selection is done by multiple hidden layers using different techniques (Lundervold, 2019). Thus the discovery of DL originated within ANNs and multilayer perceptron's itself. History and evolution and the simple description on those are tabulated in table 1.

The Requirement of Deep Learning over Machine Learning

As medical image processing is concerned, there are lots of advantages with DL instead of ML. DL have automated feature selection capability and good performance while we are dealing with large data; these features are really useful while we are dealing with medical image data. Deep Learning is an extended version of ANN where it contains more hidden layers and complex operations involved in it. Some applications of DL in medical imaging are image segmentation, annotation, content-based image retrieval, classification, detection, etc… The fact of selecting deep learning algorithms over machine learning and performance parameters (Pandya, 2019) are discussed in table 3.

Deep Learning Models

DL is also called representation learning. For example, in image recognition, it can be interpreted that feature learning is done in the order of pixel, edge, texton, motif, part, and object. Similarly, in-text recognition, features are learned in the

Table 1. History and evolution of AI related concepts

S. No.	Year of Contribution	Scientists Behind the Model	Concepts
1	1943	Walter Pitts and Warren McCulloch	Threshold logic was created which mimics the thought process
2	1950	Alan Turing	The machine learning prediction was done
3	1952	Arthur Samuel	The program of ML was created
4	1957	Frank Rosenblatt	The deep learning neural networks foundation was set
5	1959	David H. Hubel and Torsten Wiesel	The simple and complex cells were created
6	1960	Henry J. Kelley	The back propogation model was created
7	1965	Alexey Ivakhnenko and V.G. Lapa	The working deep learning networks were created
8	1962	Stuart Dreyfus.	The chain rule applicable for deep learning was created.
9	1965	Alexey Grigoryevich Ivakhnenko	*Data handling methods were identified*
10	1979	Kunihiko Fukushima	Neocognitron, a design for hierarchical models
11	1982	John Hopfield	Hopfield models came into picture
12	1985	Terry Sejnowski	English words pronouncing models were discovered
13	1986	Rina Dechter	The DL model was introduced to ML models
14	1989	Yann LeCun	Back propogation and CNN worked together
15	1995	Dana Cortes and Vladimir Vapnik	support vector machines concepts identified and used
16	2001	Gartner)	Big Data concept came into the market vigorously
17	2009	Fei-Fei Li	ImageNEt, 14 million labeled images were used
18	2011	Alex Krizhevsky	Alexnet(Rectified linear units)
19	2012	Google Brain	Cat experiment

order of character, word, word group, clause, sentence, and story. There are three categories of DL architecture, namely DNN, Convolution Neural Network (CNN), and Recurrent Neural Network (RNN). The comparison of all these Deep learning algorithms is shown in table 2.

Now, if we look into deep learning, basically we have five types of learning algorithms. Now the first type is called a fully connected network family and this is similar to a multilayer perceptron in ANN. In this model, each neuron on any

Table 2. The significance of DL versus ML algorithms.

S.No	Parameters	Significance
1.	Data dependencies	In Deep Learning its performance increases as the scale of data increases than in traditional Machine Learning.
2.	Hardware operability	Deep Learning algorithms requires high-end machines, whereas Machine Learning algorithms can work on low-end machines
3.	Feature Identification	In ML, significant features are hand-coded but in DL the learning algorithms try to learn high-level features from data.
4.	Time	A DL algorithm requires more execution time than ML because of it computational complexity. For example the ResNet takes about 2 weeks to train completely from scratch whereas ML comparatively takes much less time like hours.
5.	Problem Solving	To sort out a task, Machine Learning algorithm splits its parameters into different components and solve them individually, and combine them to get the result. In contrast, Deep Learning solves the problem end-to- end.
6.	Interpretability	As DL are automated feature pulling kind of algorithm it is hard to optimise and trace features but in ML it is easy to interpret.

layer is connected to every single neuron on the subsequent layer of the hierarchy (Mohanasundaram, 2019). So this architecture is an autoencoder which learns to basically to encode and decode. To precise, the input image given to the model can be reconstructed in the output end. An example is labeling and indexing of anatomical locations in Computed Tomography, Magnetic Resonance images. There are other sister terms for autoencoders, they are Stacked autoencoder, sparse encoders. In stacked encoders, it basically you stack down one by one auto encoders together and this creates a much deeper network. The applications like skin tumor detection etc. work on this algorithm. The next one is a Sparse autoencoder, this works by using sparsity constraints and extracting the feature. For example, In Optical Coherence Tomography images pixel labelling with anatomical and physiological significance can be solved. Added on other classes of called Denoising autoencoders are available, which uses denoisers actually to remove noise from a certain kind of an image. Most of the ultrasound images use these models. It can be scaled up with Gaussian un-speckle noise, Poisson and Multiplicative noise which are usually present in ultrasound images due to transducer and instrumentation limitations.

The next class is the Boltzmann Machines and belief network. As the name suggests a Boltzmann, it has Boltzmann distribution imposed over layers of network and can have a very good amount of memory associativity within these networks (Mohanasundaram, 2019). Deep Belief Network is basically sort of a stack version of the Restricted Boltzmann Machine. It is one kind of generative model. It mainly joins the distribution of probability.

Table 3. Comparison of DL Models

S. No.	Features Compared	Classic Neural Networks (Multilayer Perceptrons)	Convolutional Neural Networks	Recurrent neural Networks	Self-Organizing Maps	Boltzmann Machines	Autoencoders
1	YEAR OF INVENTION	1958	1994	1986	1982	1985	1980
2	LEARNING	Supervised Models	Supervised Models	Supervised Models	Unsupervised Models	Unsupervised Models	Unsupervised Models
3	ARCHITECTURE	classic neural network model consisting of more than 2 layers.	Shared weights	Connection form a directed graph.	Competitive learning	Knowledge representation, learning and solving counting problems	Learn the data codings.
4	WORKING DIRECTION	Input → Hidden Layer → Output.	Input → Hidden Layer → Output.	Input → Hidden Layer → Output.	Input → Hidden Layer → Output.	All nodes are connected to each other in a circular kind of hyperspace like in the image.	Input → Hidden Layer → Output.
5	SCIENTIST BEHIND THE MODEL	American psychologist Frank Rosenblatt.	Yann LeCun	David Rumelhart's	Kohonen 1982, Kohonen 2001	Terry Sejnowski	Hinton
6	APPLICATIONS	Tabular dataset is required and is formatted in rows along with the columns	Image Datasets are the applications, medical imaging, natural language processing	It helps in Predicting sequences.	Applied for dimensionality reduction	Monitoring a system	Dimensionality reduction and Feature detection
7	APPLICATIONS	Grouping and Regression issues where a lot of genuine values is given as the info.	Information is a 2 dimensional field yet can be changed over to 1 dimensional inside for quicker handling.	Sentiment analysis	When data provided does not contain an output or a Y column.	Recommendation system for binary values can be built.	Recommendation system(Powerful)
8	FLEXIBILITY	high	Models complex	Flexible with activation functions	Understand the framework	When working with a very specific set of data	Features in massive datasets are to be encoded.

DBNs have "learning features" that means the network can learn layer-by-layer with higher-level features that are discovered and passes through the past layer, thus more complex features that are acknowledged to get better-reflected knowledge inside the input structures.

The next is Convolutional Neural Networks. In Convolutional Neural Networks you can have generalized Conv-Nets or very specific models like as LeNet, GoogLeNet and AlexNet. So LeNet is from the) challenge with Yann LeCun was solving in 1998, and so they have a much-improvised version on top of that from Google and that is called as a GoogLeNet and the ImageNet Challenge being solved by Alex Krizhevsky, what is called as the AlexNet (Mohanasundaram, 2019). Then there are U-Nets and Res-Nets, which are basically networks where the input image is loaded and automatic segmentation of the whole image is done instead of doing it as a pixel by pixel. Example Whole to detect Intervertebral discs from whole spine images.

The other is Recurrent Neural Networks and one very famous component of that is Long short-term memory, which can try to encode temporal patterns itself within a network.All the Dl models are represented in the figure 4.An example is Cancer diagnosis and comparison to study the progression of cancer every 3 months, so that a mapping of temporal data and voxel at the same space for the patient scans can give relative clinical significance by LSTM networks.

Figure 4. Neural architectures (a) Auto-encoder, (b) restricted Boltzmann machine, (c) recurrent neural network, (d) convolutional neural network, (e) multi-stream convolutional neural network, (f) U-net (with a single downsampling stage). (Litiens, 2017)

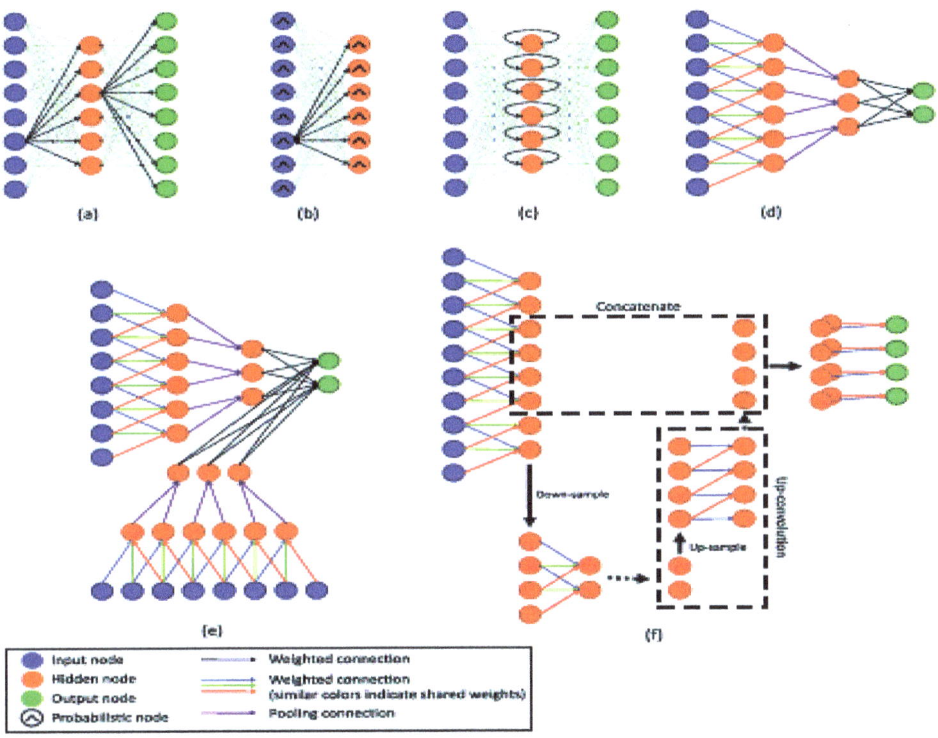

Healthcare Industries Using AI, ML and DL

The Major IT industries are investing in the health care sector to provide the best diagnostic and predictive solutions. (Medical Futurist (n.d.)

- Google- Google Deep mind and G Suite designed to maintain and transfer patient health record an insecure way.
- IBM- Watson Health was set up to translate data and knowledge into more insights to make a decision by combining human intelligence.
- CloudMedX- It utilizes NLP and DL to obtain data from electronic medical records and outputs clinical insights for health care professionals so as to improve patient outcomes.
- GE Healthcare – It is one of the leading industry in production of imaging devices. It uses AI to improve the speed of analyzing scan reports with better accuracy.
- Siemens – It uses AI for CT scan to measure and identifies orangs and lesions in thorax automatically. It generates a quantitative report to assist the radiologist in diagnosing.
- Babylon Health – It provides a remote consultation service. The free smartphone app's dynamic A.I. will begin to ask users about their complaints and subsequently match them to a relevant physician, 24/7, via video or voice call for further medical assistance.
- Corti- It is an A.I.-powered "co-pilot" for emergency medicine staffers. By listening in on patient interviews, analyzing the caller's voice and background noises, and taking insights from historical data and artificial neural networks, it can understand the context and patterns in critical conversations.
- Butterfly Network- It aims to create a new handheld medical imaging device and to automate its process through AI.
- Enlitic- uses the power of deep learning technologies, for image recognition to harvest the data stemming from radiology images.
- Oncora Medical- It simplifies the workflow, reduce documentation burden and optimize treatment with intelligent patient care software.
- Caption Health – It tends to empower healthcare providers with new capabilities to acquire and interpret ultrasound exams using AI.
- Atomwise – It discovers drug-using AI. It uses the most advanced technology for small molecule binding affinity prediction.

Applicability of DL in Medical Image Processing

The applications and trend research in AI domain changes with time to time. There were applications like diabetic retinopathy, glaucoma detections, cancer detection as a common problem statement where many, minds were working. As technology elevates, with different tools and platforms recognizing anomalies and quantifying dimensions are becoming usual applications in image analysis. Now people are shifted to other paradigms like cell motility, assay pairing, molecular diagnostic application, etc. The DL technique is systematically a useful technique that provides state-of-the-art accuracy (Litiens, 2017). DL has stepped into another dimension called medical image scrutiny. DL applications in medical domains cover a large range of complications, going from cancer detection and disease monitoring to custom-made behavior suggestions. Nowadays, numerous sources of data from medical digital imaging (X-ray, CT, and MRI scans) and genomic sequences have brought a huge quantity of clinical parameters to the physician. But the challenges associated with DL in the fields of Medical imagining remain higher. The most common among those are:

1. Resource identification and collection: The collection of data sets for medical image processing is really an ice edge task which even makes many problems statements nonfeasible. This is due to the unavailability of datasets in consideration with patient security etc. Even then De-identified patient reports are only maintained in a few hospitals. Electronic health records are rarely available in most of the developing countries.
2. Selection of models and algorithms: When DL algorithm is selected, there are lots of hyperparameters that we have to take under consideration like learning rates, the number of hidden layers, initial weight values, bias values, learning iterations, etc. because this decides the performance of the system. Even then, the same model, same algorithm the performance may vary with objective and datasets.
3. Multimodality DL: In biomedical domain, with improvement in the diagnostic and therapeutic domain, we can combine results of one or more clinical studies and train in hybrid DL models to get better results. The challenge is that the clinical relevance among the study results of two data for the same patient. This needs detailed descriptive knowledge from medical practitioners to design an intelligent system.
4. Time: In medical image applications, the size of the database becomes larger and larger. To analyze this kind of data using DL architectures require a large amount of time. To get faster result and speed up the performance, the need for GPU arises.

EXAMPLE

Brain Tumor Image Classification Using Python

In this example image classification is done to classify images of with and without brain tumors using python in the Windows operating system. Python has been installed through the anaconda package. Execution of the code is done through jupyter notebook Interface.Try running the code in google colabs.

Steps involved in Image Classification using python and keras framework as follows

- Import basic libraries used for image classification like keras, numpy, cv2
- Split the dataset as training and testing in to a separate folder & sub folder.
- Apply one hot encoding technique to represent each class of images in array format
- Represent the input images and its corresponding class label as numpy array
- Construct CNN model with convolution, pooling and fully connected layer
- Train the model
- Analyse the accuracy and redesign the network if required
- Test the model with sample image

Step 1: Import required libraries

Keras framework is used to build the model. Numpy to represent the data in the form of numpy array. Matplotlib to visualize the data in the form of graph. Timeit to calculate the total time taken to run the model.

```
from keras.models import Model
from keras.models import Sequential
from keras.layers import Input, Dense, Dropout
from keras.layers import Reshape, Flatten
from keras.layers import Conv2D, MaxPooling2D
import numpy as np
from PIL import Image
import os
from matplotlib import pyplot as plt
%matplotlib inline
import cv2
import timeit
```

Step 2: Split the dataset as training and testing in to a separate folder & sub folder.

Step 3: Apply one hot encoding technique to represent each class of images in array format

For Training Data:

```
def training_image_data():
    train_images=[]
    PATH = 'E:\\AC 2019-2020\\Brain-Tumor-Detection\\Training'
    # for each folder (holding images of with and without
cancer)
    for directory in os.listdir(PATH):
        # for each image in the folder
        DATA_PATH=PATH + '\\' + directory
        for image in os.listdir(DATA_PATH):
            img = cv2.imread(os.path.join(DATA_PATH,image))  #
convert to array
            img=cv2.cvtColor(img,cv2.COLOR_BGR2RGB)
            dim=(64,64)
            new_array=cv2.resize(img, dim, interpolation = cv2.
INTER_AREA)
            new_array=np.array(new_array)
            if directory=="no":
                ohl=np.array([1,0])
            elif directory=="yes":
                ohl=np.array([0,1])
            train_images.append([new_array,ohl])
    print(len(train_images))
    return(train_images)
```

For Testing Data:

```
def testing_image_data():
    test_images=[]
    PATH = 'E:\\AC 2019-2020\\Brain-Tumor-Detection\\Testing'
    # for each folder (holding images of with and without
cancer)
    for directory in os.listdir(PATH):
        # for each image in the folder
        DATA_PATH=PATH + '\\' + directory
        for image in os.listdir(DATA_PATH):
            img = cv2.imread(os.path.join(DATA_PATH,image))  #
convert to array
            img = cv2.cvtColor(img,cv2.COLOR_BGR2RGB)
            dim=(64,64)
            new_array=cv2.resize(img, dim, interpolation = cv2.
```

```
INTER_AREA)
            new_array=np.array(new_array)
            #print(len(new_array))
            if directory=="no":
                ohl=np.array([1,0])
            elif directory=="yes":
                ohl=np.array([0,1])
            test_images.append([new_array,ohl])
    print(len(test_images))
    return(test_images)
```

Step 4: Represent the input images and its corresponding class label as numpy array

```
training_images = training_image_data()
testing_images = testing_image_data()
#Reshape the image to size 64X64 of 3 color channels
tr_img_data = np.array([i[0] for i in training_images]).
reshape(-1,64,64,3)
tr_lbl_data = np.array([i[1] for i in training_images])
tst_img_data = np.array([i[0] for i in testing_images]).
reshape(-1,64,64,3)
tst_lbl_data = np.array([i[1] for i in testing_images])
Output display the number of training and testing images used
218
77
```

Step 5: Construct CNN model with convolution, pooling and fully connected layer

```
import timeit
np.random.seed(12)
model = Sequential()
model.add(Conv2D(32, kernel_size=(5,5),
activation='relu',strides=2, input_shape=[64,64,3]))
model.add(Conv2D(16, (5, 5),strides=2, activation='relu'))
model.add(MaxPooling2D(strides=(2, 2)))
model.add(Flatten())
```

```
model.add(Dense(32, activation='relu'))
model.add(Dropout(0.25))
model.add(Dense(2, activation='softmax'))
model.summary()
```

Step 6: Train the model

Box 1. Output: Display the model summary

Layer (Type)	Output Shape	Param #
conv2d_11 (Conv2D)	(None, 30, 30, 32)	2432
conv2d_12 (Conv2D)	(None, 13, 13, 16)	12816
max_pooling2d_6	MaxPooling2 (None, 6, 6, 16)	0
flatten_6 (Flatten)	(None, 576)	0
dense_11 (Dense)	(None, 32)	18464
dropout_6 (Dropout)	(None, 32)	0
dense_12 (Dense)	(None, 2)	66
Total params: 33,778 Trainable params: 33,778 Non-trainable params: 0		

```
start = timeit.default_timer()
model.compile(loss=keras.losses.categorical_crossentropy,
              optimizer=keras.optimizers.Adadelta(),
              metrics=['accuracy'])
history=model.fit(tr_img_data, tr_lbl_data, batch_size=128,
epochs=50,verbose=1,
          validation_data=(tst_img_data, tst_lbl_data))
end = timeit.default_timer()
print("Time Taken to run the model:",end - start, "seconds")
Train on 218 samples, validate on 77 samples
Epoch 1/50
218/218 [==============================] - 3s 12ms/step - loss:
0.8776 - acc: 0.8073 - val_loss: 1.0861 - val_acc: 0.7532
Epoch 2/50
218/218 [==============================] - 1s 2ms/step - loss:
1.1480 - acc: 0.6789 - val_loss: 0.5088 - val_acc: 0.9091
```

```
Epoch 3/50
218/218 [==============================] - 0s 2ms/step - loss:
0.7252 - acc: 0.7661 - val_loss: 0.3180 - val_acc: 0.8831
Epoch 4/50
218/218 [==============================] - 0s 2ms/step - loss:
0.4527 - acc: 0.8165 - val_loss: 0.3949 - val_acc: 0.7792
Epoch 5/50
218/218 [==============================] - 0s 2ms/step - loss:
0.4635 - acc: 0.8165 - val_loss: 0.3514 - val_acc: 0.8052
Epoch 6/50
218/218 [==============================] - 1s 2ms/step - loss:
0.3399 - acc: 0.8394 - val_loss: 0.3990 - val_acc: 0.7792
Epoch 7/50
218/218 [==============================] - 0s 2ms/step - loss:
0.3227 - acc: 0.8440 - val_loss: 0.3366 - val_acc: 0.8571
.
.
.
.
Epoch 46/50
218/218 [==============================] - 0s 2ms/step - loss:
0.0474 - acc: 0.9817 - val_loss: 0.2785 - val_acc: 0.8701
Epoch 47/50
218/218 [==============================] - 0s 2ms/step - loss:
0.0305 - acc: 1.0000 - val_loss: 0.2748 - val_acc: 0.9091
Epoch 48/50
218/218 [==============================] - 1s 3ms/step - loss:
0.0147 - acc: 1.0000 - val_loss: 0.3271 - val_acc: 0.9091
Epoch 49/50
218/218 [==============================] - 1s 3ms/step - loss:
0.0142 - acc: 1.0000 - val_loss: 0.3637 - val_acc: 0.9091
Epoch 50/50
218/218 [==============================] - 0s 2ms/step - loss:
0.0153 - acc: 1.0000 - val_loss: 0.3657 - val_acc: 0.9091
Time Taken to run the model: 28.631909300000075 seconds
```

Step 7: Analyze the accuracy and redesign the network if required

Training Accuracy:

```
score = model.evaluate(tr_img_data, tr_lbl_data, verbose=1)
print('Training loss:', score[0])
print('Training accuracy:', score[1])
Output:
218/218 [==============================] - 0s 454us/step
Training loss: 0.44881731381110096
Training accuracy: 0.8761467895376573
```

Testing Accuracy:

```
score = model.evaluate(tst_img_data, tst_lbl_data, verbose=1)
print('Validation loss:', score[0])
print('Validation accuracy:', score[1])
Output:
77/77 [==============================] - 0s 875us/step
Validation loss: 0.2672835219796602
Validation accuracy: 0.922077922077922
```

Step 8: Test the accuracy with sample image data

Figure 5.

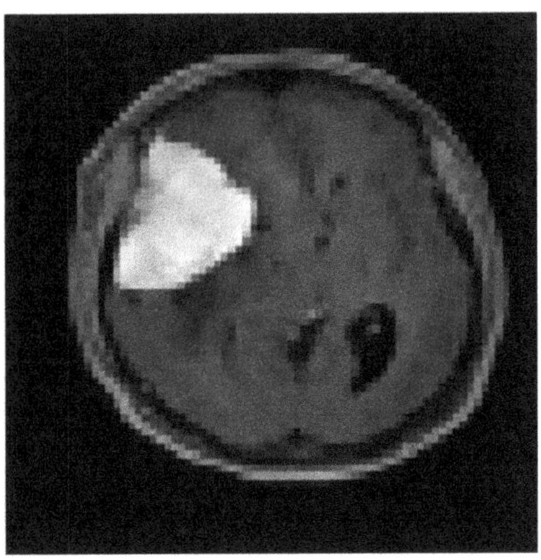

```
import pylab as plt
plt.imshow(tst_img_data[55].reshape(64,64,3))
plt.show()


import numpy as np
prediction = model.predict(tst_img_data[70:71])
print('Prediction Score:\n',prediction[0])
thresholded = (prediction>0.5)*1
print('\nThresholded Score:\n',np.array(thresholded[0]))
print('\nPrediction result is:\n')
if (list((thresholded))==[1,0]):
    print("no")
else:
    print("yes")
output:
Prediction Score:
 [5.2905566e-06 9.9999475e-01]
Thresholded Score:
 [0 1]
Prediction result is:
YES
```

REFERENCES

De Bruijne, M. (2016). *Machine learning approaches in medical image analysis: From detection to diagnosis*. Academic Press.

Goldbaum, M., Moezzi, S., Taylor, A., Chatterjee, S., Boyd, J., Hunter, E., & Jain, R. (1996, September). Automated diagnosis and image understanding with object extraction, object classification, and inferencing in retinal images. In *Proceedings of 3rd IEEE international conference on image processing* (Vol. 3, pp. 695-698). IEEE. 10.1109/ICIP.1996.560760

Krizhevsky, A., Sutskever, I., & Hinton, G. E. (2012). Imagenet classification with deep convolutional neural networks. In Advances in neural information processing systems (pp. 1097-1105). Academic Press.

Langley, P. (2011). The changing science of machine learning. *Machine Learning*, *82*(3), 275–279. doi:10.100710994-011-5242-y

Litjens, G., Kooi, T., Bejnordi, B. E., Setio, A. A. A., Ciompi, F., Ghafoorian, M., van der Laak, J. A. W. M., van Ginneken, B., & Sánchez, C. I. (2017). A survey on deep learning in medical image analysis. *Medical Image Analysis*, *42*, 60–88. doi:10.1016/j.media.2017.07.005 PMID:28778026

Lundervold, A. S., & Lundervold, A. (2019). An overview of deep learning in medical imaging focusing on MRI. *Zeitschrift fur Medizinische Physik*, *29*(2), 102–127. doi:10.1016/j.zemedi.2018.11.002 PMID:30553609

Medical Futurist. (n.d.). *Top artificial intelligence companies in healthcare*. Retrieved from https://medicalfuturist.com/top-artificial-intelligence-companies-in-healthcare/

Mohanasundaram, R., Malhotra, A. S., Arun, R., & Periasamy, P. S. (2019). Deep Learning and Semi-Supervised and Transfer Learning Algorithms for Medical Imaging. In *Deep Learning and Parallel Computing Environment for Bioengineering Systems* (pp. 139–151). Academic Press. doi:10.1016/B978-0-12-816718-2.00015-4

Pandya, M. D., Shah, P. D., & Jardosh, S. (2019). Medical image diagnosis for disease detection: A deep learning approach. In *U-Healthcare Monitoring Systems* (pp. 37–60). Academic Press. doi:10.1016/B978-0-12-815370-3.00003-7

Summers, R. M. (2003). Road maps for advancement of radiologic computer-aided detection in the 21st century. *Radiology*, *229*(1), 11–13. doi:10.1148/radiol.2291030010 PMID:14519863

Chapter 8
Deep Learning Applications in Medical Imaging:
Artificial Intelligence, Machine Learning, and Deep Learning

S. Sasikala
Velammal College of Engineering and Technology, India

S. J. Subhashini
Velammal College of Engineering and Technology, India

P. Alli
Velammal College of Engineering and Technology, India

J. Jane Rubel Angelina
Thiagarajar College of Engineering, India

ABSTRACT

Machine learning is a technique of parsing data, learning from that data, and then applying what has been learned to make informed decisions. Deep learning is actually a subset of machine learning. It technically is machine learning and functions in the same way, but it has different capabilities. The main difference between deep and machine learning is, machine learning models become well progressively, but the model still needs some guidance. If a machine learning model returns an inaccurate prediction, then the programmer needs to fix that problem explicitly, but in the case of deep learning, the model does it by itself. Automatic car driving system is a good example of deep learning. On other hand, Artificial Intelligence is a different thing from machine learning and deep learning. Deep learning and machine learning both are the subsets of AI.

DOI: 10.4018/978-1-7998-5071-7.ch008

Copyright © 2021, IGI Global. Copying or distributing in print or electronic forms without written permission of IGI Global is prohibited.

INTRODUCTION

Artificial Intelligence (AI) has gained significant attention in recent years, particularly in the context of improving health and well-being. Artificial Intelligence can help transform healthcare by improving diagnosis, treatment, and the delivery of patient care. Machine Learning (ML) is a subset of AI, and Deep Learning(DL) is a further subset of Machine Learning. Deep Learning is the process by which algorithms can learn to identify hierarchies within data that allow for truly complex understandings of data. Machine Learning for health care is a rapidly growing interdisciplinary field gaining interest in academia and practice. The purpose of this chapter was to perform quantitative and qualitative evaluations of the state of Artificial Intelligence, Machine Learning and Deep Learning for health research. As the field evolves, analyses can elucidate research trends, behaviors, and future opportunities.

A broad scientific discipline with its roots in philosophy, mathematics and computer science that aims to understand and develop systems that display properties of intelligence. A sub discipline of AI, where computers programs (algorithms) learn associations of predictive power from examples in data. Machine Learning is most simply the application of statistical models to data using computers. Machine Learning uses a broader set of statistical techniques than those typically used in medicine. Newer techniques such as Deep Learning are based on models with less assumption about the underlying data and are therefore able to handle more complex data. Trends in Machine Learning for health research indicate the importance of well-annotated, easily accessed data and the benefit from greater clinician involvement in the development of translational applications.

Deep Learning methods allow a machine to be fed with large quantities of raw data and to discover the representations necessary for detection or classification. Deep Learning methods rely on multiple layers of representation of the data with successive transformations that amplify aspects of the input that are important for discrimination and suppress irrelevant variations. Deep Learning may be supervised or unsupervised. Deep Learning methods have been responsible for many of the recent foundational advances in Machine Learning.

ARTIFICIAL INTELLIGENCE

Artificial Intelligence consists of two words Artificial and Intelligence, where Artificial defines "man-made" and Intelligence defines "thinking power," therefore AI means "man-made thinking power." Artificial Intelligence exists when a machine can have human-based skills such as learning, reasoning, and problem-solving. Holding an Artificial Intelligence is known to be a computer with the ability to perform cognitive functions such as perceiving, understanding, thinking and solving problems. With the aid of AI, software or devices that can solve real-world problems quite easily and accurately such as health issues, marketing, traffic problems etc. can be build. AI paves the way for other new technologies, for new devices.

Goals of Artificial Intelligence

The following goals are influenced by Artificial Intelligence in various fields. They include

1. Replicate human intelligence
2. Solve Knowledge-intensive tasks
3. An intelligent connection of perception and action
4. Building a machine which can perform tasks that requires human intelligence such as:
    a. Proving a theorem
    b. Playing chess
    c. Plan some surgical operation
    d. Driving a car in traffic
5. Creating some system which can exhibit intelligent behavior, learn new things by itself, demonstrate, explain, and can advise to its user.

Types of Artificial Intelligence

AI is divided into three categories based on the capabilities of Narrow AI, General AI and Strong AI.

1. **Narrow AI:** An Artificial Intelligence is said to be narrow when the computer performs a specific to ask better than a human. This focuses on a particular category of cognitive abilities and developments in that spectrum. It can be used to handle spam emails, music streaming apps, and even autonomous vehicles. Any program that uses technology such as Machine Learning, data mining, pattern recognition and natural language processing to make autonomous decisions can be known as narrow AIs.
2. **General AI:** An Artificial Intelligence enters the general state when it is able to perform any intellectual activity with the same level of precision as a human being does. Control of robots at least as dexterous and mobile as an individual would result in a new breed of machines capable of performing any human task. With the passing of time these intelligences would be able to take over every

human role. Initially, humans could be cheaper than computers, or humans working alongside AI could be more successful on their own than AI.

3. **Strong AI:** An AI is strong when it can beat humans in many tasks. Strong AI involves a system with comprehensive knowledge and cognitive capabilities so that its performance is indistinguishable from that of a human, although its data processing speed and ability is much greater.It's another perception of AI in which it equates AI to humans. It stipulates that a computer can be programmed to actually be a human mind, to be intelligent in every sense of the word, to have perceptions, beliefs and other cognitive states that are normally only ascribed to humans.

AGENTS

The AI system is made up of an agent and its environment. The agents act within their surroundings. Certain agents could be in the area. An agent is anything that can be seen as perceiving its environment through sensors, and acting through actuators on that environment. The agent may perceive their own actions.

Types of Agents

Agents can be grouped into five classes based on their degree of perceived intelligence and capability.

Simple Reflex Agents

Simple reflection agents ignore the rest of the history of perception and act only on the basis of the current perception. Percept history is the history of everything that has been perceived by an agent to date. The function of the agent is based upon the rule of condition-action. A condition-action rule is a rule mapping a condition to an action, i.e. If the condition is true then the action will be taken, otherwise not. This agent function only succeeds when it is fully observable in the environment. Infinite loops are often unavoidable for simple reflex agents which operate in partially observable environments. Escape from infinite loops may be possible if the agent can randomize his actions.

Model Based Agents

Model-based reflex agents finding a rule whose condition fits the current situation works. By using model about the world, a model-based agent can handle partially observable environments. The agent must keep track of the internal state that is changed by each percept and depends on the experience of perception. The current state is stored inside the agent which has some sort of structure that describes the part of the world that can not be seen.

Goal based Agents

Goal-based agents take decisions oriented on how far from their goal they are currently. Their every move is meant to ease their distance from the target. This allows the agent to choose between multiple possibilities, selecting the one that will reach a goal state. The knowledge which supports its decisions is explicitly represented and can be modified, making these agents more flexible. Typically they need to check and plan. The actions of the target dependent agent can be easily changed.

Utility-based Agents

The agents that are developed are called utility-based agents having their end uses as building blocks. When there are multiple possible alternatives, then use utility-based agents to decide which one is best for each state. They select actions based on a preference for each state. Achieving the desired goal sometimes isn't enough task.

Learning Agents

Learning agent in AI is the type of agent that can learn from past experiences or have learning capabilities. It starts acting with basic knowledge and then automatically acting and adapting through learning.

BROAD AREAS OF AI

The broad areas of AI includes the following,

1. Knowledge representation
2. Reasoning (logical, probabilistic)
3. Decision making (search, planning, decision theory)

Knowledge Representation

Knowledge Representation (KR) is the study of how world knowledge and facts can be interpreted, and what kinds of logic that knowledge can be used to construct.

Knowledge Representation must consider representational adequacy, quality of representation, computational cost of related inferences, default representation, commonsense, or uncertain information. Knowledge-based agent consists of base of knowledge and Inference Engine.

Knowledge Base (KB) is a set of sentences describing the world and its behaviour in some formal (representational) language. Typically domain specific but extensive knowledge corpus is built to provide general knowledge resources. Inference engine is a set of procedures using the representational language to infer new facts from known ones or answer a variety of KB queries.

Reasoning

The reasoning is the mental process of deriving logical conclusion from the available knowledge, facts and beliefs and making predictions Or it can be said that, "Reasoning is a means of inferring facts from existing data".

Reasoning can be divided into deductive reasoning, inductive reasoning, abductive reasoning, common sense reasoning, monotonous reasoning and non-monotonic reasoning

Deductive Reasoning

Deductive reasoning deduces new information from logically related known information. It is the type of valid reasoning, which implies that where the premises are true, the conclusion of the statement must be true. Deductive reasoning in AI is a type of propositional logic, and requires different rules and facts.

Inductive Reasoning

Inductive reasoning is a method of reasoning used by the generalization process to arrive at a conclusion using limited set of evidence. It begins with the series of specific facts or data and reaches a general statement or conclusion. Inductive reasoning is a type of propositional logic which is also known as cause-effect reasoning or bottom-up reasoning. In inductive reasoning, historical data or different premises to generate a general rule for which premises support the conclusion is used.

Abductive Reasoning

Abductive reasoning is a form of logical reasoning that begins with single or multiple observations and then seeks to find the most likely explanation or conclusion for observation. Abductive reasoning is an extension of deductive reasoning, but in abductive reasoning the premises do not guarantee the conclusion.

Common Sense Reasoning

The reasoning of common sense is an informal method of reasoning that can be learned from experiences. Common Sense reasoning simulates the ability of humans to make presumptions about everyday events. It is based on good judgment rather than precise logic, and operates on heuristic knowledge and heuristic rules.

Monotonic Reasoning

In monotonic reasoning, once the conclusion is reached, it will remain the same even if we apply some other information in our knowledge base to the existing information. Through monotonic logic, the application of information does not weaken the collection of prepositions to be obtained. To solve monotonic problems, we can draw the valid conclusion only from the facts available, and new facts will not impact it.For real-time systems, monotonic reasoning is not useful, as facts are changed in real time, so we cannot use monotonic reasoning. In conventional reasoning systems monotonic reasoning is used, and a system based on logic is monotonic.

Non-Monotonic Reasoning

In non-monotonic reasoning, if we add more facts to our knowledge base, certain assumptions may be invalidated. Logic will be said to be non-monotonic if the addition of more knowledge into our knowledge base can invalidate some conclusions. Non-monotonic reasoning deals with incomplete and uncertain models.A general example of non-monotonic reasoning is human perceptions for various things in daily life.

DECISION MAKING

Artificial Intelligence techniques are increasingly extending and enriching decision support through such means as coordinating data delivery, analyzing data trends, providing forecasts, developingdata consistency, quantifying uncertainty, anticipating the user's data needs, providing information to the user in the most appropriate forms, and suggesting courses of action.

APPLICATIONS OF AI: AI IN HEALTHCARE

AI helps to discover hidden insights into clinical decision-making, link patients with self-management tools, and derive value from previously inaccessible, unstructured data properties (Holden et al,2015).

Medical imaging data is one of the best, and often one of the most complex, sources of patient information. For megapixel by megapixel of data crammed into the findings of X-rays, CAT scans, MRIs and other test modalities, integrating extremely high-resolution images can be difficult for even the most skilled healthcare professional.

AI in health care applies primarily to doctors and hospitals accessing large data sets of information that could potentially save lives. It covers treatment methods and their effects, levels of recovery, and pace of care collected through millions of patients, geographic locations, and numerous, often intertwined health conditions. New computing power can detect and analyze large and small data patterns and even predict them through machine learning to identify potential health outcomes. Artificial Intelligence is said to offer significant improvements in the quality and safety of patient care at reduced costs, with some analysts also claiming that it constitutes an imminent revolution in clinical practice (Tang et al, 2018). AI provides many benefits over conventional modeling and decision making approaches in clinical practice. Learning algorithms can become more predictive and reliable as they engage with training data, allowing people to gain unparalleled insights into diagnostics, care processes, variation in treatment and outcomes for patients.

Medical practice includes diagnosis, care, and prognosis, in effect requiring judgments that need to be guided in health and clinical expertise, abilities, insight, experience, and judgment. Therefore, medical practice relies on the science and evidence-based expertise of the doctors, but also on their ability to organize and remember the experiences of their past professional activities.

Experienced physicians use less unnecessary tests to make better decisions, and determine more easily than new doctors. Medical Decision Support Systems (MDSS) are computer software designed to help doctors and other health care professionals (and patients) make decisions (Conejar & Kim, 2014).

Because medical decision-making relies on medical knowledge but also on medical experience, MDSS is required to integrate information mechanisms that promote evidence-based health care values, as well as additional frameworks to store useful past experience. One of the structures consistent with experience storage to reflect medical knowledge are decision tables. A decision table is a matrix that compares a collection of decision input variables with a set of output behavior.

Artificial Intelligence systems for advanced acute care decision making for Healthcare applications is shown in figure 1.

EXAMPLE APPLICATIONS IN HEALTHCARE

BUOY Health an Intelligent Symptom Checker

Buoy Health is a symptom and cure checker focused on AI that uses algorithms to diagnose and treat illness (Ziabari, 2018). Chatbot listens to the symptoms and health concerns of a patient, and directs the patient to get the right care based on their diagnosis. Harvard Medical School is just one of the several hospitals and healthcare providers that use Buoy's AI to help patients diagnose and treat faster.

Figure 1. AI for Advanced Acute Care Decision Making for Healthcare Applications

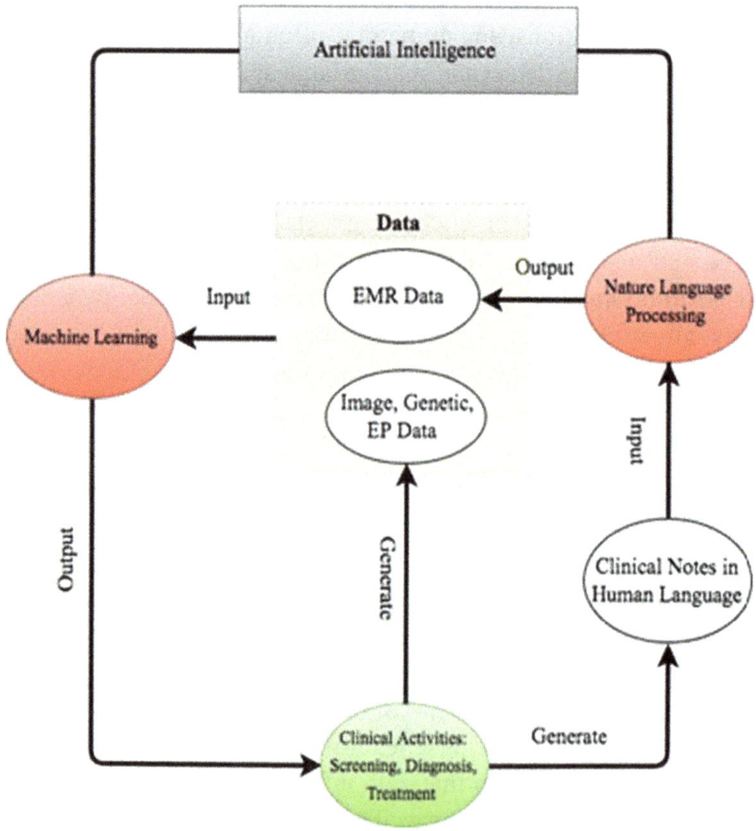

Earlier Cancer Detection with AI

Freenome uses AI to monitor (Hunter,2019) for cancer in examinations, diagnostic tests, and bloodwork. Through introducing AI at general scans, Freenome aims at identifying cancer at its earliest stage and then developing new therapies.

MEDICAL IMAGE CLASSIFICATION WITH AI

Medical image classification using Artificial Intelligence takes as input different medical images and uses AI techniques to output a diagnostic decision. Clustering techniques are used in the classification of medical images. Fuzzy C-means (FCM) clustering was used to extract the suspected tumour region from the segmented liver (Kumar & Moni, 2010). Fuzzy C-means clustering was used in cancer tumour diagnosis (Basha & Prasad, 2009). Particle swarm optimization is used along with Particle swarm optimization for detection of micro calcification in digital mammogram.

Fuzzy inference neural network that combines fuzzy systems and Radial Basis Function (RBF) was proposed in the classification of endoscopic images (Vassilis & Jonh, 2008). A fuzzy inference system incorporated with multilayer perceptron was proposed to identify women with osteoporosis (Nakamoto et al,2008). Neuro fuzzy logic was used in brain cancer detection and classification system. A fuzzy possibilistic C Mean algorithm was used for detection of lung cancer (Gomathi & Thangaraj, 2010). An adaptive neuro fuzzy system for ROI classification in mammograms dealt specifically with calcifications (Fernandes et al,2010). A fuzzy technique in conjunction with three features entropy, standard deviation, and number of pixels were used to distinguish a benign micro calcification pattern from a malignant one.

Supervised algorithms are also used in image classification. A supervised diagnosis system for digital mammogram is developed, by transforming the data of the images into a feature vector using wavelets multilevel decomposition (Essam Al-Daoud,2010). A classification based on SVM was proposed to detect breast cancer (Leonardo et al,2009). Breast cancer detection was also done by combining wavelets and Artificial Neural Network (ANN) (Sepehr et al,2005).SVM kernel classification was also performed for all types of radiographic images (Matteo, 2006).

MEDICAL IMAGE SEGMENTATION WITH AI

Accurate diagnosis and treatment of diseases is vital. Researchers have shown that incorrect analysis of images is often the result of improper segmentation. The segmentation methods depend on modality and dimension of imaging. A system was developed to detect tumours that used thresholding as the segmentation method.

Fuzzy approaches used for segmentation require a sufficient expert knowledge for the formulation of the rule base, the combination of the sets and the defuzzification. Fuzzy C means clustering was used for intensity based segmentation (Vassilis & Jonh, 2008)

Three parallel approaches such as adaptive thresholding method, Gabor filtering and fuzzy entropy were used as a form of hybrid segmentation (RiyahiAlam et al, 2009) for detection of masses in digitized mammograms.

Feature difference between neighboring pixels and relative location of the neighboring pixel are the two influential factors in segmentation. A new computational method (Nosratallah et al,2007) based on PSO was introduced to compute optimum values of these two parameters. A two-dimensional FCM was proposed by making use of the global searching ability of the predator-prey particle swarm optimization (Zhou Xian-cheng et al, 2008).

EMERGING OF MACHINE LEARNING

Machine Learning (ML) is an emerging field, which is aimed in finding patterns automatically and reason about data. Machine Learning methods have made numerous advances in healthcare domain. This chapter discusses about fundamentals and the inferences of Machine Learning in health care domain . ML enables personal care in health to promote precision medicine. In future Machine Learning (ML) and Artificial Intelligence (AI) will transform health care into safety environment and makes this, as a Decision Support Systems (DSS) to address the problems faced by patients and physicians in effective diagnosis.

Artificial Intelligence (AI) has received increased attention in recent years. Innovation, made possible through the Internet, has brought AI closer to our everyday lives. This advance, alongside interest in the technology's potential socio-economic and ethical impacts, brings AI to the forefront of many contemporary debates. Industry investments in AI are rapidly increasing and governments are trying to understand what the technology could mean for their bring revolution in citizens (Trishan et al,2018).

The collection of "Big Data" and the expansion of the Internet of Things (IoT) have made a perfect environment for new AI applications and services to grow. Applications based on AI are already visible in healthcare diagnostics, targeted treatment, transportation, public safety, service robots, education and entertainment, but will be applied in more fields in the coming years. Together with the Internet, AI changes the way we experience the world and has the potential to be a new engine for economic growth (Jabbar et al,2018).

EVOLUTION OF MACHINE LEARNING

Machine Learning is a branch of Artificial Intelligence. Using computing, we design systems that can learn from data in a manner of being trained. The systems might learn and improve with experience, and with time, refine a model that can be used to predict outcomes of questions based on the previous learning. Machine Learning is the systematic study of algorithms and systems that improve their knowledge or performance with experience (Tom,1997) .

Of specific focus is Machine Learning, a particular approach to AI and the driving force are framed behind recent developments. Instead of programming the computer every step of the way, Machine Learning makes use of learning algorithms that make inferences from data to learn new tasks.

As Machine Learning is used more often in products and services, there are some significant considerations when it comes to users' trust in the Internet. Several issues must be considered when addressing AI, including, socio-economic impacts, issues of transparency, bias, and accountability; new uses for data, considerations of security and safety, ethical issues and how AI facilitates the creation of new ecosystems (Burrell,2016).

At the same time, in this complex field, there are specific challenges facing AI, which include a lack of transparency and interpretability in decision making, issues of data quality and potential bias, safety and security implications, considerations regarding accountability, and, its potentially disruptive impacts on social and economic structures.

Machine Learning algorithms characteristically fall into two learning types such as supervised or unsupervised learning.

Supervised Learning

Supervised learning refers to working with a set of labeled training data. For every example in the training data you have an input object and an output object. An example would be classifying Twitter data. There are issues with supervised learning that must be taken into account. The *bias-variance dilemma* is one of them: how the Machine Learning model performs accurately using different training sets. High bias models contain restricted learning sets, whereas high variance models learn with complexity against noisy training data. There is a trade-off between the two models.

The key is where to settle with the trade-off and when to apply which type of model.

Unsupervised Learning

On the opposite end of this spectrum is unsupervised learning, where you let the algorithm find a hidden pattern in a load of data. With unsupervised learning there is no right or wrong answer; it is just a case of running the Machine Learning algorithm and seeing what patterns and outcomes occur.

Unsupervised learning might be more a case of data mining than of actual learning. Clustering data spends a lot of time with unsupervised learning. Figure 2 depicts the learning types of Machine Learning algorithms.

Figure 2. Learning Types of Machine Learning Algorithms

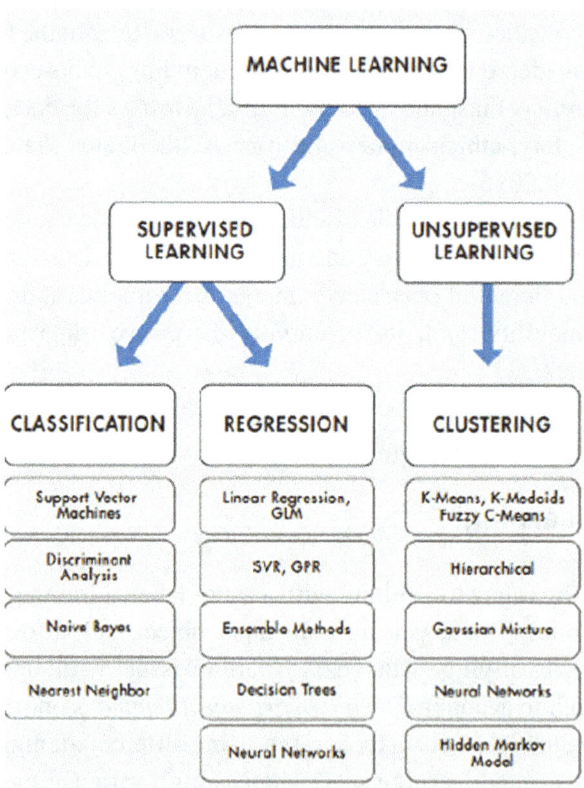

Data mining and Machine Learning have been around for a number of years already, and the huge media push surrounding. Big Data has to do with data volume (Obermeyer & Emanuel 2016) (Shimabukuro et al,2017) .

A computer program is said to learn from experience E with respect to some class of tasks T and performance measure P, if its performance at tasks in T, as measured by P, improves with the experience E(Tom, 1997). The important thing here is that you now have a set of objects to define Machine Learning:

- Task (T), either one or more
- Experience (E)
- Performance (P)

So, with a computer running a set of tasks, the experience should be leading to performance increases. As Machine Learning algorithms are used in more and more products and services, there are some serious factors must be considered when addressing AI, particularly in the context of people's trust in the Internet:

- **Socio-economic impacts:** The new functions and services of AI are expected to have significant socio-economic impacts. The ability of machines to exhibit advanced cognitive skills to process natural language, to learn, to plan and to perceive, makes it possible for new tasks to be performed by intelligent systems, sometimes with more success than humans could open up exciting opportunities for more effective medical care, safer industries and services, and boost productivity on a massive scale.
- **Transparency, bias and accountability:** AI-made decisions can have serious impacts in people's lives. AI may discriminate against some individuals or make errors due to biased training data. How a decision is made by AI is often hard to understand, making problems of bias harder to solve and ensuring accountability much more difficult.
- **New uses for data:** Machine Learning algorithms have proved efficient in analyzing and identifying patterns in large amounts of data, commonly referred to as "Big Data". Big Data is used to train learning algorithms to increase their performance (Tom,1997). This generates an increasing demand for data, encouraging data collection and raising risks of over sharing of information at the expense of user privacy.
- **Security and safety:** Advancements in AI and its use will also create new security and safety challenges. These include unpredictable and harmful behavior of the AI agent, but also adversarial learning by malicious actors.

- **Ethics**: AI may make choices that could be deemed unethical, yet also be a logical outcome of the algorithm, emphasizing the importance to build in ethical considerations into AI systems and algorithms.
- **New ecosystems:** Like the impact of mobile Internet, AI makes new applications, services, and new means of interacting with the network possible. For example, through speech and smart agents, which may create new challenges to how open or accessible the Internet becomes.

An overview of how Machine Learning is used to address a given task is shown in figure 3. A task requires an appropriate mapping a model from data described by features to outputs. Obtaining such a mapping from training data is what constitutes a learning problem.

Figure 3. General framework for Machine Learning Model

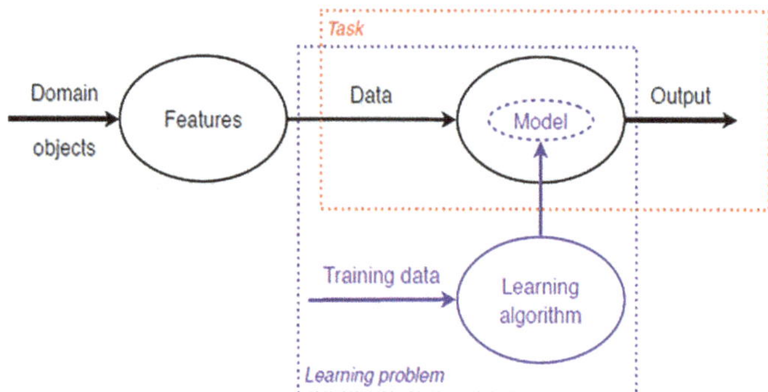

Models address tasks, whereas learning problems are solved by learning algorithms that produce models. Machine Learning is concerned with using the right features to build the right models that achieve the right tasks. Models lend the machine learning field diversity, but tasks and features give it unity.Table 1 shows basic model built with supervised and unsupervised learning.

Table 1. Outcomes of supervised and unsupervised learning

	Predictive model	*Descriptive model*
Supervised learning	classification, regression	subgroup discovery
Unsupervised learning	predictive clustering	descriptive clustering, association rule discovery

The rows refer to whether the training data is labeled with the target value, while the columns indicate whether the models learned are used to predict a target variable or rather describe the given data.

Machine Learning models can be distinguished according to their main intuition:

- Geometric models use intuitions from geometry such as separating (hyper) planes, linear transformations and distance metrics.
- Probabilistic models view learning as a process of reducing uncertainty, modelled by means of probability distributions.
- Logical models are defined in terms of easily interpretable logical expressions.

Alternatively, they can be characterized by their modus operand as

- Grouping models divide the instance space into segments; in each segment a very simple (e.g., constant) model is learned.
- Grading models learning a single, global model over the instance space.

With Artificial Intelligence performing tasks ranging from self-driving cars to managing insurance payouts, it's critical we understand decisions made by an AI agent. But transparency around algorithmic decisions is sometimes limited by things like corporate or state secrecy or technical literacy. Machine Learning further complicates this since the internal decision logic of the model is not always understandable, even for the programmer.

The algorithm can produce bad predictions. The common causes of this are over fitting and under fitting. In case of over fitting, the algorithm performs well on the training data, but underperforms on the new data because instead of finding a general pattern explaining the variation, it has found some random patterns in the training data. Under fitting means that the algorithm does not fully exploit the data provided for its training; this happens in case of choosing an insufficiently complex model. Over fitting and under fitting come together. If one decreases, the other one will increase. It is therefore important to find a balance between those - then the total prediction error is minimal.

MODELS: THE OUTPUT OF MACHINE LEARNING

Models form the central concept in Machine Learning as they are what is being learned from the data, in order to solve a given task. There is a considerable not to say bewildering the range of machine learning models to choose from. One reason for this is the ubiquity of the tasks that machine learning aims to solve: classification, regression, clustering, association discovery, to name but a few. Examples of each of these tasks can be found in virtually every branch of science and engineering. Mathematicians, engineers, psychologists, computer scientists and many others have discovered and sometimes rediscovered the ways to solve these tasks. They have all brought their specific background to bear, and consequently the principles underlying these models are also diverse.

Geometric Models

The *instance space* is the set of all possible or describable instances, whether they are present in our data set or not. Usually this set has some geometric structure. For instance, if all features are numerical, then we can use each feature as a coordinate in a Cartesian coordinate system. A *geometric model* is constructed directly in instance space, using geometric concepts such as lines, planes and distances. It is important to keep in mind, though, that a Cartesian instance space has as many coordinates as there are features, which can be tens, hundreds, thousands, or even more. Such high-dimensional spaces are hard to imagine but are nevertheless very common in Machine Learning. Geometric concepts that potentially apply to high-dimensional spaces are usually prefixed with 'hyper-': for instance, a decision boundary in an unspecified number of dimensions is called a *hyper plane*. If there exists a linear decision boundary separating the two classes, then the data is *linearly separable*.

Probabilistic Models

The second type of models are probabilistic in nature, like the Bayesian classifier.Many of these models are based around the following idea. Let *X* denote the variables we know about, e.g., our instance's feature values; and let *Y* denote the *target variables* we're interested in, e.g., the instance's class. The key question in Machine Learning is how to model the relationship between *X* and *Y* . The statistician's approach is to assume that there is some underlying random process that generates the values for these variables, according to a well-defined but unknown probability distribution. We want to use the data to find out more about this distribution.

Logical Models

The third type of model we distinguish is more algorithmic in nature, drawing inspiration from computer science and engineering. Logical models can be easily translated into rules that are understandable by humans. The idea of feature tree is that features are used to iteratively partition the instance space. The leaves of the tree therefore correspond to rectangular areas in the instance space which we will call *instance space segments*, or segments for short. Depending on the task we are solving, we can then label the leaves with a class, a probability, a real value, and so on. Feature trees whose leaves are labeled with classes are commonly called *decision trees*.

Grouping and Grading

The key difference between *grouping models* and *grading models* is the way they handle the instance space. Grouping models do this by breaking up the instance space into groups or *segments*, the number of which is determined at training time. One could say that grouping models have a fixed and finite 'resolution' and cannot distinguish between individual instances beyond this resolution. What grouping models do at this finest resolution is often something very simple, such as assigning the majority class to all instances that fall into the segment. The main emphasis of training a grouping model is then on determining the right segments so that we can get away with this very simple labeling at the local segment level. Grading models, on the other hand, do not employ such a notion of segment. Rather than applying very simple, local models, they form one global model over the instance space. Consequently, grading models are (usually) able to distinguish between arbitrary instances, no matter how similar they are. Their resolution is, in theory, infinite, particularly when working in a Cartesian instance space. A good example of grouping models are the tree-based models we have just considered. They work by repeatedly splitting the instance space into smaller subsets. Because trees are usually of limited depth and don't contain all the available features, the subsets at the leaves of the tree partition the instance space with some finite resolution. Instances filtered into the same leaf of the tree are treated the same, regardless of any features not in the tree that might be able to distinguish them. Support Vector Machines and other geometric classifiers are examples of grading models. Because they work in a Cartesian instance space, they are able to represent and exploit the minutest differences between instances. As a consequence, it is always possible to come up with a new test instance that receives a score that has not been given to any previous test instance.

CHALLENGES OF MACHINE LEARNING IN HEALTHCARE DECISION MAKING

Machine Learning systems differ from traditional software systems. Machine Learning uses self-learning, continuously improving algorithms. Before implementation in real-world conditions, the system must be trained on local data. Each algorithm has its strengths and weaknesses, therefore, it is important to try several algorithms to find out which one works best on the current problem. The strategy for developing a machine-learning system for healthcare should involve mapping of clinical needs and technological capabilities to identify good cases for pilot projects. Pilots showing good results can then be scaled up.

Machine Learning has been tested in many research projects with promising results. If Machine Learning is going to be used for clinical decision support, a ready-trained model and access to individual patient data is needed. This means that the system must be integrated With Electronic Health Record (EHR) or other systems where data is stored. This can be done in several ways, either 1) by incorporating with the EHR system/ radiology system, 2) as a cloud service provided by a third party, or 3) as a service in a private cloud.

The use of Machine Learning can convert data to knowledge, which will lead to disruptions in at least three healthcare areas, with different time horizons (Devinsky et al,2016):

1. **Interpretation of medical images:** This area is most developed. Many projects have proven their effectiveness, showing results as good or even better than medical specialists. In the next few years, the area will develop rapidly.
2. **Prognostics:** Algorithms for prognostics are not so developed. It will take about five years before this area becomes mature enough.
3. **Diagnostics:** This is the most complicated of the areas. It will take about ten years before such solutions are ready for use in practice.

The algorithm becomes a "black box" when the process behind the results is too complex to understand. Personal health information must be treated in a privacy-preserving manner. According to Healthcare, data must be sufficient, relevant and limited to what is necessary to achieve the purpose for which the data is processed. Patients must be fully informed about the cause of data processing to be able to choose whether or not allow the use of their data in an algorithm.

COMPETENCE OF MACHINE LEARNING IN MEDICINE AND HEALTHCARE

Machine Learning algorithms can analyze large amounts of varied data with accurate results. Three disruption areas for Machine Learning in healthcare are:

- Interpretation of medical images (eye diseases, radiology, pathology)
- Prognostics (dementia, metastatic cancer, stroke)

- Diagnostics (oncology, pathology, rare diseases)

The health service is becoming more proactive using AI, however, more research and development is needed before the potential of the technology can be fully realized.

The race is on for Machine Learning to be used in healthcare analytics. A number of startups are looking at the advantages of using Machine Learning with big data to provide healthcare professionals with better-informed data to enable them to make better decisions.

IBM's famed Watson supercomputer, once used to win the television quiz program *Jeopardy* against two human contestants, is being used to help doctors.

Using Watson as a service on the cloud, doctors can access learning on millions of pages of medical research and hundreds of thousands of pieces of information on medical evidence.

With the number of consumers using smart phones and the related devices for collating a range of health information such as weight, heart rate, pulse, pedometers, blood pressure, and even blood glucose levels. It's now possible to track and trace user health regularly and see patterns in dates and times.

Machine Learning systems can recommend healthier alternatives to the user via the device. Although it's easy enough to analyze data, protecting the privacy of user health data is another story. Obviously, some users are more concerned about how their data is used, especially in the case of it being sold to third-party companies.

The increased volume of analytics in healthcare and medicine is new, but the privacy debate will be the deciding factor about how the algorithms will ultimately be used.

Machine Learning, yields better results in health care domain. As per McKinsey report Machine Learning and big data in pharmacy and medicine could generate revenue up to $100B annually. This is due to the faster decision-making, improved efficiency clinical trials, optimized innovation. Figure 4 shows the types of health data.

There are various applications of Machine Learning in pharmacy. They are broadly classified into following

1. Disease Identification/Diagnosis
2. Personalized Treatment/Behavioral Modification
3. Drug Discovery/Manufacturing
4. Clinical Trial Research
5. Radiology and Radiotherapy
6. Smart Electronic Health Records
7. Epidemic Outbreak Prediction

Figure 4. Types of health data

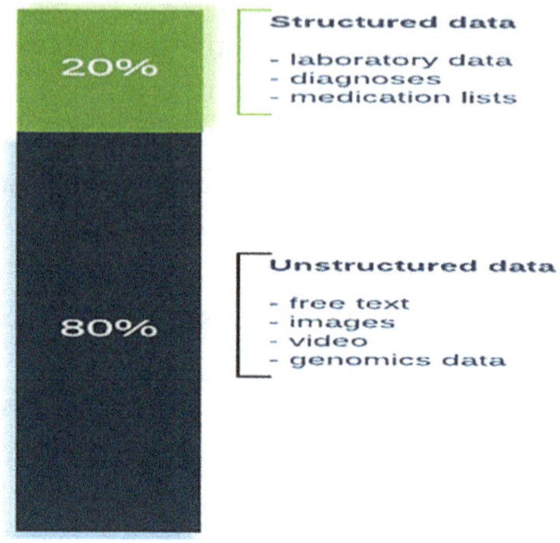

The application of Machine Learning approach in regimen treatment is focused in figure 5 and Figure 6.

Figure 5. Cognitive Computing Approach in Regimen Treatment

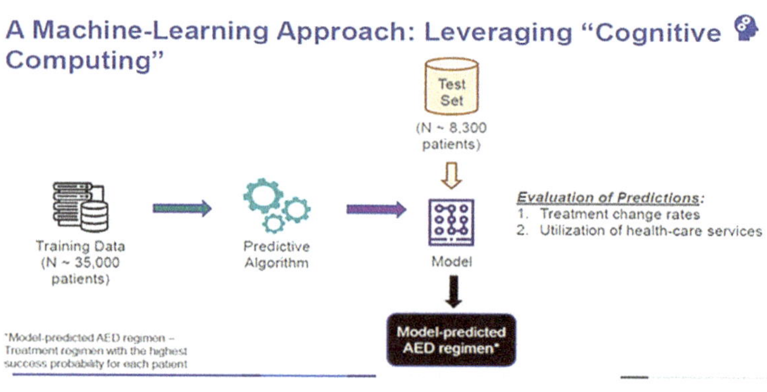

From the figure 5 and figure 6, it is clear the data has a high potential in provision of healthcare services (primary use) as well as quality improvement, research, public health, management and planning (secondary use).

The combination of large amounts of varied data, increased computing power and better methods enables fast and automated production of machine-learning algorithms able to analyze complex data with accurate results.

Figure 6. Impact of Machine Learning Approach in Regimen Treatment

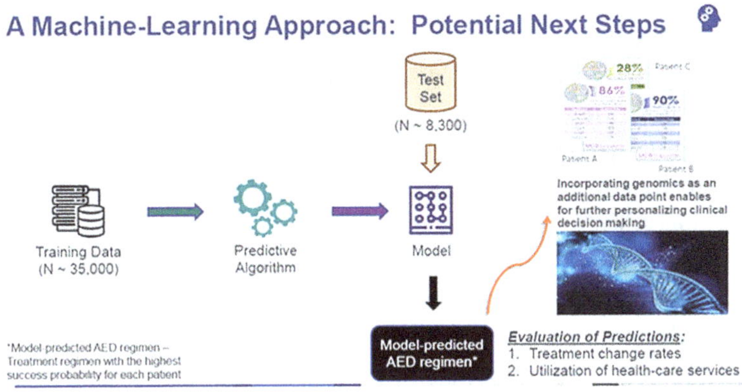

DEEP LEARNING

This section emphasizes the significance and characterization of deep learning. A brief discussion on the use of Deep Learning techniques in medical imaging is also presented.

Basics of Deep Learning

In this section, we explain the fundamental concepts involved in deep learning.

Neural Networks

Neural networks form the basis for deep learning. The goal of a neural network is to find a similarity to an unknown entity. It is formed from neurons connected to each other. Such neurons have weights and bias which are changed during network training, depending on the error. The activation function places the linear combination in a nonlinear transformation that produces the output.

A neural network is a device or hardware designed to function just like a human brain. Typically, a neural network is described as having different strata. The first layer is the input layer; it receives and transfers the input signals to the next layer. The next layer does all kinds of measurements and extractions of features— it is called the hidden layer. There'll often be more than one hidden layer there. And then, there's an output layer that produces the final outcome.

Multi Layer Perceptron

A Multil Layer Perceptron (MLP) is an Artificial Neural Network (ANN) feedforward type. Increasing layer has several neurons and all the neurons in each layer are connected to all the neurons in the next layer. MLP uses the supervised learning method for instruction, called backpropagation.

As we construct a neural network, our nodes are assigned random weights and bias values. Once we've obtained the output for a single iteration, the network error can be determined. This error is then fed back to the network along with the cost function gradient for updating the network's weights. Then, these weights are modified to reduce the errors in the subsequent iterations.

Gradient Descent is a process that takes place in the backpropagation step, where the aim is to continuously resample the gradient of the parameter of the model in the opposite direction depending on the weight w, constantly updating until we hit the global minimum.

Convolutional Neural Network (CNN)

A convolutionary neural network (CNN, or ConvNet) in Deep Learning is a subset of deep neural networks, most widely applicable to visual image research. These are also classified as change invariant or Space Invariant Artificial Neural Networks (SIANN), focused on the features of their shared-weights design and invariance translation. Multilayer perceptrons are regularized variants of CNNs.

A Convolutionary Neural Network (CNN) is designed to use spatial and structure information more effectively by using each 2-D or 3-D construct as data. Structural, in a typical multilayer neural network, CNNs include convolutionary layers interspersed with pooling layers accompanied by fully connected layers.

Recurrent Neural Network (RNN)

A Recurrent Neural Network (RNN) is a type of artificial neural networks in which node-to-node links shape a directed graph along a time continuum. It allows it to show transient dynamic actions. Recurrent Neural Networks(RNN) is a form of Neural Network, where the output from the previous step is fed to the current phase as data. Like feedforward neural networks, RNNs can use its internal state (memory) to process input sequences of variable lengths. It makes them specific to functions such as unsegmented identification, linked handwriting, or speech recognition.

APPLICATION OF DEEP LEARNING IN MEDICAL IMAGING

Deep Learning approaches have become a favored tool for examining medical images.This section describes the use of Deep Learning for image classification, segmentation and registration.

Use of Deep Learning in Medical Image Classification

Classification of photographs or tests was one of the first fields where insightful understanding made a significant contribution to the study of medical pictures. In the grouping of tests, each usually has one or more photos (an exam) as input with a specific descriptive attribute as output (e.g., current or not present disease). In such an environment, each test analysis is a snapshot, and usually, data set sizes are small compared to those in computer vision.

Two transfer learning techniques were identified: (1) the use of a pre-trained network as an extractor function, and (2) the fine tuning of a pre-trained medical data network. The former approach has the additional advantage of not needing one to build a deep network at all, enabling the extracted features to be conveniently inserted into established pipelines for study of image.

In the case of (Antony et al,2016), fine tuning significantly outperformed function extraction, reaching 57.6% precision in multi-class osteoarthritis classification evaluation versus 53.4%. Nevertheless, (Kim et al,2016) found that using CNN as a function extractor outperformed fine-tuning in the consistency classification of cytopathology picture (70.5 per cent versus 69.1 per cent). In 2013, the first studies using such methods for analysis classification emerged and based on neuroimaging. (Brosch, & Tam, 2013), (Plis et al,2014) and (Suk, & Shen, 2013) used DBNs and SAEs to identify patients as Alzheimer's based on brain MRI.

Both approaches use fields are very diverse, varying from brain MRI to retinal imaging, and optical anatomy to lung Computed Tomography (CT). A strong change towards CNNs could be noticed recently. Also in the more recent papers use CNN writers frequently build from scratch their own network structures instead of using pre-trained networks. (Menegola et al,2016) published several studies relating programming from scratch to pretrained network fine tuning.

Image grouping usually focuses on classifying a small part of the visual picture (previously identified) into two or more sections. Some systems use several CNNs each taking a nodule patch as feedback at a different scale. The corresponding characteristic outputs of the three CNNs are then concatenated to form the final matrix.

(Kawahara & Hamarneh,2016) pursued a somewhat similar approach which used a multi-stream CNN to identify skin lesions, where each stream operates on a specific image resolution. A combinationation of CNNs and RNNs can be used to assess nuclear cataracts in slit-lamp pictures, where CNN filters can be pre-trained. The 3D complexity of MRI can be manipulated by using a 3D CNN to test survival in patients with high-grade gliomas.

Use of Deep Learning in Medical Image Segmentation

Image segmentation subdivides the image based on physically distinct regions that have a conceptual meaning for the issue in question. Usually, each of these areas has standardized features of either the gray level, texture, or colour. A majority of Deep Learning approaches for the segmentation of biomedical images are based on a convolutionary neural network. (Moeskops et al,2016) suggested a single CNN for various image segmentation tasks including six tissues in MR brain images, pectoral muscles in MR breast images, and coronary arteries. CNN describes the form of imaging, anatomical structure and type of tissue. A complete convolutionary 3D network can be coupled with a 3D deep-surveillance mechanism to segment liver from 3D CT scans. The technique is also used to segment entire heart and large vessels from 3D MR images. Certain techniques use a CNN method that would conduct 2D segmentation of multiple organs from fetal MR slices using two annotations of organs for research. Alternatively, annotated tumor core is used to perform 3D segmentation of the brain tumor core from MR sequences

The segmentation process of brain tumors can be automated based on multiple CNN architectural variations. (Xu et al,2019) suggested a CNN method that would segment breast ultrasound images into four major tissues: skin, glandular fibrous tissue, mass, and fatty tissue, using 3 orthogonal image planes. Convolutional Neural Networks can be used to segment endoscopic OCT images automatically using the parallel architecture of qualified deep neural networks.

Few studies are present on segmentation of medical images using Restricted Boltzmann Machine(RBM). Restricted Boltzmann Machine can be used for Unattended Feature Learning. Random Forest Classifier can be used that combines existing correlations between image data, features, and target variables. This approach can be used to improve the interpretability of the Machine Learning features that were automatically extracted.

(Agn et al,2015) suggested a fully automated generative approach for the segmentation of healthy brain tissues, where Gaussian mixture models model the tissues. Convolutionary Restricted Boltzmann Machines (cRBMs) were used to model tumor core form as well as total tumor shape, which includes edema and heart. The cRBMs are specialized in expert image segmentation. Segmentation can be done for the left ventricle's endocardial and epicardial boundaries.

Use of Deep Learning in Medical Image Registration

Image registration is the method of converting multiple image databases into one coordinate system with compatible image material that has significant medical imaging applications. Authentication may be needed when examining a pair of images obtained from different points of view, or at different times. Automatic intensity-based image registration requires both a metric quantifying the similarity between a moving image and a fixed image and an optimization algorithm that updates the parameters of the transformation to optimize the similarity between the images. Registration based on similarity allows use of Deep Learning to learn a similarity metric. This similarity metric is introduced into a classical intensity-based registration system with a given strategy of interpolation, model of transformation and algorithm of optimization. Certain works used a Convolutional-stacked Auto Encoder (CAE) to extract the features that are used for unimodal, deformable registration. Later, the processing was carried out using gradient descent (Wu et al,2015). Certain works use a stacked denoising autoencoder to learn a similarity metric for multimodal registration. Certain other works use CNN to learn the dissimilarity for multimodal registration (Cheng et al,2018).

In a registration based on reinforcement learning, a qualified agent is used instead of a predefined optimization algorithm to perform the registration. Many works train a single agent to conduct rigid enrolment(Ma et al,2017). In a reinforcement learning model some other works (Miao et al, 2018) perform used a multi-agent method to perform rigid registration.

CHALLENGES AND OPPORTUNITIES IN MEDICAL IMAGING

It is noteworthy that the techniques of Deep Learning seem to have achieved considerable efficiency. Notwithstanding this, Medical Imaging poses many challenges and opportunities when implementing deep learning. The shortage of large data sets for preparation is often cited as an obstacle. This downside can however be resolved by referring to large public data sets which are made available. The real challenge for these images is therefore not the availability of the image data itself, but the collection of appropriate annotations / labelling. The model obtained through a Deep Learning approach can be likened to a black box that can be interpreted in terms of its inputs and outputs without understanding its internal functions. No Deep Learning network can adequately explain its decision-making process at the present time. Acceptance within the medical industry is therefore also a concern. A difficulty in the classification of medical images is the presence of systems which are extremely good at excluding the most common standard subclasses but which fail miserably on several rare ones.

CONCLUSION

In this chapter we briefly discuss the concepts of Artificial Intelligence, Machine Learning and Deep Learning that are used in healthcare. It also describes methods used for medical image operations such as image detection and segmentation. The healthcare industry has been captivated by Artificial Intelligence, Machine Learning and Deep Learning, as these ground-breaking computing approaches become more effective and relevant to a variety of tasks. This chapter provides the key factors about the powerful techniques, approaches and their applications in health care.

REFERENCES

Agn, M., Puonti, O., afRosenschöld, P. M., Law, I., & Van Leemput, K. (2015). Brain tumor segmentation using a generative model with an RBM prior on tumor shape. In *BrainLes* (pp. 168–180). Springer.

Al-Daoud, E. (2010). Cancer diagnosis using modified fuzzy network. *Universal J. Comput. Sci.&Engg. Technol.*, *1*(2), 73–78.

Antony, J., McGuinness, K., O'Connor, N. E., & Moran, K. (2016). Quantifying radiographic knee osteoarthritis severity using deep convolutional neural networks. In *Proceedings of International Conference on Pattern Recognition (ICPR)* (pp. 1195-1200). IEEE. 10.1109/ICPR.2016.7899799

Basha, S. S., & Prasad, K. S. (2009). Automatic detection of breast cancer mass in mammograms using morphological operators and fuzzy c—means Clustering. *Journal of Theoretical & Applied Information Technology*, *5*(6), 1–6.

Brosch, T., & Tam, R. (2013).Alzheimer's Disease Neuroimaging Initiative. Manifold learning of brain MRIs by deep learning. In *Proceedings of International Conference on Medical Image Computing and Computer-Assisted Intervention* (pp. 633-640). Springer.

Burrell, J. (2016). How the machine 'thinks': Understanding opacity in Machine Learning algorithms. *Big Data & Society*, 1-12.

Cheng, X., Zhang, L., & Zheng, Y. (2018). Deep similarity learning for multimodal medical images. *Computer Methods in Biomechanics and Biomedical Engineering. Imaging & Visualization*, *6*(3), 248–252. doi:10.1080/21681163.2015.1135299

Conejar, R. J., & Kim, H. K. (2014). A medical Decision Support System (DSS) for ubiquitous healthcare diagnosis system. *International Journal of Software Engineering and Its Applications*, *8*(10), 237–244.

Devinsky, O., Dilley, C., Ozery-Flato, M., Aharonov, R., Goldschmidt, Y., Rosen-Zvi, M., Clark, C., & Fritz, P. (2016). Changing the approach to treatment choice in epilepsy using big data. *Epilepsy & Behavior*, *56*(1), 32–37. doi:10.1016/j.yebeh.2015.12.039 PMID:26827299

Fernandes, F. C., Brasil, L. M., Lamas, J. M., & Guadagnin, R. (2010). Breast cancer image assessment using an adaptative network based fuzzy inference system. *J. Pattern Recognition and Image Analysis*, *20*(2), 192–200. doi:10.1134/S1054661810020112

Forghani, Forouzanfar, & Fourouzanfar. (2007). MRI fuzzy segmentation of brain tissue using IFCM Algorithm with particle swarm optimization. *IEEE Intl. Sym. Comput. & Information Sci.*, 113-121.

Gomathi, M., & Thangaraj, P. (2010). Computer aided diagnosis system for detection of lung cancer nodules using extreme learning machine. *International Journal of Engineering Science and Technology*, *2*(10), 5770–5779.

Holden, R. J., Schubert, C. C., & Mickelson, R. S. (2015). The patient work system: An analysis of self-care performance barriers among elderly heart failure patients and their informal caregivers. *Applied Ergonomics*, *47*(1), 133–150. doi:10.1016/j.apergo.2014.09.009 PMID:25479983

Hunter, P. (2019). The advent of AI and Deep Learning in diagnostics and imaging: Machine Learning systems have potential to improve diagnostics in healthcare and imaging systems in research. *EMBO Reports*, 548–559. PMID:31267716

Jabbar, Samreen & Aluvalu. (2018). The Future of Health care: Machine Learning. *IACSIT International Journal of Engineering and Technology*, *7*(4), 23–25. doi:10.14419/ijet.v7i4.6.20226

Kawahara, J., & Hamarneh, G. (2016). Multi-resolution-tract CNN with hybrid pretrained and skin-lesion trained layers. In *Proceedings of International workshop on Machine Learning in medical imaging* (pp. 164-171). Springer. 10.1007/978-3-319-47157-0_20

Kim, E., Corte-Real, M., & Baloch, Z. (2016). A deep semantic mobile application for thyroid cytopathology. In Medical Imaging 2016: PACS and Imaging Informatics: Next Generation and Innovations (Vol. 9789). International Society for Optics and Photonics.

Kodogiannis & Lygouras. (2008). Neuro-fuzzy classification system for wirelesscapsule endoscopic images. *J. WorldAcad. Sci.Engg. & Technol*, *45*, 620–628.

Kumar, S. S., & Moni, R. S. (2010). Diagnosis of liver tumor from CT images using curvelet transform. *International Journal on Computer Science and Engineering*, *2*(4), 1173–1178.

Lee, S. I., Celik, S., & Logsdon, B. A. (2018). A Machine Learning approach to integrate big data for precision medicine in acute myeloid leukemia. *Nature Communications*, *9*(42), 1–15. PMID:29298978

Leonardo de Oliveira, M., Silva, A. C., Cardoso de Paiva, A., & Gattass, M. (2009). Detection of breast masses in mammogram images using growing neural gas algorithm and ripley's K function. *J. Signal Processing Sys*, *55*(1), 77–90. doi:10.100711265-008-0209-3

Ma, K., Wang, J., Singh, V., Tamersoy, B., Chang, Y. J., Wimmer, A., & Chen, T. (2017). Multimodal image registration with deep context reinforcement learning. In *Proceedings of International Conference on Medical Image Computing and Computer-Assisted Intervention* (pp. 240-248). Springer. 10.1007/978-3-319-66182-7_28

Masotti, M. (2006). A ranklet –based image representation for mass classification in digital mammograms. *Journal of Medical Physics / Association of Medical Physicists of India*, *33*(10), 3951–3961. PMID:17089857

Menegola, A., Fornaciali, M., Pires, R., Avila, S., & Valle, E. (2016). *Towards automated melanoma screening: Exploring transfer learning schemes*. arXiv preprint arXiv:1609.01228

Miao, S., Piat, S., Fischer, P., Tuysuzoglu, A., Mewes, P., Mansi, T., & Liao, R. (2018). Dilated fcn for multi-agent 2d/3d medical image registration. *Thirty-Second AAAI Conference on Artificial Intelligence.*

Moeskops, P., Wolterink, J. M., van der Velden, B. H., Gilhuijs, K. G., Leiner, T., Viergever, M. A., & Išgum, I. (2016). Deep Learning for multi-task medical image segmentation in multiple modalities. In *Proceedings of International Conference on Medical Image Computing and Computer-Assisted Intervention* (pp. 478-486). Springer. 10.1007/978-3-319-46723-8_55

Nakamoto, T., Taguchi, A., Ohtsuka, M., Suei, Y., Fujita, M., Tsuda, M., Sanada, M., Kudo, Y., Asano, A., & Tanimot, K. (2008). A computer-aided diagnosis system to screen for osteoporosis using dental panoramic radiographs. *J. Dento Maxillo Facial Radiology*, *37*(5), 274–281. doi:10.1259/dmfr/68621207 PMID:18606749

Obermeyer, Z., & Emanuel, E. J. (2016). Predicting the Future - Big Data, Machine Learning, and Clinical Medicine. *The New England Journal of Medicine*, *375*(13), 1216–1219. doi:10.1056/NEJMp1606181 PMID:27682033

Panch, T., Szolovits, P., & Atun, R. (2018). Artificial Intelligence, Machine Learning and health systems. *Journal of Global Health*, *8*(2), 1–8. doi:10.7189/jogh.08.020303 PMID:30405904

Plis, S. M., Hjelm, D. R., Salakhutdinov, R., Allen, E. A., Bockholt, H. J., Long, J. D., & Calhoun, V. D. (2014). Deep Learning for neuroimaging: A validation study. *Frontiers in Neuroscience*, *8*(229), 1–11. PMID:25191215

RiyahiAlam, N., Younesi, F., & RiyahiAlam, M.S. (2009). Computer-Aided mass detection on digitized mammograms using a novel hybrid segmentation system. *Intl. J. Biol. & Biomedical Engg.*, *3*(4), 51–58.

Sepehr, M. H., Jamarani, B. H., & Rezai rad, G. A. (2005). Multiwavelet based neural network for breast cancer diagnosis. *Proceedings of Intl. Conf. Graphics, Vision & Image Processing*, 29-34.

Shimabukuro, D., Barton, C. W., Feldman, M. D., Mataraso, S. J., & Das, R. (2017). Effect of a Machine Learning-based severe sepsis prediction algorithm on patient survival and hospital length of stay: Randomised clinical trial. *BMJ Open Respiratory Research*, *4*(1), e000234. doi:10.1136/bmjresp-2017-000234 PMID:29435343

Suk, H. I., & Shen, D. (2013). Deep learning-based feature representation for AD/MCI classification. In *Proceedings of International Conference on Medical Image Computing and Computer-Assisted Intervention* (pp. 583-590). Springer. 10.1007/978-3-642-40763-5_72

Tang, A., Tam, R., Cadrin-Chênevert, A., Guest, W., Chong, J., Barfett, J., & Poudrette, M. G. (2018). Canadian Association of Radiologists white paper on Artificial Intelligence in radiology. *Canadian Association of Radiologists Journal*, *69*(2), 120–135. doi:10.1016/j.carj.2018.02.002 PMID:29655580

Tom, M. (1997). *Mitchell, Machine Learning*. McGraw-Hill.

Wu, G., Kim, M., Wang, Q., Munsell, B. C., & Shen, D. (2015). Scalable high-performance image registration framework by unsupervised deep feature representations learning. *IEEE Transactions on Biomedical Engineering*, *63*(7), 1505–1516. doi:10.1109/TBME.2015.2496253 PMID:26552069

Xu, Y., Wang, Y., Yuan, J., Cheng, Q., Wang, X., & Carson, P. L. (2019). Medical breast ultrasound image segmentation by Machine Learning. *Ultrasonics*, *91*, 1–9. doi:10.1016/j.ultras.2018.07.006 PMID:30029074

Zhou, X., Shen, Q., & Liu, L. (2008). New two-dimensional fuzzy C-means clustering algorithm for image segmentation. *J.Central South Univ. Technol*, *15*(6), 882–887. doi:10.100711771-008-0161-1

Ziabari, M. K. (2018). *Mobile Self-Triage Applications: A Usability Perspective* (Doctoral dissertation). University of Ottawa.

Chapter 9
Malaria Parasites Detection Using Deep Neural Network

Biswajit Jena
International Institute of Information Technology, Bhubaneswar, India

Pulkit Thakar
International Institute of Information Technology, Bhubaneswar, India

Vedanta Nayak
International Institute of Information Technology, Bhubaneswar, India

Gopal Krishna Nayak
International Institute of Information Technology, Bhubaneswar, India

Sanjay Saxena
https://orcid.org/0000-0002-8288-1010
International Institute of Information Technology, Bhubaneswar, India

ABSTRACT

Malaria is a dreadful infectious disease caused by the bite of female Anopheles mosquito, by the protozoan parasites of the genus Plasmodium. It's an epidemic disease and demands rapid and accurate diagnosis for proper intervention. Microscopic test on the thick and thin blood smear to detect the malaria and counts the infected cells is the gold standard for diagnosis of this disease. An automation process in the form of computer-aided diagnosis is much needed as it plays a vital role in fully or semi-automated diagnosis of diseases based on medical image information. Deep learning has vast ranging applications. This work is to build a convolutional neural network to expertly detect the presence of malaria parasitized cells in the thin blood smear. The authors construct the model as small and computationally efficient to obtain the highest level of accuracy possible.

DOI: 10.4018/978-1-7998-5071-7.ch009

Copyright © 2021, IGI Global. Copying or distributing in print or electronic forms without written permission of IGI Global is prohibited.

INTRODUCTION

Malaria is caused by protozoan parasites of the genus *Plasmodium*, single celled organisms that cannot survive outside of their host. It is a life-threatening infectious disease caused by parasites that are transmitted to individuals through the bite, mainly at night time of contaminated female Anopheles mosquitoes. The parasites grow within the vertebrate body, especially in liver, before entering the bloodstream to infect red blood cells (RBC). This ensuing destruction of host RBC can results in disease, called malaria. Over last 20th century, various species of malaria were discovered in various host and classified. The five species regularly infect humans are: *P. falciparum*, *P. malariae*, *P. ovale*, *P. knowlesi* and *P. vivax*. Among these, *P. falciparum* is the most dominant species of parasites and lethal in humans, resulting in hundreds of thousands of deaths per year. Typical symptoms of malaria include fever, fatigue, headaches, and, in severe cases, seizures and coma, leading to death .Most of the cases, it is preventable and curable with immunity to malaria increases after each malaria attack. According to the latest *World malaria report,* unleashed in November 2018 by World Health Organization (WHO), there were 219 million cases of malaria in 87 countries in the year 2017 and 217 million cases recorded in 2016. The estimated number of malaria deaths stood at 435000 in 2017, a comparable number to the previous year. Majority of these deaths are children from Sub-Saharan Africa. Approximately half of the world's population is at risk of malaria and most cases occur in sub-Saharan Africa, where 20% of childhood deaths result from this disease. African children have between 1.6 and 5.4 episodes of fever caused by malaria each year. Malaria is also an important cause of prenatal anemia, miscarriage, abortion, stillbirths and of preventable low birth weight. The WHO African region carries an excessively high share of the global malaria burden and in 2017; the area was home to 92% of malaria cases and 93% death due to malaria. This is because of the fact that, the habitat over there are suitable for breeding of mosquitoes, furthermore, the poor socio-economic situation which make difficult to access the health care and disease prevention resources (WHO, n,d; South Sudan, n.d.)

Hundreds of millions of blood films are examined every year for malaria, which involves manual counting of parasites and infected red blood cells by a trained microscopist. Accurate parasite counts are essential not only for malaria diagnosis. They are also important for testing for drug resistance, measuring drug-effectiveness, and classifying disease severity (Poostchi et al. 2018). Conventional microscopy, which is at present the gold standard for malaria diagnosis has sometimes proved inefficient since it is time consuming and results are difficult to reproduce. This method follows the blood film examination under the microscope. There are two kinds of blood films: thick and thin. The thick film is used for quick identification and quantification of parasites and the thin film is used for differentiation of parasite species. The generally used microscopy method so far is inspecting thin blood smears under a microscope, and visually observing for infected cells. The patient's blood is smeared on a glass slide and stained with contrasting agents to identify infected parasites in a better way in their red blood cells. After that, a paramedical professional manually counts the number of malaria parasites cells present in the RBC. The presence (or count) of malaria parasites cells in the image of thin blood smear are shown in fig 1, 2 and 3 with stained parasites are deep purple in color [2]. The life cycle stages of all the five different species of Plasmodium are Ring, Trophozoite, Schizont and Gametocyte (Poostchi et al. 2018), where shape, size, border of the infected cells changes. This methodology not only difficult and time consuming but sometimes gives fatal result due human error (Ghate and Jadhav, 2012).

Figure 1. Ring stage of P. falciparum with multicity of ring within RBCs

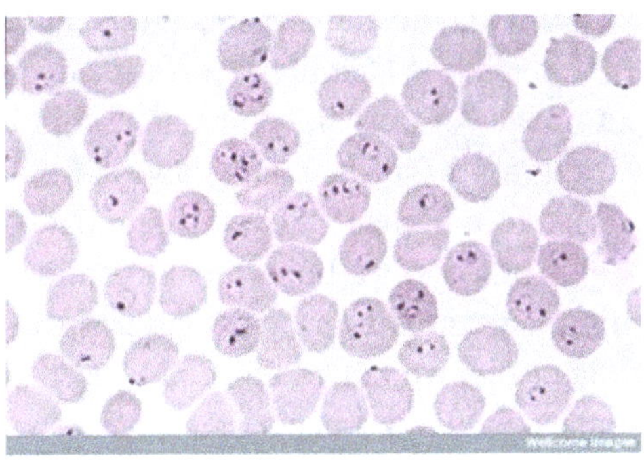

Figure 2. Ring stage of P. falciparum with schizont in the center.

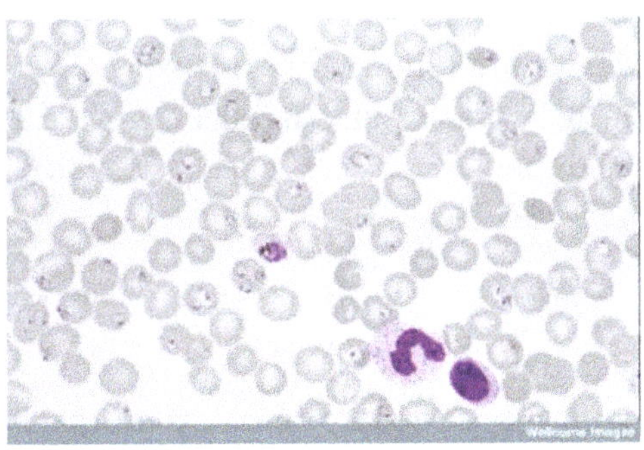

Figure 3. P. ovale with affected cells is oval, enlarged, irregular border.

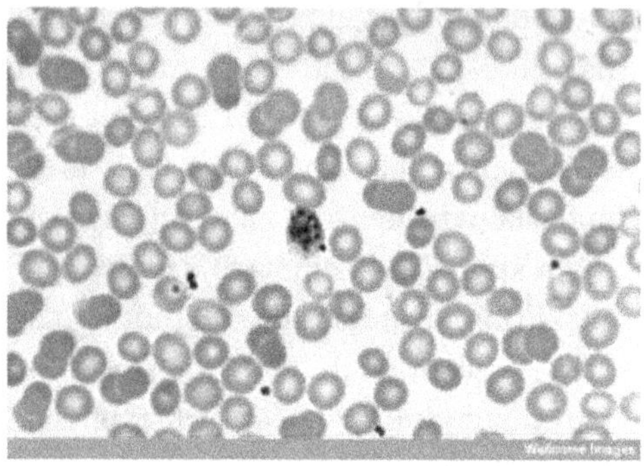

As it represents a genuine global health issue, automation of the assessment process is of highly required. So we proposed a convolution neural network based solution to combat the current diagnosing process of this disease which is tiresome and time-consuming. A Convolution Neural Network is a deep Learning algorithm which can take an input images of thin blood smear, assign importance learnable weights and biases to various objects in the image, have the ability to extract features from image and learn itself from it, then able to differentiate infected images from the uninfected one. By this process, we build an automatic malaria classification system using deep learning. Time is of the most essential aspect in disease outbreaks. To reduce the time of diagnosis, we utilize the CNN based pre-trained models to correctly classify the infected cells in image. Hence, we are able to help doctors and clinicians working in this field, to detect the positive samples of disease with much faster.

Further the works in this paper is divided into different sections. Section 2 discusses about relates works in the area of malaria parasite detection. Section 3 discusses about the architecture followed for this work. Section 4 presents about datasets implemented in this work. Results and analysis of the architecture is given in section 5. Discussions and conclusion is presented in section 6. Finally, the valuable references are given in last sections.

Related Work

Till dates, various works have been done to detect malaria parasite in image of blood sample through automation process. Some of the important and helpful works that are used to progress in our research direction are cited here. The prominent research work for the detection of malaria parasites in the images of thin blood smear includes are image processing methodology, artificial neural network, machine learning and deep learning techniques. The work on (Ghate and Jadhav, 2012) is based on automatic detection of malaria by image processing methodology of image segmentation. Their procedure includes image segmentation, thinning algorithms, thresholding and labeling algorithms. In the similar fashion, the literature on (Suradkar, 2013) follows the methods of edge detection, thresholding, gray scale image conversion, binary image, thinning and labeling of binary image algorithms. A content based image retrieval (CBIR) approach of image processing algorithm for detection is discussed in (Khan et al. 2011). The novel threshold selection and morphological technique are used to identify the parasite present. Apart from this, a two stage tree classifier with back propagation feed forward neural network used to distinguish the true positive and false positive cases present. Related work on (Bashir et al. 2017), in which a set of features based on intensity have been proposed, and the performance of these features on the red blood cell samples from the dataset have been evaluated using an artificial neural network (ANN) classifier. The work in (Pandit et al. 2016) is based on feature extracted from the holographic images of thin blood smear and is given as input to ANN for classification of images as infected or not. The machine learning way of malaria parasite detection is described in this research work (Poostchi et al. 2018). Starting from the description of malaria, various staining methods, various image acquisition techniques, pre-processing and finally various techniques for parasite detection are mentioned in a well-organized way. For each of the section, the method for thick blood smear and thin blood smear also described. The various image processing techniques they have followed are noise reduction, low image contrast, uneven illumination and cell staining variation for both thin and thick image respectively. Some of the image segmentation techniques mentioned are Ostu thresholding (Vala et al. 2013), histogram thresholding (Vala et al. 2013), edge detection algorithms etc. The feature that are considered for computation are color, texture and morphological. Some of the supervised and unsupervised classification models for classification between infected and non-infected are mentioned again for both thin and thick blood smear. The supervised models for thin blood smear are Bayesian classifier, Naive Bayes tree, K-nearest neighbours classifier, Ada-boost, Euclidean distance classifier, Fuzzy interface system are important ones. The unsupervised models for thin and thick blood smear are K-mean clustering and Quaternion Fourier transform. Like that for thick blood smear the supervised models mentioned are Naive Bayes tree, Randomized tree classifier, Nearest mean classifier (NM), Thresholding, Support vector machine (SVM)(Yang et al. 2017), Neural network, Genetic algorithm. The future work regarding deep learning and Android based mobile application is briefly mentioned. This article(Vala et al. 2013) presents a comparative experimental analysis of visual detection of infected erythrocytes malaria parasites via the most efficient morphological techniques from gold standard blood smear images . Twelve different widely-used morphological algorithms are evaluated followed by a random forest classifier for detecting infected erythrocytes based on their performance vis-a-vis microscopic blood smear Images. Rajaraman et.al on (Rajaraman et al. 2018) applied deep learning pre-trained models to detect infected red blood cells in images.

The Architecture

The proposed methodology of our work is based on deep neural network and medical image analysis, which is the thin blood smear of malaria parasites. The network model we will be using a customized convolutional neural network(CNN)(LeCun et al. 1998), which give better result for performance metric like accuracy that are considered important in healthcare application. The Convolutional Neural Network is one of the most effective neural networks to work with medical images and also give result for classification problem. This CNN model is based on the AlexNet model (Krizhevsky et al. 2012), which was the winner of ImageNet(ILSVRC) challenge in 2012. The basic block diagram this model is depicted in figure 4.

Convolutional Layers stand out to be one among the best to build a machine learning model where the model itself extracts the features from the given inputs. One such machine learning model involving Convolutional neural network (LeCun et al. 1998). It is a precious machine learning solutions, features like size, color, the morphology of the cells had to be manually programmed. Utilizing convolutional neural networks (CNN) will greatly speed up prediction time while mirroring (or even exceeding) the accuracy of clinicians. For the malaria diagnosis we use a model that is smaller and more compact. The main reason to do so is to be able to run the model on small devices such as smartphone which is being used to capture images of the blood samples and reduce the storage size for the model. The main advantage of CNN compared to its predecessors is that it automatically detects the important features without any human supervision. The various layers of this model always play vital roles in achieving this. The different layers, which are the building blocks this model are input layer, convolutional layer, activation layer, pooling layer, fully connected layer, hidden layers and output layer.

Convolution layer started functioning with input layer. An input layer is a matrix of pixel values in the shape of width, height, channels.

Convolutional layers are the major building blocks used in convolutional neural networks. The utmost intention of convolution layer is to obtain the feature maps. Convolution is the first layer to extract features from an input image. It is a mathematical operation that takes two inputs such as image matrix and a filter or kernel. Convolution preserves the relationship between pixels by learning image features using small squares of input data. Normally, we begin with few numbers of filters for low-level feature detection. Gradually we go deep inside the CNN, then more number of filters (usually they are also smaller) are required to detect high-level features. The procedure of convolution requires sliding a filter window through the image to calculate the sum of the product under the window and the underlying image before down sampling (Pandit et al. 2016).

ReLU layer work as an activation function. We will use ReLU activation function that gives 0 for each negative pixel values in the input image while the value remain same for each positive values of pixel. So shape of the feature matrix will remain unchanged in this layer.

Pooling layer will accomplish to down sampling functions along the spatial dimensions (width, height), giving the output over a pooling size. So, this layer is just used to reduce the image dimension size.

Hence, the job of this pooling layer is to impart spatial variance, which clearly measures that the system will be competent to acknowledge an object as an object truly when its appearance differ in some aspect.

In the fully connected layer, we flatten the output of the last convolution layer and connect each node of the present layer with the every other nodes of the subsequent layer. Neurons in a fully connected layer have full connections to all activations in the previous layer, as seen in regular neural networks and it operates in a analogous manner. The last layer or softmax layer or output layer of our CNN will compute the class probability scores. So the probability scores are computed in the last layer of our CNN.

For implementation, we are using keras library with Tensorflow as backend. The important modules necessary for this model to work are Numpy, Scikit-learn, Matplotlib, argparse, sklearn and imutils.

Figure 4. Basic block diagram of AlexNet Model
(Krizhevsky et al. 2012)

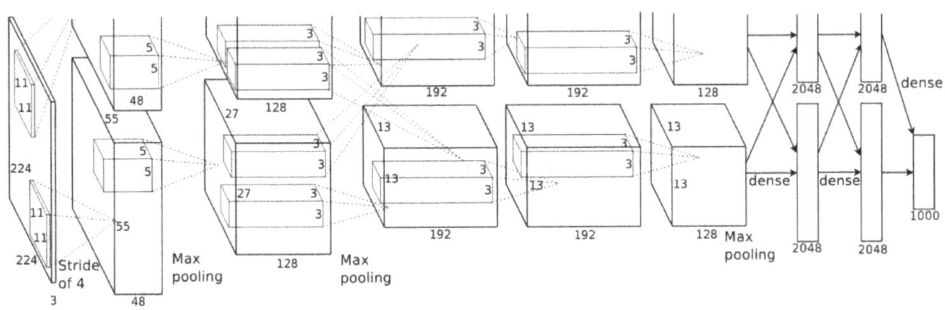

The summery of network structure of our model is described as follows.

Images of dimension of 64 x 64 x 3 (length, width, and depth with 3 channel of RGB images) are used as input to the models. Two input classes of parasitized and un-parasitized are used to train the model and hence to get the result that our test images of blood smear is infected or uninfected. The various layers of this model include two 2-dimentional Convolution layer, two 2-dimentional max polling layer and two fully connected layers and one softmax layer. Some basic features of the network to enhance the efficiency of the model are used as batch normalization, dropout as the regularization technique.

The optimizer we'll be using is stochastic gradient descent (SGD). Our learning rate is set to 0.1 and the momentum term as 0.9. Finally, we compile our model. Our loss function is set as binary_crossentropy as we are performing binary, 2-class classification and evaluation metric as accuracy.

The result of the model on the particular dataset will give us satisfactory level. Its gives approximately 96% classification result, which is standard till dates to detect malaria parasite from the image of blood sample.

Dataset and Pre-processing

The most common method used to diagnose Malaria is Light Microscopy. In this, a microscopist is specifically trained to manually read the blood specimen of the patient to give the reports. This process is arduous in nature. Henceforth, a new technique had to be developed to replace the previous one. The researchers at Lister Hill National Center of Biomedical Communications (LHNCBC) found a breakthrough for the same. The National Library of Medicine (NLM) of LHNCBC holds a repository of segmented cells from the thin blood smear slide images from the Malaria Screener research activity. The method that they introduced involves the development of a mobile application that can be run on a standard Andriod smartphone. The smartphone is attached to a conventional Light Microscope and the in-built camera of the phone captures the images of slides for each microscopic field of view. Giesma-stained thin blood smear slides from 150 Plasmodium falciparum infected and 50 healthy patients were collected and photographed. The captured images were then manually annotated by an expert slide reader. The de-identified images and annotations are archived at NLM. Images of positive samples contained plasmodium cells while images of negative samples does not have these cells, but may contain other types of objects including staining artifacts and impurities, that present in both cases.

So, we have an incredible dataset of labeled and preprocessed images to train and assess the model. This Dataset is taken from the official NIH Website: https://ceb.nlm.nih.gov/repositories/malaria-datasets/ . This dataset has been made available publicly. NIH (National Institute of Health), United States of America has a malaria dataset of 27,558 with same number of infected and uninfected cell images. To detect and segment the red blood cells in the image, a level-set based algorithm was applied. The images of the dataset were collected and annotated by well-trained medical professionals.

The dataset also undergoes preprocessing task to remove the artifacts and impurities present in it. Pre-processing is mainly applied to improve the quality of the image and to reduce variations in the images that would unnecessarily complicate the subsequent processing steps. Three key objectives can be identified: noise removal, contrast improvement, illumination and staining correction. For noise removal, the most popular approaches have been well-established filters, such as mean and median filters, or Gaussian low-pass filtering. In addition, applying morphologic operations is very popular. For contrast improvement, contrast stretching techniques and histogram equalization in particular, have been the most popular approaches. For illumination and staining variations, color normalization techniques have been applied, including the popular use of grayscale colors [8, 16].

Experimentation and Result Analysis

Dataset

The dataset consists of segmented cells from the thin blood smear slide images from the Malaria Screener research activity. Giemsa-stained thin blood smear slides from 150 P. falciparum-infected and 50 healthy patients were collected and photographed at Chittagong Medical College Hospital, Bangladesh. The dataset contains a total of 27,558 cell images with equal instances of parasitized and uninfected cells.

Languages

All of the programming has been done on Python with the help packages such as scikit-learn, numpy, pandas, matplotlib, opencv and keras with tensorflow as the backend.

Image Processing

All the images were read in openCV. These were resized to 64x64. Parasitized images were saved with label 0 and uninfected cells were saved with label 1.

Data Visualization

Five parasitized and five uninfected cells were chosen randomly and visualized with matplotlib as shown in Fig 5 and Fig 6.

Figure 5. Parasitized cells

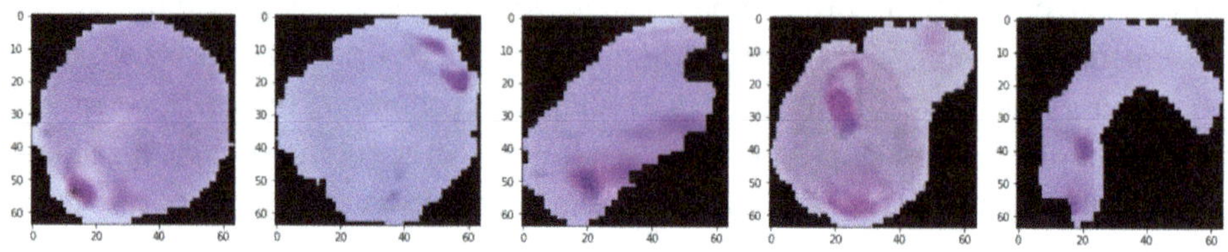

Figure 6. Uninfected cells

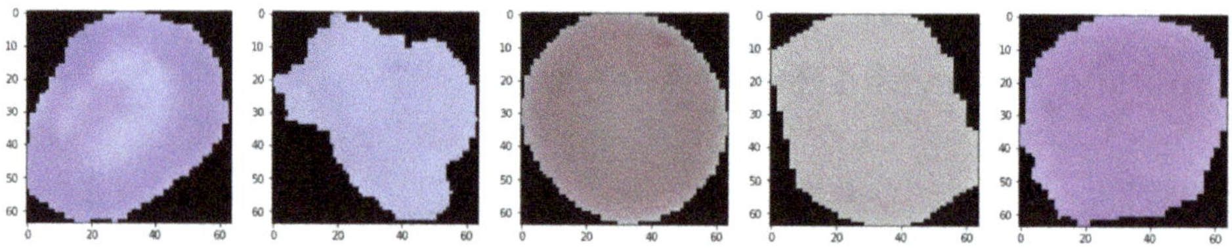

Applying Convolutional Neural Network

A convolution network was created from the following modules. A *sequential* CNN model was used to process the images. First, a *Convolution2D* layer was created and was followed by a *MaxPooling* layer. After passing through a *BatchNormalization* layer and a *Dropout* layer, another set of layers is appended. The combination of these layers are then *Flattened* and sent into the neural network. The model was compiled with stochastic gradient descent optimizer.

1. *Convolution2D*: This creates a two-dimensional convolution kernel. The kernel size was kept as 3x3.The number of kernel is set to 32 in both of convolutional layer of this model. Since the images comprise of RGB channels, the input size was set as (64, 64, 3). The activation function used was the RELU function.
2. *MaxPool2D*: This function is used to downscale the images. It was set to 2x2, so that an image of size 64x64 would be downscaled to 32x32.
3. *BatchNormalization*: This function normalizes the output of the previous activation option.

4. *Dropout*: This function selects some of the values at random and sets them to 0 so as to prevent overfitting of the model. The rate was kept at 0.2
5. *Flatten*: This function converts a n-dimensional matrix into a single array. In our model, it will flatten the image from a 64x64x3 matrix to a single array of 12,288. The output of this function acts as the input for the neural network.
6. *Dense*: This defines a dense interconnected neural network. Three layers of 512, 256 and 2 neurons were set up, with RELU as the activation functions of the first two and Sigmoid for the last layer.

Training and Test Results

Initially, our malaria dataset does not have pre-split data for training, validation, and testing. So we will need to perform the splitting the dataset ourselves. The dataset was divided into training and test sets in the ratio 4:1. A total of 50 epochs were used for train the model. Each epoch tales approximately 60 seconds on a single NVIDIA Tesla K80 GPU provided by Google Colab. 0.1 validations was also added so that the model trained on 90% training data and validated on 10% training data. An accuracy of 95.75% was obtained from the convolutional neural network.

Data Augmentation and Further Testing

The available dataset was only of 27,558 images, so to increase the amount of images the model trained on, data augmentation was used. Keras' ImageDataGenerator was used to rescale the image by dividing by 255, zooming in with a range of 0.3, flipping horizontally and rotating by 30. The model was then trained on this dataset. After data augmentation, an accuracy of 96.41% was achieved by the convolutional neural network Our malaria classifier model training/testing accuracy and loss plot shows that we've achieved high accuracy and low loss. The model isn't exhibiting signs of either over or underfitting (Fig.7).

CONCLUSION

The customized CNN model used in this research work to detect the presence of malaria parasites in the blood sample is achieving a state-of-the-art result. As we go through different literature in previous section, our proposed model definitely resulting better result than merely used image processing tools and technique based methodology. While comparing with some of the deep leaning based pre-trained models, even our proposed customized model giving better with data augmentation

Figure 7. Accuracy and Loss curve

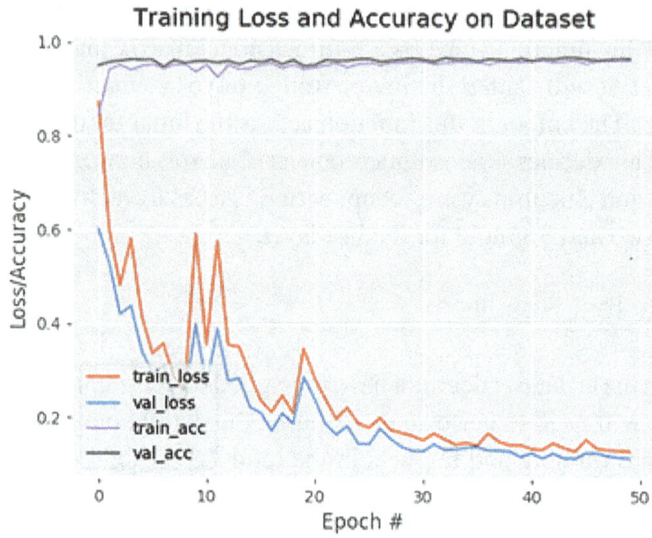

process. Hence we are reducing the complexity of training, validating the CNN model as compared to the pre-trained model, which takes lots of times in this aspect.

In this article, we learnt how to take convolutional deep learning and apply it in the field of medicine. Malaria is a life-threatening disease, if not detected in the early stage and malaria has become a true endemic in some areas of the world specifically in African regions with an epidemic in other parts of world. A dataset of 27,588 RBC cell images both parasitized and uninfected was used for this paper. A customized convolution neural network was applied, using the sigmoid and RELU functions for activation. The accuracy of the model was 95.75% before data augmentation and the accuracy increased to 96.41% with after this data augmentation process, as demonstrated a larger dataset increases the accuracy of the model. This shows the practicality of detecting malaria through deep learning applications.

REFERENCES

Bashir, A. (2017). Detection of malaria parasites using digital image processing. In *2017 International Conference on Communication, Control, Computing and Electronics Engineering (ICCCCEE)*. IEEE. 10.1109/ICCCCEE.2017.7867644

Ghate, D. A., & Jadhav, P. C. (2012). Automatic Detection of Malaria Parasite from Blood Images. *International Journal of Advancements in Computing Technology*, *1*(3), 66–71.

Jena, B., Nayak, G. K., & Saxena, S. (2019). Maximum Payload for Digital Image Steganography Obtained by Mixed Edge Detection Mechanism. In *2019 International Conference on Information Technology (ICIT)*. IEEE. 10.1109/ICIT48102.2019.00043

Khan. (2011). Content based image retrieval approaches for detection of malarial parasite in blood images. *International Journal of Biometrics and Bioinformatics, 5*(2), 97.

Krizhevsky, A., Sutskever, I., & Hinton, G. E. (2012). Imagenet classification with deep convolutional neural networks. *Advances in Neural Information Processing Systems*.

LeCun, Y., Bottou, L., Bengio, Y., & Haffner, P. (1998). Gradient-based learning applied to document recognition. *Proceedings of the IEEE, 86*(11), 2278–2324. doi:10.1109/5.726791

Pandit, P., & Anand, A. (2016). *Artificial neural networks for detection of malaria in RBCs*. arXiv preprint arXiv:1608.06627

Pattanaik, P. A., & Swarnkar, T. (2018). Comparative analysis of morphological techniques for malaria detection. *International Journal of Healthcare Information Systems and Informatics, 13*(4), 49–65. doi:10.4018/IJHISI.2018100104

Poostchi, M., Silamut, K., Maude, R. J., Jaeger, S., & Thoma, G. (2018). Image analysis and machine learning for detecting malaria. *Translational Research; the Journal of Laboratory and Clinical Medicine, 194*, 36–55. doi:10.1016/j.trsl.2017.12.004 PMID:29360430

Rajaraman, S., Antani, S. K., Poostchi, M., Silamut, K., Hossain, M. A., Maude, R. J., Jaeger, S., & Thoma, G. R. (2018). Pre-trained convolutional neural networks as feature extractors toward improved malaria parasite detection in thin blood smear images. *PeerJ, 6*, e4568. doi:10.7717/peerj.4568 PMID:29682411

South Sudan Medical Journal. (n.d.). Retrieved from http://www.southsudanmedicaljournal.com/archive/february-2011/malaria-in-south-sudan-1.-introduction-and-pathophysiology.html

Suradkar, P. T. (2013). Detection of malarial parasite in blood using image processing. *International Journal of engineering and innovative Technology, 2*(10), 124-126.

Toward Data Science. (n.d.). Retrieved from https://towardsdatascience.com/understanding-and-coding-a-resnet-in-keras-446d7ff84d33

Vala, H. J., & Baxi, A. (2013). A review on Otsu image segmentation algorithm. *International Journal of Advanced Research in Computer Engineering & Technology*, *2*(2), 387–389.

World Health Organization. (n.d.). *Malaria*. https://www.who.int/news-room/fact-sheets/detail/malaria

Yang, D., Subramanian, G., Duan, J., Gao, S., Bai, L., Chandramohanadas, R., & Ai, Y. (2017). A portable image-based cytometer for rapid malaria detection and quantification. *PLoS One*, *12*(6), e0179161. doi:10.1371/journal.pone.0179161 PMID:28594960

Chapter 10
Automatic Lung Tuberculosis Detection Model Using Thorax Radiography Image

Sudhir Kumar Mohapatra
https://orcid.org/0000-0003-3065-3881
Addis Ababa Science and Technology University, Ethiopia

ABSTRACT

Tuberculosis (TB) is a communal disease with high death and disease rates worldwide. The chest radiograph (CXR) is commonly used in diagnostic solutions for lung TB. Automatic computer-aided solutions to identify TB using CXRs and can advance the efficiency of the diagnostic of TB. In this chapter, an automatic TB detection model using CXR image is proposed. By identifying open issues include how detect the lung region automatically and what are the features, one can identify if a given CXR image is infected or normal using three public datasets such as Schengen, Montgomery Country (MC), and JSRT. The possible textural features of a lung object are obtained from the first-order and second-order gray level co-occurrence matrix (GLCM) statistical features. The performance of the proposed model was evaluated using accuracy, sensitivity, and specificity, and the model achieved AUC 91%, 62%, 71%, and 81% on Schengen, JSRT, MC, and combined datasets.

INTRODUCTION

The beginning of image processing methods times back to the late 1960s and early 1970s and was used in medical imaging, astronomy and remote earth resources observation. Meanwhile, digital image processing has been growing dynamically.

DOI: 10.4018/978-1-7998-5071-7.ch010

Copyright © 2021, IGI Global. Copying or distributing in print or electronic forms without written permission of IGI Global is prohibited.

Almost all application areas are now using digital image processing techniques ranging from robotic vision, product inspection to scientific research (Gonzales et al., 2002). In medical field image processing has a plays a vital role. Image processing is used for disease detection, identification, prevention and prediction.

The preventive medication can be characterized as primary, secondary, or else tertiary (McPhee et al.,2017). Primary prevention goals to eliminate or decrease disease threat factors or vulnerability. For example, vaccination, giving up or not starting something to the danger that used in activities or actions for both individual and public. Secondary prevention practices inspire timely discovery of disease or ancestor states at the subclinical stage. For example, Papsmear to detect certain biological infections, measurement of blood pressure. Such methods focus on the subclinical and the early clinical stage. Tertiary prevention measures contain the caution of established disease, with efforts made to restore to maximum function, minimalize the dangerous effects of a disease, and avoid disease correlated difficulties. Beyond these above levels of preventive medication, developing population centered information systems create it highly probable to combine prevention and care giving that new attention on the opportunities for realizing well and more reasonable delivery of healthiness (Starfield et al.,2008). The tool for supplementary examination is focus on the level of the competence where the action takes place (McPhee et al.,2017). Once there is no test center available, either for outpatient or inpatient care, fast analysis tests may be made obtainable (for malaria, HIV, etc.). A laboratory and material necessity is a system for certain diseases, such as TB.

The secondary prevention mechanism can be automated for early detection and diagnosis when if the occurrence of primary prevention is unsuccessful. According to the World Health Organization (WHO)(World Health Organization, 2013), TB is the second most communal cause of death in the globe along with HIV/AIDS. A great occurrence of TB anywhere in the world poses dangers to the healthiness of people elsewhere. While the application of current knowledge and methods for the diagnosis, handling, and prevention of TB can create an influence (Kwan et al,,2011). TB is a highly contagious, persistent disease considered by the development of tough grimy nodules, or tubercles because it spread by air. The disease is most often produced by the bacterium Mycobacterium TB; typically happens in the lungs, but it also can spread to the other organs like skeleton or bone. Since its signs and symptoms are simply confused with those of many other mainly respiratory diseases, TB can be hard to diagnose. Communal symptoms are cough, night sweats, chest pain, and breathlessness. 90% of those infected with TB mount a real immune response and certainly not develop the disease (H. Communities,2019).

In general and radiological point of view (Burrill et al., 2007), TB has exposed a renaissance in non-endemic residents in current years, a case that has indorsed to influences such as increased relocation or migration and the HIV widespread.

While the thorax is most often involved, TB may involve any of a number of organ systems (like respiratory, central nervous, cardiac, gastrointestinal, musculoskeletal, and genitourinary systems), and appropriate analysis of the disease is extremely risky and challenging, meanwhile, late action is allied with severe sickness.

TB is hard to diagnose since the signs and symptoms are alike to those produced by other diseases like lung cancer, pneumonia, allergic broncho pulmonaryaspergillosis, sarcoidosis, allergic alveolitis, pneumoconiosis, silicosis, anorexia nervosa, diabetes mellitus, hyperthyroidism, and Mediastinial.

The challenges during TB test or diagnosis and can be non-technical or technical (Dheda et al.,2013).

Technical aspects:-

- Antibody information in patients through active TB overlay with patients with presumed latent TB infection (a significant facet of TB control in low drain locations),
- Antigens can be differentially stated in different body sections,
- Overlap TB symptoms with others' diseases symptoms like coughing and night sweet,
- Test correctness may vary in HIV infested against uninfected individuals and individuals with pulmonary alongside extra-pulmonary TB,
- HIV infected individuals,
- Samples like saliva or sputum may not be willingly available, and
- Lack of appropriate or incomplete antigenic targets are some issues included under technical aspects.

Related Works

The section primary intention is image processing stages using CXR image. So the related work focused on the literature based on the segmentation, the feature extraction, and the overall TB screening using CADe.

First the relevant articles related to the lung segmentation using CXR image are reviewed. Karargyris et al.(2016),built a system that can bring about population screening in resource-limited areas wherein the use of CXR image by improving their previous similar work by joining texture and shape features of the image to notice pulmonary anomalies (Candemir et al.,2013). In order to accomplish the objective which is to build a TB screening system and improve their previous contribution, the researchers were identified three main agendas:

1. *Difficulty of tasks to construct a robust automated application used to detect TB and still it is an open research area.*

2. *The variability of image quality, size, shape, and texture of CXR image.*
3. *Texture information is not sufficient to screen and geometrical shape information is needed especially for classification that used to acquire overall performance.*

Similarly, Kiran et al.(2019), proposed a flexible lung segmentation techniques called Sauvola thresholding-Gaussian derivatives using CXR image. The technique is used four Gaussian derivatives responses. As reported, using Sauvola image thresholding which typically places of interest the inner area of the lung region. To highlight the lung region completely the Sauvola threshold image and gradient average image is combined then remove the noisy area such as trachea, clavicle region and outer body, XOR is applied between similar CXR average image and combined image are basic tasks. The proposed solution was tested on the two public datasets JSRT, Montgomery, and one private set and achieved 94.57%, 90.75%, and 65.25% accuracy respectively using Jaccard coefficient.

Next the focus is on extracted lung features from CXR image for the purpose of TB detection. Primary,Singh et al.(2019), implemented an approach for lung's feature extraction methodology from CXR image for TB detection, the study also examined the two pertinent image descriptors which are shape and texture using different descriptors and the Gray-Level Co-occurrence Matrix (GLCM) followed by the log Gabor filtering techniques. Finally, by applying SVM classifier, the ROC curve and confusion matrix of classifier shown an AUC of 0.98 and 0.96 on MC and Schengen dataset, respectively, with 100% specificity. But, limited instances were considered from the two datasets.

Likewise, Szilard et al.(2018), established a feature extraction methodology to find the optimum feature set from a greater pool of common image features, which is used originally for problems such as object recognition, image retrieval, etc. they used about seven different shape and texture descriptors like: Intensity Histogram, Gradient Magnitude Histogram, Shape Descriptor Histogram, etc. For performance assessment measures such as AUC and ACC were considered. Using a CNN classifier on two publicly available data collections, MC and the Shenzhen dataset, they achieved the AUC and ACC of 0.99 and 97.03%, respectively.

Lastly this section focus on the article related to general TB detection or screening mechanisms using CXR. Rajaraman et al.(2018), attained TB detection models using CXR image. The study was proposed two different proposals such as: feature extraction using local and global feature descriptors and classification using SVM, and feature extraction using pre-trained CNNs and classification using SVM. Similarly, Jaeger et al.(2018), developed new methodology for the purpose of implementing a timely diagnosis of drug-resistant TB. For the development, about 135 instance dataset was used aside patients' day to day follow-up as patient history attachment. Thus, the solution attained area under curve (AUC) >66% performance.

Table 1. Summary of Related Works

Author	Title	Performance	Dataset	Open Issue
Karargyris et al. (2016)	Combination of texture and shape features to detect pulmonary abnormalities in digital chest X-rays	AUC 85.4%	Shenzhen and JSRT datasets	Manual segmentation made by Experts
Kiran et al. (2019)	Chest X-ray segmentation using Sauvola thresholding and Gaussian derivatives responses	AUC 94.57%, 90.75%, and 65.25% on three different datasets	JSRT, MC, and one private set	Not attractive because of overlapping with other organs like trachea the obvious case
Singh et al.(2019)	Tuberculosis Detection Using Shape and Texture Features of Chest X-Rays	AUC of 0.98 and 0.96 on MC and Schengen dataset	Part of MC and Schengen dataset	Selected images, they may ignored low quality images. Because standard datasets are prepared intentionally by adding images with different defects by expertise.
Szilard et al.(2018)	Feature selection for automatic tuberculosis screening in frontal chest radiographs	AUC and ACC of 0.99 and 97.03%, respectively	MC and Schengen dataset	Applied lung model for best fitting for the segmentation task, thus, the performance is depend on the lung model
Rajaraman et al. (2018)	A novel stacked generalization of models for improved TB detection in chest radiographs	Variable	JSRT, Montgomery and others two from Kenya and India a total of 2073	Used manual boundary box in order to get ROI and this may not effective for image with improper acquisition.
Jaeger et al.(2018)	Detecting drug-resistant (DR) tuberculosis in chest radiographs	AUC up to 66% among drug-resistant cases	The 135 cases consist of 45% sensitive (61) and 54% DR (74) cases	Too low performance even if supported by patient history. Small dataset and limited coverage or location.

Proposed Model

The typical image processing steps may works for image processing application but in medical the challenge is different. Unlike the normal image acquisition mechanism like photo camera, medical imaging is very tedious task and the image will be interference by different human organs. Thus, the image processing task in medical image processing is more challenging. Based on the aim of this chapter i.e. TB detection model using CXR image, all digital image processing stages are accumulated as shown in Figure 1.

Next the following subsections will discuss in details about the indivisual stages of the proposed model.

Figure 1. The Proposed Model

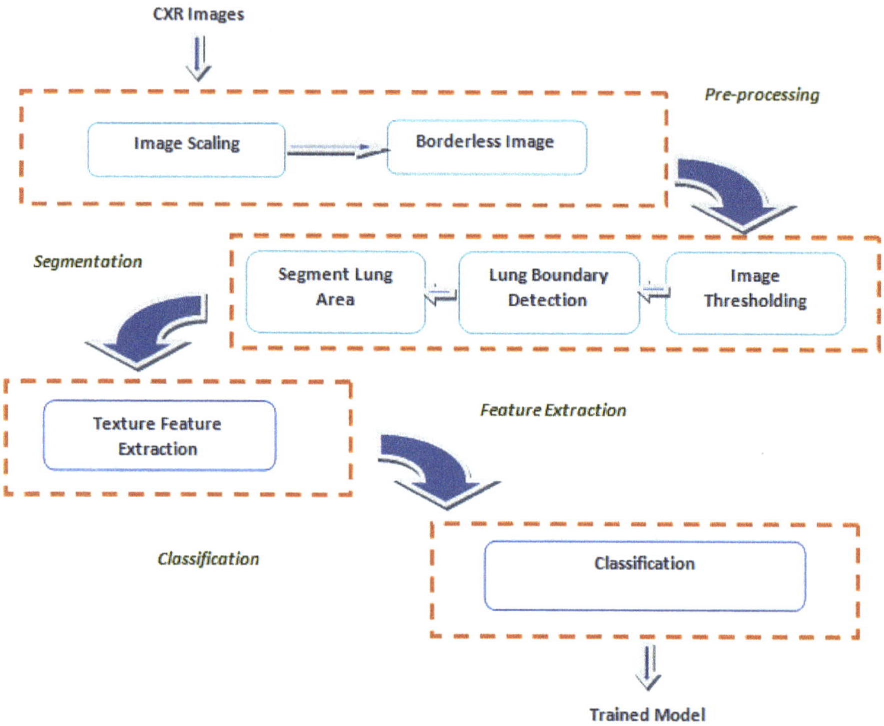

Preprocessing

Each dataset have different resolution, even if under the same dataset the resolutions between images are different. Therefore, image normalization should be attained. The preprocessing section does basic and intensive tasks such as: image scaling from variable resolution to one uniform size removing non-zero pixels which are connected with the border, etc.. In most of articles, the normalization task shown that the image normalization is to low up to 128 x 128 to attain best performance during implementation, especially, in medical image analysis. But, if the work is on the statistical or textural feature, too low resolution or size is not effective. Thus, to achieve the intended result from this study the images are normalized to 1024 x 1024.

Detection of Lung Region

At this level the majority of the preprocessing tasks are over, but, the approximate lung area is detected. Furthermore, in order to sharpen the lung objects (left and right side lungs) from CXR image, object sharpening algorithms is needed which includes: dilation and erosion (Van Den Boomgaard et al.,1992). Using Matlab image processing toolbox, built-in functions *imdilate*, and *imerode* are taken for the object sharpening.

Segmentation

Segmentation of CXR images has several challenges such as: the distortion produced by the medical or personal equipment, poor contrast, diverse size of lungs and basic shape varieties due to an infection or age as shown in Figure 2.

Figure 2. Some distorted images from the datasets

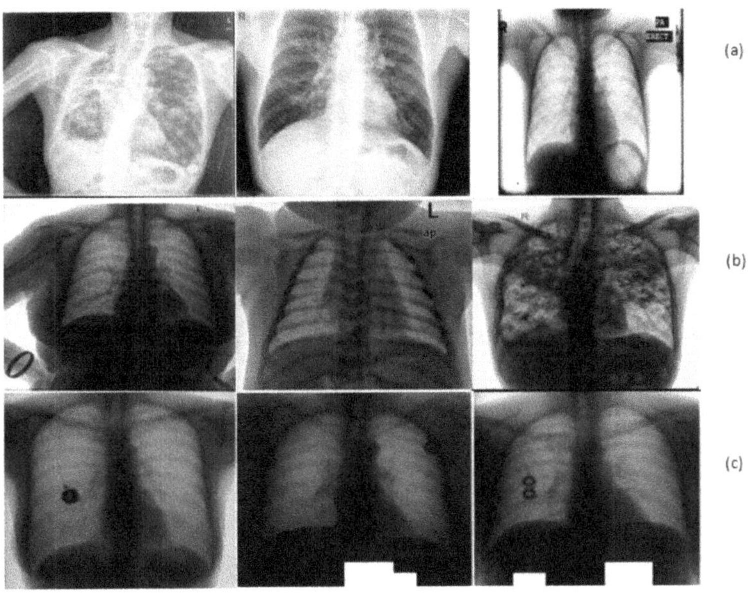

The graphical view of some of the challenges is shown in Figure 2, labeled as (a), (b) and (c) that are sampled from MC, Shenzhen and JSRT dataset respectively.

Usually, the input CXR image contains both foreground i.e. lung region and background information. To remove the background information that are lighter than the neighboring from a given image, researchers were proposed several solutions. But, using gray-level image the extraction of the foreground information is challenging. In CXR image most of the background information are connected to the border.

In this proposed model, the clear border algorithm is applied (Soille, 2013) . This algorithm is used to destroy the structures that are brighter than their surrounds which are associated to the image border. Due to its implementation, using Matlab image processing toolbox, the input can be either binary or an intensity image and the output is binary or intensity respectively. To make the removal of information from the image, there are two possible connectivity in 2d image: 4 or 8 and the default is 8, but in 3d image 6, 18 and 26are possible connectivity and the default is 26. In this chapter, the default connectivity in 2d i.e. 8 is applied. The process of extracting the lung objects from CXR image, image thresholding methods was applied using both global i.e. Otsu thresholding (Otsu, 1979; Bradley et al.,2007) and local thresholding methods independently, then after, the result with best fitting is used for further implementation processes as an input. In CXR, it is difficult to isolate out lung fields using pure pixel-based approaches. In the Segmentation field, there are many techniques are there that used to segment the images. Thresholding centered on visual appearance does not work due to extremely mingled intensities. In above scenarios, the relative lung objects are detected. Here, the actual lung area is detected using the overlapping technique to extract the lung area from the background.

Textural Feature Extraction

Obviously the textural profile of the normal and abnormal images are relatively different in depth of their gray-level. Especially in CXR images, i.e. the abnormality can be expressed by depth of the actual color than the normal one, because, parts of the organs could be affected by the infections like lung TB in lung organ. In this proposed model, the texture of a segmented region is analyzed using different statistical methods which are a combination of first-order and second-order textural features extraction parameters. Texture analysis methods can be categorized into statistical, structural, transform and model-based. The effect of basic statistical methods clues to high representations of textures in an image and the gray-level histogram labels the texture of an image. The proposed model adapted the textural feature analysis techniques with ten parameters which are the first five from the first-order and another five also from the grey level co-occurrence matrix (GLCM) features extraction parameters applied as described below.

The statistical technique of considering the texture of an image is that it reflects pixel phenomenon relationship with grey level. The GCLM was primary proposed (Haralick et al.,1973) with four second-order parameters such as contrast, energy, correlation and entropy then it enriched (Soh et al., 1999) by adding extra feature extraction up to 22 parameters. This GCLM technique also adapted in many technical procedures starting from image segmentation to textural feature analysis (Tuceryan et al.,1998; Hiremath et al.,2007; Palanivel et al.,2012). The texture features using GLCM are determined by seeing the rate of pixel pairs with the values which agrees the grey level in spatial connection of an image and extracting the factors from the matrix (Tsaneva et al.,2008).As proposed on consecutive articles (Karargyris et al.,2016) on textural feature extraction methods i.e. GLCM, beside the above five main parameters of GLCM, this study considered and used the seventeen GLCM parameters namely: the contrast, correlation, cluster prominence, cluster shade, difference-entropy, difference-variance, dissimilarity, energy, entropy, homogeneity, maximum probability, information measure of correlation, sum average, sum entropy, sum of squares: variance and sum variance. Hence, parameters except the main are second-order parameters that are taken based on the main parameters of the GLCM.

Classification

The aim of this study is to distinguish the lung area is infected by TB or not using CXR image i.e. need to acquire two classes which are infected and non-infected case. Among classifiers which are reported by researchers (Kotsiantis et al.,2006), the Support Vector Machine (SVM)(Hears et al.,1998) which is restricted to consider two-classes is selected. SVM, which is a supervised learning algorithm, is used as a classifier in this study to detect CXR with TB manifestations.

The SVM produces hyperplane with principal margin to differentiate samples within two classes which are either normal or abnormal. In order to classify then train the machine for this study and acquire the SVM classification algorithm, the Matlab Classification Learner is considered.

In order to evaluate the performance of the proposed model, the dataset is segmented in to two subsets: train and test sets. Using cross-validation (Golub et al.,1979), the k-folds technique was used i.e. 10-folds, because each instance has a chance to consider as in test and train set in different occasion.

Experiments and Results

Based on the specified propped model in section 3, lets discuss step by step implementation events of the proposed model staring from the image preprocessing task to evaluation of the model. As mentioned in the proposed model, each step has its own separate sub processes and in, process and out sessions. Therefore, in this section, the implementation of the proposed model at each basic image processing steps is shown how and what look like.

Dataset Preparation

The CXRs dataset is the only data that can be used in this proposed model. The two public datasets reported are considered (Jaeger et al.2014). The first one is the

Montgomery County chest X-ray set (MC) has 138 frontal chest X-rays with the size of either 4,020×4,892 or 4,892×4,020 pixels and Portable Network Graphics (PNG) format as 12-bit gray level images, which 80 are normal cases and 58 are cases with signs of TB. Also, the second set is the Shenzhen chest X-ray set has 662 frontal chest X-rays with PNG format and the size can vary, but approximately 3K × 3K pixels.

Among the datasets, the third dataset i.e. JSRT is cannot be access directly in Matlab unlike others two. Because, the dataset or each image was formatted with IMG type. Due to this, the image slicing task was done and used PNG image format with an appropriate resolution (2048 x 2048). The process was yielded as shown in Figure 3 below that the sliced, rotated but mirrored and un-mirrored images labeled as (a), (b) and (c) respectively.

Figure 3. Slicing image in JSRT dataset

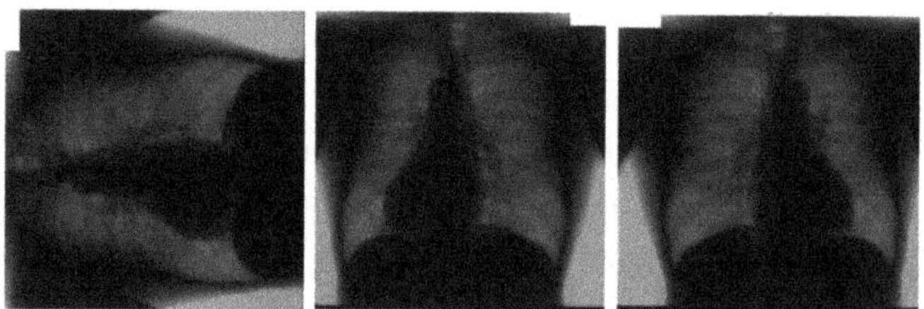

(a) (b) (c)

Preprocessing

First all the images should be standardized. Including the obtained JSRT sliced images, all images are normalized to the size 1024 x 1024 using Matlab built-in imresize function. Subsequently, the removal of lighter information by considering as background information which are connected with the border is applied. In this case, the Matlab image processing toolbox, explicitly, imclear border was used with 4 connectivity. In, the sample images are shown after normalization and removal of bordered pixel values, the left side column is the original image and the right side also the borderless version of each corresponding image: (a), (b) and (c) from JSRT, Shenzhen and MC dataset respectively.

Thus, with the obtained borderless intensity image from the previous task the intensity image was changed to binary using imbinarize function with three different threshold values which are 0.01, 0.001, and Otsu threshold algorithm independently (Otsu, 1979; Cheremkhin et al.,2019). Then, based on best fit selection, the expected

Figure 4. Sample Image from Each Dataset

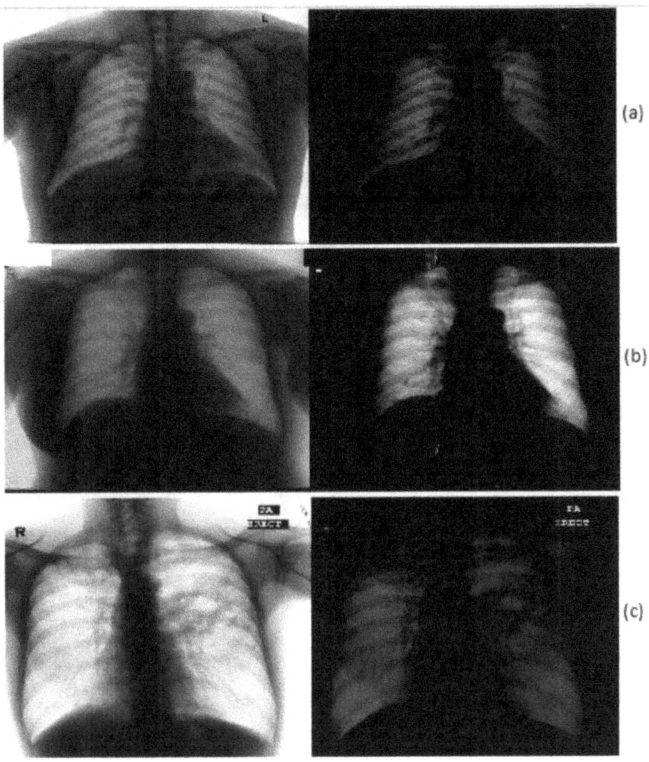

lung objects are filtered using Matlab bwareafilt by passing value 2 to select 2 top objects only. Here, the selected objects may contain a hole like area surrounded by somewhere by the object. The hole surrounded by the lung object is definitely the lung part which it may lose its intensity by infection and distortion. To tackle such problems the hole fill function which is imfill is applied.

The Figure 5 shown below is tabulated as the rows: (1), (2) and (3) are represented sample image from datasets Shenzhen, JSRT and MC respectively and the columns represents the original image, borderless, binaries then thresholding with local threshold value 0.01, reopen the binary image with two biggest objects among objects, another local threshold value 0.001 and the last one is global Otsu's threshold method i.e. 'adaptive' using the same input image respectively.

Detection of Lung Region

Now the lung objects are clearly identified but the objects' boundary may not sharpen. In order to keep the edge sharpen of the expected lung region, the imdilate

Figure 5. Image binarization and thresholding with different threshold values

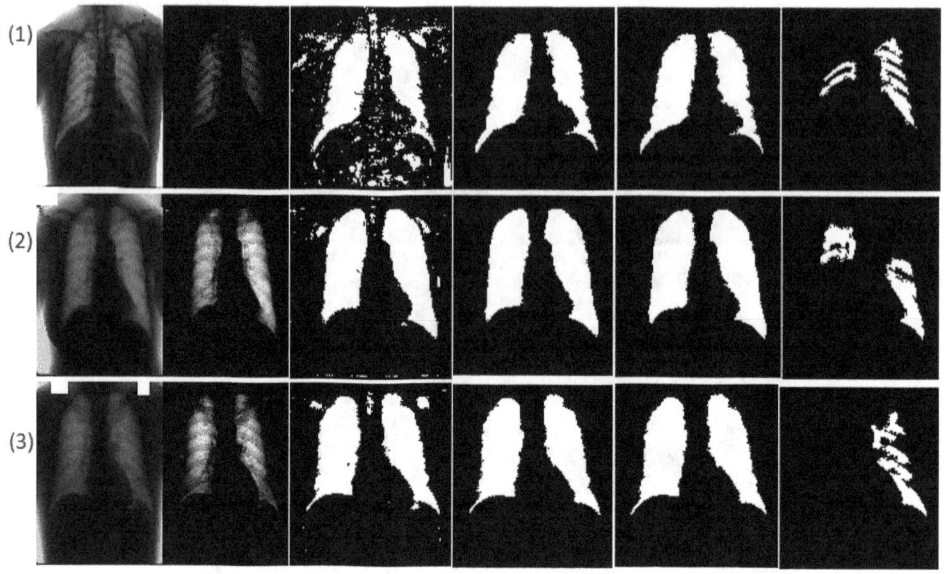

is applied. The Figure 6 shown below is tabulated as the rows: (1), (2) and (3) are represented sample image from datasets Shenzhen, JSRT and MC respectively and

Figure 6. Sharpening lung area using image dilation technique

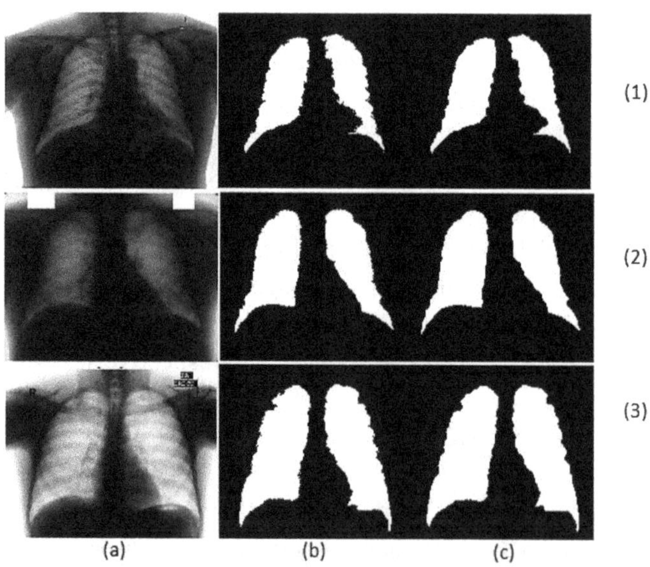

the columns: (a), (b) and (c) are also represented the original image, the detected objects and sharpened or dilated image respectively.

Segmentation

The segmentation is a process of taking a desired object from an object. Shortly, it is a process of filtering desired object and remove unwanted area i.e. treated as background information. The background of detected lung image is in binary format with while color. The aim of the process is extracting the white equivalent region from the original intensity image with the actual intensity value at detected region only otherwise make it 0 or black. The Figure 7 shown below is tabulated as the rows: (1), (2) and (3) are represented sample image from datasets Shenzhen, JSRT and MC respectively and the columns represents the original image and segmented image respectively.

Figure 7. Sample segmented images from all datasets

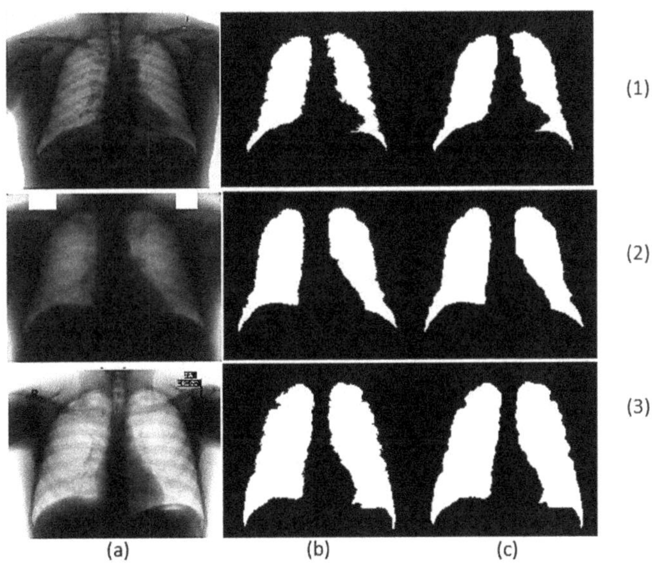

Feature Extraction

In this chapter, the textural feature extraction technique was applied using Matlab image processing toolbox, specifically, graycomatrix which is a GLCM function includes all the four second-order statistics parameters as already describe in section

3 and Five features from first-order statistics totally 9 parameters was extracted. During the implementation the first and the second order statistical features was extracted. In the case of the first-order i.e. Kurtosis, skewness, mean, variance and standard deviation and the Matlab hardcode is implemented, calculated, and stored in local permanent storage with excel (.xlsx) format and the second-order or GLCM features are also calculated using Matlab graycomatrix function,the default file type is struct and it needs some conversion task from struct to array then excel as shown the Matlab code in as stated. The sample extracted features are shown in Figure 8.

Figure 8. Sample features extracted data

	A	B	C	D	E	F	G	H	I	J	K	L	M	N
1	Mean	STD	Variance	Kurtosis	Skewness	Contrast_LungA	Contrast_LungB	Correlation_LungA	Correlation_Lu	Energy_LungA	Energy_LungB	Homogeneity_Lu	Homogeneity_Lu	Indicator
2	0.801703	0.210457	0.01109	415.9765	-6.24571	0.078465907	0.082901654	0.970828173	0.969179063	0.642606095	0.640978152	0.972199279	0.972442699	0
3	0.82543	0.227558	0.012155	225.3785	-7.16978	0.063610376	0.068326235	0.974756234	0.972884746	0.681749034	0.680331837	0.977455617	0.977410291	0
4	0.778831	0.236393	0.013601	372.9256	-10.0232	0.071795019	0.074104984	0.969787586	0.968815518	0.609417018	0.607893706	0.97086419	0.971416261	0
5	0.792253	0.231673	0.012847	124.2969	-2.9146	0.070129696	0.077092207	0.975311422	0.972860328	0.632309639	0.630383234	0.975167396	0.974639867	0
6	0.758869	0.24077	0.014304	99.97811	-4.85655	0.077790568	0.083933848	0.974369946	0.972345889	0.584956074	0.583378721	0.971935075	0.972073053	0
7	0.788416	0.225239	0.012458	280.9971	-6.42384	0.078039983	0.084662906	0.972141574	0.969777347	0.626338264	0.624631326	0.97260242	0.972700027	0
8	0.743512	0.228463	0.013232	179.3313	-5.24848	0.063621887	0.062965734	0.97111191	0.971409842	0.560485147	0.559486595	0.97095876	0.971467423	0
9	0.826325	0.216961	0.010818	270.5043	-6.07876	0.056732282	0.055611834	0.975274114	0.975762444	0.681674799	0.681019414	0.976366106	0.977328751	0
10	0.804154	0.21892	0.011444	230.4832	-7.07903	0.047594106	0.049148152	0.973463867	0.972597407	0.649269177	0.64785892	0.977863154	0.977121945	0
11	0.857297	0.224601	0.011272	108.859	-4.83975	0.053806454	0.055655961	0.97195637	0.970992418	0.733578698	0.732499465	0.980780588	0.981467758	0
12	0.79551	0.223895	0.012242	251.8641	-6.39153	0.072848317	0.075469092	0.971597163	0.970575349	0.634415232	0.633175515	0.971985198	0.972411921	0
13	0.74681	0.236798	0.013373	249.5024	-9.10593	0.088231457	0.103794943	0.973298872	0.968588958	0.569079965	0.566322679	0.970053033	0.967441132	0
14	0.809267	0.208155	0.010643	201.7783	-5.56495	0.07609071	0.073214765	0.972974289	0.97399576	0.654717788	0.654299179	0.97262992	0.97485179	0
15	0.816236	0.227463	0.012127	251.4172	-5.71216	0.070626607	0.071246307	0.972292034	0.972048915	0.666469836	0.665500312	0.974045349	0.975143334	0
16	0.786554	0.229515	0.012884	515.1321	-8.30419	0.073017152	0.071844902	0.969050628	0.969547503	0.621364137	0.620566467	0.971595328	0.97315457	0
17	0.839931	0.228614	0.011886	396.3559	-9.55878	0.063942289	0.064517862	0.972268464	0.97201884	0.704219769	0.703320374	0.97769432	0.978698454	0
18	0.772927	0.219998	0.012181	292.5407	-7.63806	0.076211581	0.079952803	0.971192263	0.969778092	0.601285603	0.599785542	0.969062008	0.969387527	0
19	0.734484	0.228315	0.012717	119.8843	-4.70869	0.091287748	0.101394804	0.973556834	0.970629141	0.548460059	0.546252997	0.967338888	0.966507585	0

The Performance Evaluation

Of course in order to evaluate the performance of the proposed model, the dataset should be segmented in to two subset: train and test sets. Using cross-validation (Golub et al.,1979), the k-folds technique was used i.e. 10-folds, because each instance has a chance to consider as in test and train set in different occasion.

Result

In previous sub-sections, the implementation of proposed mode is done. Of course each major step has its own result then the overall result can characterized by the performance measurement given below.

The proposed model was implemented using three previously discussed dataset. Each dataset has its own and different intensity value than others two. This implication gives different results between datasets and a total set also affect the performance of the model. Statistically, Table 2 shows the row facts regarding truly-detected and incorrectly-detected i.e. among 1047 instances 780 instances are detected as same

Table 2. Confusion Matrix of SVM on Each Dataset

Dataset		Positive	Negative	Total
Shenzhen	Normal	280	46	662
	Abnormal	64	272	
JSRT	Normal	23	70	247
	Abnormal	20	134	
MC	Normal	62	18	138
	Abnormal	26	32	
Total	Normal	375	124	1047
	Abnormal	143	405	

as human expertise and the remaining 267 are detected incorrectly which are from normal and abnormal cases . When analyzing the true and false detection on each dataset, gives different result and one set can achieve better performance than other.

Depend on the above statistical information obtained by the SVM classification, the overall performance is better on Schengen dataset, then MC, and JSRT is slightly low than others. Table 3 present the details of SVM classifier.

Table 3. Classification Performance Analysis on Each Dataset

Dataset	AUC	Accuracy (%)	Sensitivity (%)	Specificity (%)
Shenzhen	0.91	83.4	86	81
JSRT	0.62	63.6	25	87
MC	0.71	68.1	78	55
Combined	0.81	74.5	75	74

The following Figure 9 shown the overall performance characterized by AUC on Schengen dataset.

Figure 9. AUC on Shenzhen Dataset

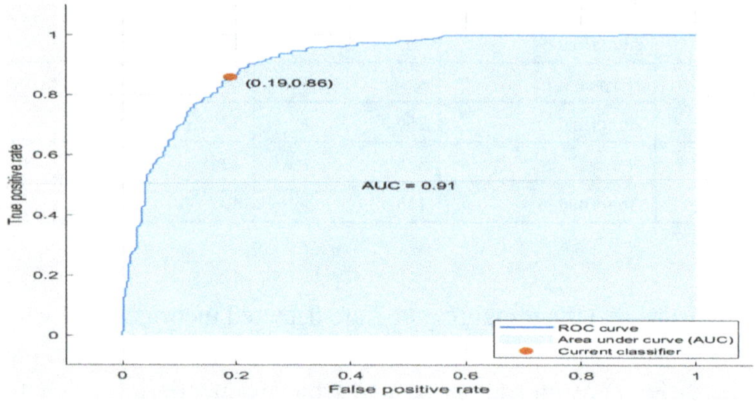

The following Figure 10 shown the overall performance characterized by AUC on JSRT dataset.

Figure 10. Class based AUC on JSRT Dataset

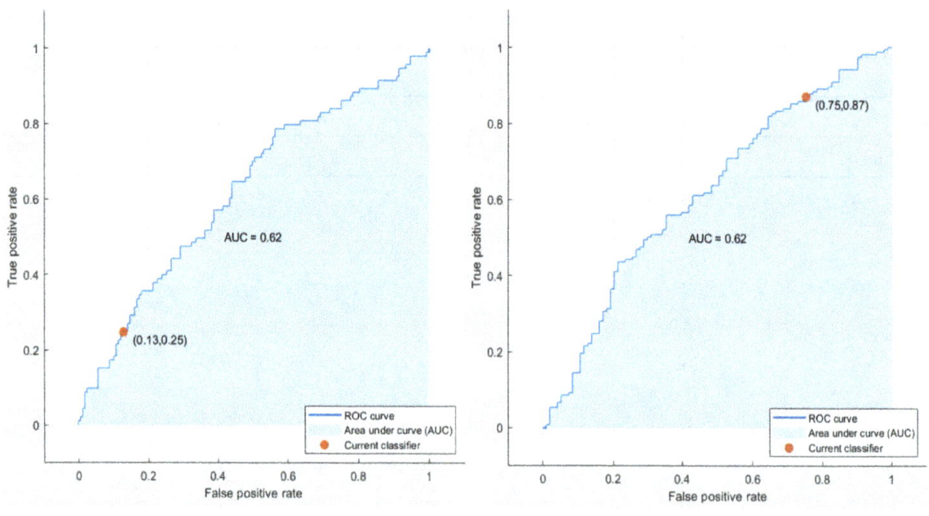

The following Figure 11 shown the overall performance characterized by AUC on combined dataset.

Figure 11. AUC on a combination use of all datasets

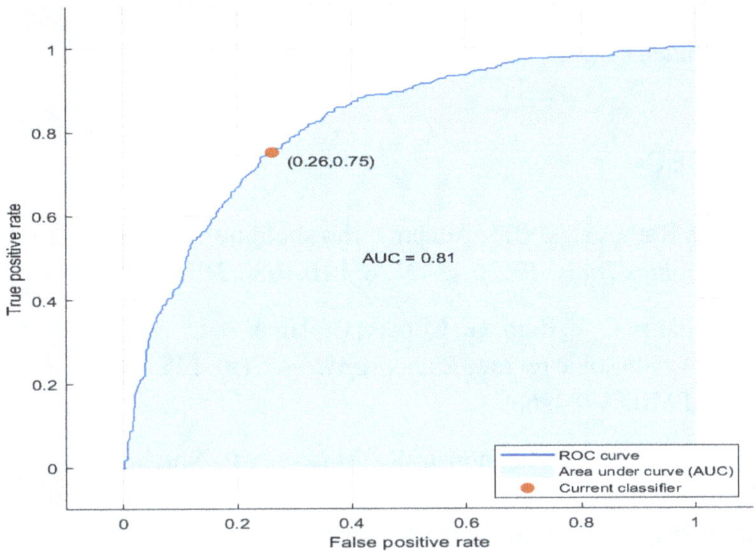

CONCLUSION

TB is one of dominant infectious disease in the world, especially, in developing countries. Like its domination, the detection or diagnosis of TB is tedious step in medical service. When the occurrences of dependent cases like HIV/AIDS, the diagnosis make it more difficult. Nowadays, like any service, medical services are supporting by computer systems, CADe or CADx in medical term with the input of patient medical information and/or medical imaging. The CADx system may accept one or both of the inputs during the implementation.

In order to support lung TB detection using CXR image in health sector, this model is proposed. Based on the survey of the related work, the open issues are identified which may respond by researchers as well. Similarly, the proposed system initiate a novel approach, especially at lung area detection by creating the background portion of CXR image.

By identifying open issues include how detect the lung region automatically, and what are the features can identify a given CXR image is infected or normal are considered using three public datasets such as Schengen, Montgomery Country (MC), and JSRT set a total of 1047 CXR images. As part of model proposal a new approach which is clear the intensities that interconnected with the border CXR image then continue to normal and further processes in image processing. The possible textural features of a lung object is obtained from the first-order and second-order Gray Level co-occurrence Matrix (GLCM) statistical features. The performance of the proposed model was evaluated using accuracy, sensitivity and specificity. The proposed model was achieved AUC 91%, 62%, 71%, and 81% on Schengen, JSRT, MC and Combined set.

REFERENCES

Bradley, D., & Roth, G. (2007). Adaptive thresholding using the integral image. *Journal of Graphics Tools*, *12*(2), 13–21. doi:10.1080/2151237X.2007.10129236

Burrill, J., Williams, C. J., Bain, G., Conder, G., Hine, A. L., & Misra, R. R. (2007). Tuberculosis: A radiologic review. *Radiographics*, *27*(5), 1255–1273. doi:10.1148/rg.275065176 PMID:17848689

Candemir, S., Jaeger, S., Palaniappan, K., Musco, J. P., Singh, R. K., Xue, Z., ... McDonald, C. J. (2013). Lung segmentation in chest radiographs using anatomical atlases with nonrigid registration. *IEEE Transactions on Medical Imaging*, *33*(2), 577–590. doi:10.1109/TMI.2013.2290491 PMID:24239990

Cheremkhin, P. A., & Kurbatova, E. A. (2019). Comparative appraisal of global and local thresholding methods for binarisation of off-axis digital holograms. *Optics and Lasers in Engineering*, *115*, 119–130. doi:10.1016/j.optlaseng.2018.11.019

Communities, H. (2019). *Basics of Tuberculosis*. http://www. healthcommunities. com /tuberculosis/pathology.shtml

Dheda, K., Ruhwald, M., Theron, G., Peter, J., & Yam, W. C. (2013). Point?of?care diagnosis of tuberculosis: Past, present and future. *Respirology (Carlton, Vic.)*, *18*(2), 217–232. doi:10.1111/resp.12022 PMID:23190246

Golub, G. H., Heath, M., & Wahba, G. (1979). Generalized cross-validation as a method for choosing a good ridge parameter. *Technometrics*, *21*(2), 215–223. doi: 10.1080/00401706.1979.10489751

Gonzales, R. C., & Woods, R. E. (2002). *Digital image processing*. Academic Press.

Haralick, R. M., Shanmugam, K., & Dinstein, I. H. (1973). Textural features for image classification. *IEEE Transactions on Systems, Man, and Cybernetics*, *SMC-3*(6), 610–621. doi:10.1109/TSMC.1973.4309314

Hearst, M. A., Dumais, S. T., Osuna, E., Platt, J., & Scholkopf, B. (1998). Support vector machines. *IEEE Intelligent Systems & their Applications*, *13*(4), 18–28. doi:10.1109/5254.708428

Hiremath, P. S., & Pujari, J. (2007). Content Based Image Retrieval based on Color, Texture and Shape features using Image and its complement. *International Journal of Computer Science and Security*, *1*(4), 25–35.

Jaeger, S., Candemir, S., Antani, S., Wáng, Y. X. J., Lu, P. X., & Thoma, G. (2014). Two public chest X-ray datasets for computer-aided screening of pulmonary diseases. *Quantitative Imaging in Medicine and Surgery*, *4*(6), 475. PMID:25525580

Jaeger, S., Juarez-Espinosa, O. H., Candemir, S., Poostchi, M., Yang, F., Kim, L., Ding, M., Folio, L. R., Antani, S., Gabrielian, A., Hurt, D., Rosenthal, A., & Thoma, G. (2018). Detecting drug-resistant tuberculosis in chest radiographs. *International Journal of Computer Assisted Radiology and Surgery*, *13*(12), 1915–1925. doi:10.100711548-018-1857-9 PMID:30284153

Karargyris, A., Siegelman, J., Tzortzis, D., Jaeger, S., Candemir, S., Xue, Z., Santosh, K. C., Vajda, S., Antani, S., Folio, L., & Thoma, G. R. (2016). Combination of texture and shape features to detect pulmonary abnormalities in digital chest X-rays. *International Journal of Computer Assisted Radiology and Surgery*, *11*(1), 99–106. doi:10.100711548-015-1242-x PMID:26092662

Kiran, M., Ahmed, I., Khan, N., & Reddy, A. G. (2019). Chest X-ray segmentation using Sauvola thresholding and Gaussian derivatives responses. *Journal of Ambient Intelligence and Humanized Computing*, *10*(10), 4179–4195. doi:10.100712652-019-01281-7

Kotsiantis, S. B., Zaharakis, I. D., & Pintelas, P. E. (2006). Machine learning: A review of classification and combining techniques. *Artificial Intelligence Review*, *26*(3), 159–190. doi:10.100710462-007-9052-3

Kwan, C. K., & Ernst, J. D. (2011). HIV and tuberculosis: A deadly human syndemic. *Clinical Microbiology Reviews*, *24*(2), 351–376. doi:10.1128/CMR.00042-10 PMID:21482729

McPhee, S. J., Papadakis, M. A., & Tierney, L. M. (2017). *Current Medical Diagnosis & Treatment*. McGraw-Hill Medical New York.

Otsu, N. (1979). A threshold selection method from gray-level histograms. *IEEE Transactions on Systems, Man, and Cybernetics*, *9*(1), 62–66. doi:10.1109/TSMC.1979.4310076

Palanivel, M., & Duraisamy, M. (2012). Adaptive Color Texture Image Segmentation Using α-Cut Implemented Interval Type-2 Fuzzy C-Means. *Res. J. Appl. Sci*, *7*(5), 258–265. doi:10.3923/rjasci.2012.258.265

Rajaraman, S., Candemir, S., Xue, Z., Alderson, P. O., Kohli, M., Abuya, J., Thoma, G. R., & Antani, S. (2018, July). A novel stacked generalization of models for improved TB detection in chest radiographs. In *2018 40th Annual International Conference of the IEEE Engineering in Medicine and Biology Society (EMBC)* (pp. 718-721). IEEE. 10.1109/EMBC.2018.8512337

Singh, N., & Hamde, S. (2019). Tuberculosis detection using shape and texture features of chest X-rays. In *Innovations in Electronics and Communication Engineering* (pp. 43–50). Springer. doi:10.1007/978-981-13-3765-9_5

Soh, L. K., & Tsatsoulis, C. (1999). Texture analysis of SAR sea ice imagery using gray level co-occurrence matrices. *IEEE Transactions on Geoscience and Remote Sensing*, *37*(2), 780–795. doi:10.1109/36.752194

Soille, P. (2013). *Morphological image analysis: principles and applications*. Springer Science & Business Media.

Starfield, B., Hyde, J., Gérvas, J., & Heath, I. (2008). The concept of prevention: A good idea gone astray? *Journal of Epidemiology and Community Health*, *62*(7), 580–583. doi:10.1136/jech.2007.071027 PMID:18559439

Tsaneva, M. (2008). Texture features for segmentation of satellite images. *Cybernetics and Information Technologies*, *8*(3), 73–85.

Tuceryan, M., & Jain, A. K. (1998). The Handbook of Pattern Recognition and Computer Vision, chapter 2.1. Texture Analysis. World Scientific Co.

Vajda, S., Karargyris, A., Jaeger, S., Santosh, K. C., Candemir, S., Xue, Z., Sameer, A., & Thoma, G. (2018). Feature selection for automatic tuberculosis screening in frontal chest radiographs. *Journal of Medical Systems*, *42*(8), 146. doi:10.100710916-018-0991-9 PMID:29959539

Van Den Boomgaard, R., & Van Balen, R. (1992). Methods for fast morphological image transforms using bitmapped binary images. *CVGIP. Graphical Models and Image Processing*, *54*(3), 252–258. doi:10.1016/1049-9652(92)90055-3

World Health Organization. (2013). *Global tuberculosis report 2013*. World Health Organization.

Compilation of References

Aaron van den Oord, S. D. (2016). *WaveNet: A Generative Model for Raw Audio.* arXiv:1609.03499 [cs.SD]

Abobakr, Hossny, Abdelkader, & Nahavandi. (2018). *RGB-D Fall Detection via Deep Residual Convolutional LSTM Networks*. IEEE.

Abràmoff, M. D., Lou, Y., Erginay, A., Clarida, W., Amelon, R., Folk, J. C., & Niemeijer, M. (2016). Improved automated detection of diabetic retinopathy on a publicly available dataset through integration of deep learning. *Investigative Ophthalmology & Visual Science*, *57*(13), 5200–5206. doi:10.1167/iovs.16-19964 PMID:27701631

Aerts, HJ, Velazquez, ER, & Leijenaar, RT, etal. (2014). Decoding tumour phenotype by non invasive imaging using a quantitative radiomics approach. *Nature Communications*, *5*(4006), 1–8.

Agn, M., Puonti, O., afRosenschöld, P. M., Law, I., & Van Leemput, K. (2015). Brain tumor segmentation using a generative model with an RBM prior on tumor shape. In *BrainLes* (pp. 168–180). Springer.

Al-Daoud, E. (2010). Cancer diagnosis using modified fuzzy network. *Universal J. Comput. Sci.&Engg. Technol.*, *1*(2), 73–78.

Alex Krizhevsky, I. S. (2012). *Imagenet classification with deep convolutional*. Academic Press.

Altunay, Telatar, Erogul, & Aydur. (2009). A New Approach to urinary system dynamics problems: Evaluation and classification of uroflowmeter signals using artificial neural networks. *Expert Systems with Applications*, *36*(3), 4891–4895.

Ameer. (2019). Brain tumor classification using deep CNN features via transfer learning. *Computers in Biology and Medicine*, *111*, 103345. PMID:31279167

Angel, Arevalo, Judkins, Madabhushi, & Gonzalez. (n.d.). A method for Medulloblastoma Tumor Differentiation based on Convolutional Neural Networks and Transfer Learning. *Conference: Proc. SPIE 9681, 11th International Symposium on Medical Information Processing and Analysis*. DOI: 10.1117/12.2208825

Antony, J., McGuinness, K., O'Connor, N. E., & Moran, K. (2016). Quantifying radiographic knee osteoarthritis severity using deep convolutional neural networks. In *Proceedings of International Conference on Pattern Recognition (ICPR)* (pp. 1195-1200). IEEE. 10.1109/ICPR.2016.7899799

Avendi, M. R., Kheradvar, A., & Jafarkhani, H. (2016). A combined deep learning and deformable-model approach to fully automatic segmentation of the left ventricle in cardiac MRI. *Medical Image Analysis*, *30*, 108–119. doi:10.1016/j.media.2016.01.005 PMID:26917105

Ayala, G., León, T., & Zapater, V. (2005). Different averages of a fuzzy set with an application to vessel segmentation. *IEEE Transactions on Fuzzy Systems*, *13*(3), 384–393. doi:10.1109/TFUZZ.2004.839667

Badrinarayanan, V., & Kendall, A. (2017). *Segnet: A deep convolutional encoder-decoder architecture for image segmentation*. ieeexplore.ieee.org

Baessler, B., Mannil, M., Oebel, S., Maintz, D., Alkadhi, H., & Manka, R. (2018). Subacute and chronic left ventricular myocardial scar: Accuracy of texture analysis on nonenhanced cineMR images. *Radiology*, *286*(1), 103–112. doi:10.1148/radiol.2017170213 PMID:28836886

Bai, W., Sinclair, M., Tarroni, G., Oktay, O., Rajchl, M., Vaillant, G., Lee, A. M., Aung, N., Lukaschuk, E., Sanghvi, M. M., Zemrak, F., Fung, K., Paiva, J. M., Carapella, V., Kim, Y. J., Suzuki, H., Kainz, B., Matthews, P. M., Petersen, S. E., ... Rueckert, D. (2018). Automated cardiovascular magnetic resonance image analysis with fully convolutional networks. *Journal of Cardiovascular Magnetic Resonance*, *20*(65), 1–12. doi:10.118612968-018-0471-x PMID:30217194

Bakator & Radosav. (2018). Deep Learning and Medical Diagnosis: A Review of Literature. *Multimodal Technologies and Interact*, *2*, 47. doi:10.3390/mti2030047

Basha, S. S., & Prasad, K. S. (2009). Automatic detection of breast cancer mass in mammograms using morphological operators and fuzzy c—means Clustering. *Journal of Theoretical & Applied Information Technology*, *5*(6), 1–6.

Bashir, A. (2017). Detection of malaria parasites using digital image processing. In *2017 International Conference on Communication, Control, Computing and Electronics Engineering (ICCCCEE)*. IEEE. 10.1109/ICCCCEE.2017.7867644

Bello, G., Dawes, T. J., Duan, J., Biffi, C., de Marvao, A., Howard, L. S. G. E., Gibbs, J. S. R., Wilkins, M. R., Cook, S. A., Rueckert, D., & O'Regan, D. P. (2019). Deep learning cardiac motion analysis for human survival prediction. *Nat Mach Intell*, *1*(2), 95–104. doi:10.103842256-019-0019-2 PMID:30801055

Bhuvaneswari, P., & Therese, A. B. (2015). Detection of cancer in lung with k-nn classification using genetic algorithm. *Procedia Materials Science*, *10*, 433–440. doi:10.1016/j.mspro.2015.06.077

Bolboca. (2019). *Medical diagnosis tests: a test anatomy, phases and statistical treatment of data*. Hindawi.

Boykov, Y., Veksler, O., & Zabih, R. (2001). approximate energy minimization via graph cuts. *IEEE Transactions on Pattern Analysis and Machine Intelligence*, *23*(11), 1222–1239. doi:10.1109/34.969114

Bradley, D., & Roth, G. (2007). Adaptive thresholding using the integral image. *Journal of Graphics Tools*, *12*(2), 13–21. doi:10.1080/2151237X.2007.10129236

Bratt, A., Kim, J., Pollie, M., Beecy, A. N., Tehrani, N. H., Codella, N., Perez-Johnston, R., Palumbo, M. C., Alakbarli, J., Colizza, W., Drexler, I. R., Azevedo, C. F., Kim, R. J., Devereux, R. B., & Weinsaft, J. W. (2019). Machine learning derived segmentation of phase velocity encoded cardiovascular magnetic resonance for fully automated aortic flow quantification. *Journal of Cardiovascular Magnetic Resonance*, *21*(1), 1–11. doi:10.118612968-018-0509-0 PMID:30612574

Brosch, T., & Tam, R. (2013).Alzheimer's Disease Neuroimaging Initiative. Manifold learning of brain MRIs by deep learning. In *Proceedings of International Conference on Medical Image Computing and Computer-Assisted Intervention* (pp. 633-640). Springer.

Buckley, Brock, & Oliver.(2009). Interactive segmentation for manipulation in unstructured environments. *ICRA'09: Proceedings of the 2009 IEEE international conference on Robotics and Automation*.

Budoff, M. J., Dowe, D., Jollis, J. G., Gitter, M., Sutherland, J., Halamert, E., Scherer, M., Bellinger, R., Martin, A., Benton, R., Delago, A., & Min, J. K. (2008). Diagnostic performance of 64-multidetector row coronary computed tomographic angiography for evaluation of coronary artery stenosis in individuals without known coronary artery disease. *Journal of the American College of Cardiology*, *52*(21), 1724–1732. doi:10.1016/j.jacc.2008.07.031 PMID:19007693

Burlina, P., Freund, D. E., Joshi, N., Wolfson, Y., & Bressler, N. M. (2016, April). Detection of age-related macular degeneration via deep learning. In *2016 IEEE 13th International Symposium on Biomedical Imaging (ISBI)* (pp. 184-188). IEEE. 10.1109/ISBI.2016.7493240

Burrell, J. (2016). How the machine 'thinks': Understanding opacity in Machine Learning algorithms. *Big Data & Society*, 1-12.

Burrill, J., Williams, C. J., Bain, G., Conder, G., Hine, A. L., & Misra, R. R. (2007). Tuberculosis: A radiologic review. *Radiographics*, *27*(5), 1255–1273. doi:10.1148/rg.275065176 PMID:17848689

Cancer treatment center of America. (2020). *About lung cancer.* Retrieved from https://www.cancercenter.com/cancer-types/lung-cancer/symptoms

Candemir, S., Jaeger, S., Palaniappan, K., Musco, J. P., Singh, R. K., Xue, Z., ... McDonald, C. J. (2013). Lung segmentation in chest radiographs using anatomical atlases with nonrigid registration. *IEEE Transactions on Medical Imaging*, *33*(2), 577–590. doi:10.1109/TMI.2013.2290491 PMID:24239990

Cao, C. X. L. (2015). Look and think twice: Capturingtop-down visual attention with feedback convolutional neural networks. *Proceedings of the International Conference on Computer Vision (ICCV)*, 2956–2964.

Carneiro, G., & Nascimento, J. C. (2013). Combining multiple dynamic models and deep learning architectures for tracking the left ventricle endocardium in ultrasound data. *IEEE Transactions on Pattern Analysis and Machine Intelligence*, *35*(11), 2592–2607. doi:10.1109/TPAMI.2013.96 PMID:24051722

Catalogna, Cohen, Fishman, Halpern, Nevo, & Ben-Jacob. (2012). ANN based controller for gloucose monitoring during, clamp test. *PLoS One*, *7*, e44587.

Cesar, R. M., Jr., & Jelinek, H. F. (2003). Segmentation of retinal fundus vasculature in nonmydriatic camera images using wavelets. In J. S. Suri & S. Laxminarayan (Eds.), Angiography and Plaque Imaging: Advanced Segmentation Techniques (pp. 193–224). Academic Press.

Cetiner, Sari, & Aburas. (2009). Recognition of dengue disease patterns using artificial neural networks. *Proceedings of the 5th International Advanced Technologies Symposium (IATS'09)*, 359–362.

Chaudhuri, S., Chatterjee, S., Katz, N., Nelson, M., & Goldbaum, M. (1989). Detection of blood vessels in retinal images using two-dimensional matched filters. *IEEE Transactions on Medical Imaging*, *8*(3), 263–269. doi:10.1109/42.34715 PMID:18230524

Chen, H., Zhang, Y., & Zhang, W. (2017). Low-dose CT via convolutional neural network. *Biomed Opt Express*, *8*(2), 679-94.

Chen, Xu, Wong, Wong, & Liu. (2015). Glaucoma Detection based on Deep Convolutional Neural Network. *2015 37th Annual International Conference of the IEEE Engineering in Medicine and Biology Society (EMBC)*. Doi:10.1109/EMBC.2015.7318462

Cheng, X., Zhang, L., & Zheng, Y. (2018). Deep similarity learning for multimodal medical images. *Computer Methods in Biomechanics and Biomedical Engineering. Imaging & Visualization*, *6*(3), 248–252. doi:10.1080/21681163.2015.1135299

Chen, L.-C., G. P. (2015). Semantic image segmentation with deep convolutional netsand fully connected crfs. *Proceedings of the International Conference on Learning Representations (ICLR)*.

Cheremkhin, P. A., & Kurbatova, E. A. (2019). Comparative appraisal of global and local thresholding methods for binarisation of off-axis digital holograms. *Optics and Lasers in Engineering*, *115*, 119–130. doi:10.1016/j.optlaseng.2018.11.019

Coenen, A., Kim, Y. H., Kruk, M., Tesche, C., De Geer, J., Kurata, A., Lubbers, M. L., Daemen, J., Itu, L., Rapaka, S., Sharma, P., Schwemmer, C., Persson, A., Schoepf, U. J., Kepka, C., Hyun Yang, D., & Nieman, K. (2018). Diagnostic accuracy of a machine-learning approach to coronary computed tomographic angiography-based fractional flow reserve result from the MACHINE Consortium. *Circulation: Cardiovascular Imaging*, *11*(6), 1–11. doi:10.1161/CIRCIMAGING.117.007217 PMID:29914866

Colaboratory. (n.d.). Retrieved from https://colab.research.google.com/notebooks/welcome.ipynb#scrollTo=xitplqMNk_Hc

Communities, H. (2019). *Basics of Tuberculosis*. http://www.healthcommunities.com/tuberculosis/pathology.shtml

Conejar, R. J., & Kim, H. K. (2014). A medical Decision Support System (DSS) for ubiquitous healthcare diagnosis system. *International Journal of Software Engineering and Its Applications*, *8*(10), 237–244.

D'Cruz, J., Jadhav, A., Dighe, A., Chavan, V., & Chaudhari, J. (2016). Detection of lung cancer using backpropagation neural networks and genetic algorithm. *Computer Technology and Application*, *6*(5), 823–827.

Daojun, Feng, Tian, & Peter. (2018). Understanding mixup training methods. *IEEE Access*, *6*, 58774- 58783.

Das, Acharya, Panda, & Sabut. (2019). Deep learning based liver cancer detection using watershed transform and Gaussian mixture model techniques. *Cognitive Systems Research*, *54*, 165–175.

Das, Turkoglu, & Sengur. (2009). Effective diagnosis of heart disease through neural networks ensembles. *Expert Systems with Applications*, *36*(4), 7675–7680.

Dawes, T. J. W., de Marvao, A., Shi, W., Fletcher, T., Watson, G. M. J., Wharton, J., Rhodes, C. J., Howard, L. S. G. E., Gibbs, J. S. R., Rueckert, D., Cook, S. A., Wilkins, M. R., & O'Regan, D. P. (2017). Machine learning of three-dimensional right ventricular motion enables outcome prediction in pulmonary hypertension: A cardiac MR imaging study. *Radiology*, *283*(2), 381–390. doi:10.1148/radiol.2016161315 PMID:28092203

De Bruijne, M. (2016). *Machine learning approaches in medical image analysis: From detection to diagnosis*. Academic Press.

De la Calleja, J., Tecuapetla, L., Medina, M. A., Bárcenas, E., & Nájera, A. B. U. (2014, September). LBP and machine learning for diabetic retinopathy detection. In *International Conference on Intelligent Data Engineering and Automated Learning* (pp. 110-117). Springer. 10.1007/978-3-319-10840-7_14

Deborah Oakley, MRC London Institute of Medical Sciences. (2017). *Putting people at the heart of research*. Available at: https://lms.mrc.ac.uk/putting-people-heartresearch/

Devinsky, O., Dilley, C., Ozery-Flato, M., Aharonov, R., Goldschmidt, Y., Rosen-Zvi, M., Clark, C., & Fritz, P. (2016). Changing the approach to treatment choice in epilepsy using big data. *Epilepsy & Behavior*, *56*(1), 32–37. doi:10.1016/j.yebeh.2015.12.039 PMID:26827299

Dey, D., Gaur, S., Ovrehus, K. A., Slomka, P. J., Betancur, J., Goeller, M., Hell, M. M., Gransar, H., Berman, D. S., Achenbach, S., Botker, H. E., Jensen, J. M., Lassen, J. F., & Norgaard, B. L. (2018). Integrated prediction of lesion-specific ischaemia from quantitative coronary CT angiography using machine learning: A multicentre study. *European Radiology*, *28*(6), 2655–2664. doi:10.100700330-017-5223-z PMID:29352380

Dheda, K., Ruhwald, M., Theron, G., Peter, J., & Yam, W. C. (2013). Point?of?care diagnosis of tuberculosis: Past, present and future. *Respirology (Carlton, Vic.)*, *18*(2), 217–232. doi:10.1111/resp.12022 PMID:23190246

Dirvanauskas, Maskeli, Raudonis, Damaševi˘cius, & Scherer. (2019). *HEMIGEN: Human Embryo Image Generator Based on Generative Adversarial Networks Sensors*. Academic Press.

Dutta. (2014). Neural network-based models for software effort estimation: a review. *Artif. Intell. Rev., 42*(2), 295-307.

Ege, B. M., Hejlesen, O. K., Larsen, O. V., Møller, K., Jennings, B., Kerr, D., & Cavan, D. A. (2000). Screening for diabetic retinopathy using computer based image analysis and statistical classification. *Computer Methods and Programs in Biomedicine*, *62*(3), 165–175. doi:10.1016/S0169-2607(00)00065-1 PMID:10837904

Elliott, P.M., Anastasakis, A., & Borger, M.A. (2014). ESC guidelines on diagnosis and management of hypertrophic cardiomyopathy: the task force for the diagnosis and management of hypertrophic cardiomyopathy of the european society of cardiology (ESC). *Eur Heart J, 35*(39), 2733-79.

Espona, L., Carreira, M. J., Ortega, M., & Penedo, M. G. (2007, June). A snake for retinal vessel segmentation. In *Iberian Conference on Pattern Recognition and Image Analysis* (pp. 178-185). Springer. 10.1007/978-3-540-72849-8_23

Fang, H. S., Sun, J., Wang, R. M., Gou., Y.L., Li, C., & Lu. (2019). Instaboost: Boosting instance segmentation via probability map guided copy-pasting. ICCV 2019.

Feigenbaum, H. (1996). Evolution of echocardiography. *Circulation*, *93*(7), 1321–1327. doi:10.1161/01.CIR.93.7.1321 PMID:8641018

Fenwa, O. D., Ajala, F. A., & Adigun, A. (2016). Classification of cancer of the lungs using SVM and ANN. *International Journal of Computers and Technology*, *15*(1), 6418–6426. doi:10.24297/ijct.v15i1.1715

Fernandes, F. C., Brasil, L. M., Lamas, J. M., & Guadagnin, R. (2010). Breast cancer image assessment using an adaptative network based fuzzy inference system. *J. Pattern Recognition and Image Analysis*, *20*(2), 192–200. doi:10.1134/S1054661810020112

Ferreira, V. M., Robson, M. D., & Karamitsos, T. D. (2015). Magnetic resonance imaging. In K. Nieman, O. Gaemperli, P. Lancellotti, & S. Plein (Eds.), *Advanced cardiac imaging. Sawston* (pp. 127–169). Woodhead. doi:10.1016/B978-1-78242-282-2.00006-8

Forghani, Forouzanfar, & Fourouzanfar. (2007). MRI fuzzy segmentation of brain tissue using IFCM Algorithm with particle swarm optimization. *IEEE Intl. Sym. Comput. & Information Sci.*, 113-121.

Francisco, Manuel, Antonio, & Daniel. (2008). A robust model of the neuronal regulator of the lower urinary tract based on artificial neural networks. *Neurocomputing*, *71*(4-6), 743–754.

Freiman, M., Nickisch, H., Prevrhal, S., Schmitt, H., Vembar, M., Maurovich-Horvat, P., Donnelly, P., & Goshen, L. (2017). Improving CCTA based lesions' hemodynamic significance assessment by accounting for partial volume modeling in automatic coronary lumen segmentation. *Medical Physics*, *44*(3), 1040–1049. doi:10.1002/mp.12121 PMID:28112409

Fu, H., Xu, Y., Wong, D. W. K., & Liu, J. (2016, April). Retinal vessel segmentation via deep learning network and fully-connected conditional random fields. In *2016 IEEE 13th international symposium on biomedical imaging (ISBI)* (pp. 698-701). IEEE. 10.1109/ISBI.2016.7493362

Fu, H., Xu, Y., Lin, S., Wong, D. W. K., & Liu, J. (2016, October). Deepvessel: Retinal vessel segmentation via deep learning and conditional random field. In *International conference on medical image computing and computer-assisted intervention* (pp. 132-139). Springer. 10.1007/978-3-319-46723-8_16

Fukushima, K. S. M. (1982). Neocognitron: A self-organizing neural network model for a mechanism of visual pattern recognition. Competition and cooperation in neural nets, 267–285.

Galie, N., Humbert, M., & Vachiery, J. L. (2015). ESC/ERS guidelines for the diagnosis and treatment of pulmonary hypertension: the joint task force for the diagnosis and treatment of pulmonary hypertension of the European Society of Cardiology (ESC) and the European Respiratory Society (ERS): endorsed by: Association for European Paediatric and Congenital Cardiology (AEPC), International Society for Heart and Lung Transplantation (ISHLT). *Eur Heart J, 37*(1), 67-119.

Gao, X., Lin, S., & Wong, T. Y. (2015). Automatic feature learning to grade nuclear cataracts based on deep learning. *IEEE Transactions on Biomedical Engineering*, *62*(11), 2693–2701. doi:10.1109/TBME.2015.2444389 PMID:26080373

Geyer, L. L., Schoepf, U. J., & Meinel, F. G. (2015). State of the art: iterative CT reconstruction techniques. *Radiology*, *276*(2), 339-57.

Ghate, D. A., & Jadhav, P. C. (2012). Automatic Detection of Malaria Parasite from Blood Images. *International Journal of Advancements in Computing Technology*, *1*(3), 66–71.

Gil, Johnsson, Garicia Chemizo, Paya, & Fernandez. (2009). Application of Artificial Neural Networks in the Diagnosis of Urological Dysfunctions. *Expert Systems with Applications*, *36*(3), 5754–5760.

Goldbaum, M., Moezzi, S., Taylor, A., Chatterjee, S., Boyd, J., Hunter, E., & Jain, R. (1996, September). Automated diagnosis and image understanding with object extraction, object classification, and inferencing in retinal images. In *Proceedings of 3rd IEEE international conference on image processing* (Vol. 3, pp. 695-698). IEEE. 10.1109/ICIP.1996.560760

Golub, G. H., Heath, M., & Wahba, G. (1979). Generalized cross-validation as a method for choosing a good ridge parameter. *Technometrics*, *21*(2), 215–223. doi:10.1080/00401706.1979.10489751

Gomathi, M., & Thangaraj, P. (2010). Computer aided diagnosis system for detection of lung cancer nodules using extreme learning machine. *International Journal of Engineering Science and Technology*, *2*(10), 5770–5779.

Gonzales, R. C., & Woods, R. E. (2002). *Digital image processing*. Academic Press.

Goodfellow, I. J., D. W.-F. (2013). Maxout networks. *Proceedings of the 30th International Conference on Machine Learning (ICML 2013)*, 28, 1319– 1327.

Gulshan, V., Peng, L., Coram, M., Stumpe, M. C., Wu, D., Narayanaswamy, A., ... Kim, R. (2016). Development and validation of a deep learning algorithm for detection of diabetic retinopathy in retinal fundus photographs. *Journal of the American Medical Association*, *316*(22), 2402–2410. doi:10.1001/jama.2016.17216 PMID:27898976

Han, Hwang, & Lee. (2019). The Classification of Renal Cancer in 3-Phase CT Images Using a Deep Learning Method. *Journal of Digital Imaging*, *32*, 638–643. doi:10.100710278-019-00230-2]

Han, D., Lee, J. H., Rizvi, A., Gransar, H., Baskaran, L., Schulman-Marcus, J., ó Hartaigh, B., Lin, F. Y., & Min, J. K. (2018). Incremental role of resting myocardial computed tomography perfusion for predicting physiologically significant coronary artery disease: A machine learning approach. *Journal of Nuclear Cardiology*, *25*(1), 223–233. doi:10.100712350-017-0834-y PMID:28303473

Haralick, R. M., Shanmugam, K., & Dinstein, I. H. (1973). Textural features for image classification. *IEEE Transactions on Systems, Man, and Cybernetics*, *SMC-3*(6), 610–621. doi:10.1109/TSMC.1973.4309314

Hassan, Elmogy, & Sallam. (2017). Diagnosis of Focal Liver Diseases Based on Deep Learning Technique for Ultrasound Images. *Arabian Journal for Science and Engineering*. Advance online publication. doi:10.100713369-016-2387-9]

He & Garcia. (2009). Learning from imbalanced data. *IEEE Trans. Knowl. Data Eng.*, *21*(9), 1263-1284.

He, Gkioxari, Dollár, & Girshick. (2017). *Mask R-CNN International Conference on Computer Vision (ICCV)*. Academic Press.

He, K., Zhang, X., Ren, S., & Sun, J. (2016). Deep Residual Learning for Image Recognition. *2016 IEEE Conference on Computer Vision and Pattern Recognition (CVPR)*, 770–778. 10.1109/CVPR.2016.90

He, X., & Zhang, S. R. (2015). *Deep residual learning for image recognition.* ArXiv preprint arXiv:1512.03385

Hearst, M. A., Dumais, S. T., Osuna, E., Platt, J., & Scholkopf, B. (1998). Support vector machines. *IEEE Intelligent Systems & their Applications*, *13*(4), 18–28. doi:10.1109/5254.708428

Hecht-Nielsen, R. (1988). Theory of the backpropagation neural network. *Neural Networks*, *1*, 445–448. doi:10.1016/0893-6080(88)90469-8

Heckerling, Canaris, Flach, Tape, Wigton, & Gerber. (2007). Predictors of urinary tract infection based on artificial neural networks and genetic algorithms. *International Journal of Medical Informatics*, *76*(4), 289–296. PMID:16469531

Hiremath, P. S., & Pujari, J. (2007). Content Based Image Retrieval based on Color, Texture and Shape features using Image and its complement. *International Journal of Computer Science and Security*, *1*(4), 25–35.

Holden, R. J., Schubert, C. C., & Mickelson, R. S. (2015). The patient work system: An analysis of self-care performance barriers among elderly heart failure patients and their informal caregivers. *Applied Ergonomics*, *47*(1), 133–150. doi:10.1016/j.apergo.2014.09.009 PMID:25479983

Hong, Lin, Yang, Zeng, Cai, Gou, & Yang. (2019). Predicting Alzheimer's Disease Using LSTM. *IEEE Access: Practical Innovations, Open Solutions*. Advance online publication. doi:10.1109/ACCESS.2019.2919385

Hoover, A. D., Kouznetsova, V., & Goldbaum, M. (2000). Locating blood vessels in retinal images by piecewise threshold probing of a matched filter response. *IEEE Transactions on Medical Imaging*, *19*(3), 203–210. doi:10.1109/42.845178 PMID:10875704

Hubel, D. H., & Wiesel, T. N. (1968). Receptive fields and functional architecture of monkey striate cortex. *The Journal of Physiology*, *195*(1), 215–243. doi:10.1113/jphysiol.1968.sp008455 PMID:4966457

Hunter, P. (2019). The advent of AI and Deep Learning in diagnostics and imaging: Machine Learning systems have potential to improve diagnostics in healthcare and imaging systems in research. *EMBO Reports*, 548–559. PMID:31267716

Ibrahim, Taib, Abas, Guan, & Sulaiman. (2005). A novel dengue fever (DF) and dengue haemorrhagi fever (DHF) analysis using artificial neural network (ANN). *Computer Methods and Programs in Biomedicine*, *79*(3), 273–281. PMID:15925426

Ioffe, S., & Christian, S. (2015). *Batch normalization: Accelerating deep network training by reducing internal covariate shift.* arXiv preprint arXiv:1502.03167

Itu, L., Rapaka, S., Passerini, T., Georgescu, B., Schwemmer, C., Schoebinger, M., Flohr, T., Sharma, P., & Comaniciu, D. (2016). A machine-learning approach for computation of fractional flow reserve from coronary computed tomography. *Journal of Applied Physiology (Bethesda, Md.)*, *121*(1), 42–52. doi:10.1152/japplphysiol.00752.2015 PMID:27079692

Izeboudjen, Larbes, & Farah. (2014). A new classification approach for neural networks hardware: from standards chips to embedded systems on chip. *Artif. Intell. Rev.*, *41*(4), 491-534.

Jabbar, Samreen & Aluvalu. (2018). The Future of Health care: Machine Learning. *IACSIT International Journal of Engineering and Technology*, *7*(4), 23–25. doi:10.14419/ijet.v7i4.6.20226

Jaeger, S., Candemir, S., Antani, S., Wáng, Y. X. J., Lu, P. X., & Thoma, G. (2014). Two public chest X-ray datasets for computer-aided screening of pulmonary diseases. *Quantitative Imaging in Medicine and Surgery*, *4*(6), 475. PMID:25525580

Jaeger, S., Juarez-Espinosa, O. H., Candemir, S., Poostchi, M., Yang, F., Kim, L., Ding, M., Folio, L. R., Antani, S., Gabrielian, A., Hurt, D., Rosenthal, A., & Thoma, G. (2018). Detecting drug-resistant tuberculosis in chest radiographs. *International Journal of Computer Assisted Radiology and Surgery, 13*(12), 1915–1925. doi:10.100711548-018-1857-9 PMID:30284153

Jakimovski & Davcev. (2019). Using Double Convolution Neural Network for Lung Cancer Stage Detection. *Applied Sciences (Basel, Switzerland), 9*, 427. doi:10.3390/app9030427]

Jason Brownlee. (2016). *Machine learning Mastery.* Retrieved 18 November 2016, from https://machinelearningmastery.com/confusion-matrix-machine-learning/

Jena, B., Nayak, G. K., & Saxena, S. (2019). Maximum Payload for Digital Image Steganography Obtained by Mixed Edge Detection Mechanism. In *2019 International Conference on Information Technology (ICIT)*. IEEE. 10.1109/ICIT48102.2019.00043

Jiang, X., & Mojon, D. (2003). Adaptive local thresholding by verification-based multithreshold probing with application to vessel detection in retinal images. *IEEE Transactions on Pattern Analysis and Machine Intelligence, 25*(1), 131–137. doi:10.1109/TPAMI.2003.1159954

Karargyris, A., Siegelman, J., Tzortzis, D., Jaeger, S., Candemir, S., Xue, Z., Santosh, K. C., Vajda, S., Antani, S., Folio, L., & Thoma, G. R. (2016). Combination of texture and shape features to detect pulmonary abnormalities in digital chest X-rays. *International Journal of Computer Assisted Radiology and Surgery, 11*(1), 99–106. doi:10.100711548-015-1242-x PMID:26092662

Karegowda, A. G., Nasiha, A., Jayaram, M. A., & Manjunath, A. S. (2011). Exudates detection in retinal images using back propagation neural network. *International Journal of Computers and Applications, 25*(3), 25–31. doi:10.5120/3011-4062

Karim, R., Bhagirath, P., Claus, P., James Housden, R., Chen, Z., Karimaghaloo, Z., Sohn, H.-M., Lara Rodríguez, L., Vera, S., Albà, X., Hennemuth, A., Peitgen, H.-O., Arbel, T., Gonzàlez Ballester, M. A., Frangi, A. F., Götte, M., Razavi, R., Schaeffter, T., & Rhode, K. (2016). Evaluation of state of-the-art segmentation algorithms for left ventricle infarct from late gadolinium enhancement MR images. *Medical Image Analysis, 30*, 95–107. doi:10.1016/j.media.2016.01.004 PMID:26891066

Karthika, D., & Marimuthu, A. (2014, February). Retinal image analysis using contourlet transform and multistructure elements morphology by reconstruction. In *2014 World Congress on Computing and Communication Technologies* (pp. 54-59). IEEE. 10.1109/WCCCT.2014.15

Kass, M., Witkin, A., & Terzopoulos, D. (1988). Snakes: Active contour models. *International Journal of Computer Vision, 1*(4), 321–331. doi:10.1007/BF00133570

Kavitha, S., & Duraiswamy, K. (2011). Automatic detection of hard and soft exudates in fundus images using color histogram thresholding. *European Journal of Scientific Research, 48*(3), 493–504.

Kawahara, J., & Hamarneh, G. (2016). Multi-resolution-tract CNN with hybrid pretrained and skin-lesion trained layers. In *Proceedings of International workshop on Machine Learning in medical imaging* (pp. 164-171). Springer. 10.1007/978-3-319-47157-0_20

Keras Documentation. (n.d.). *Keras-The Python Deep Learning Library.* Retrieved from https://keras.io/

Khamis, H., Zurakhov, G., Azar, V., Raz, A., Friedman, Z., & Adam, D. (2017). Automatic apical view classification of echocardiograms using a discriminative learningdictionary. *Medical Image Analysis*, *36*, 15–21. doi:10.1016/j.media.2016.10.007 PMID:27816858

Khan. (2011). Content based image retrieval approaches for detection of malarial parasite in blood images. *International Journal of Biometrics and Bioinformatics, 5*(2), 97.

Kim, E., Corte-Real, M., & Baloch, Z. (2016). A deep semantic mobile application for thyroid cytopathology. In Medical Imaging 2016: PACS and Imaging Informatics: Next Generation and Innovations (Vol. 9789). International Society for Optics and Photonics.

Kiran, M., Ahmed, I., Khan, N., & Reddy, A. G. (2019). Chest X-ray segmentation using Sauvola thresholding and Gaussian derivatives responses. *Journal of Ambient Intelligence and Humanized Computing*, *10*(10), 4179–4195. doi:10.100712652-019-01281-7

Knackstedt, C., Bekkers, S. C. A. M., Schummers, G., Schreckenberg, M., Muraru, D., Badano, L. P., Franke, A., Bavishi, C., Omar, A. M. S., & Sengupta, P. P. (2015). Fully automated versus standard tracking of left ventricular ejection fraction and longitudinal strain: The FAST-EFs Multicenter Study. *Journal of the American College of Cardiology*, *66*(13), 1456–1466. doi:10.1016/j.jacc.2015.07.052 PMID:26403342

Kodogiannis & Lygouras. (2008). Neuro-fuzzy classification system for wirelesscapsule endoscopic images. *J. World Acad. Sci.Engg. & Technol*, *45*, 620–628.

Kolossváry, M., Karády, J., Szilveszter, B., Kitslaar, P., Hoffmann, U., Merkely, B., & Maurovich-Horvat, P. (2017). Radiomic features are superior to conventional quantitative computed tomographic metrics to identify coronary plaques with napkin- ring sign. *Circulation: Cardiovascular Imaging*, *10*(12), 1–9. doi:10.1161/CIRCIMAGING.117.006843 PMID:29233836

Komodakis, S. Z. (2016). Wide residual networks. *BMVC.*

Kotsiantis, S. B., Zaharakis, I. D., & Pintelas, P. E. (2006). Machine learning: A review of classification and combining techniques. *Artificial Intelligence Review*, *26*(3), 159–190. doi:10.100710462-007-9052-3

Krizhevsky, A., Sutskever, I., & Hinton, G. (2012). ImageNet Classification with Deep Convolutional Neural Networks. NIPS 2012: Neural Information Processing Systems.

Krizhevsky, A., Sutskever, I., & Hinton, G. E. (2012). Imagenet classification with deep convolutional neural networks. In Advances in neural information processing systems (pp. 1097-1105). Academic Press.

Krizhevsky, Sutskever, & Hinton. (2012). Imagenet classification with deep convolutional neural networks. Advances in Neural Information Processing Systems, 1097-1105.

Krizhevsky, A., Sutskever, I., & Hinton, G. E. (2012). Imagenet classification with deep convolutional neural networks. *Advances in Neural Information Processing Systems.*

Kumar, S. S., & Moni, R. S. (2010). Diagnosis of liver tumor from CT images using curvelet transform. *International Journal on Computer Science and Engineering*, *2*(4), 1173–1178.

Kwan, C. K., & Ernst, J. D. (2011). HIV and tuberculosis: A deadly human syndemic. *Clinical Microbiology Reviews*, *24*(2), 351–376. doi:10.1128/CMR.00042-10 PMID:21482729

Langley, P. (2011). The changing science of machine learning. *Machine Learning*, *82*(3), 275–279. doi:10.100710994-011-5242-y

Le Cun, B. B., J. S. (1989). Handwritten digit recognition with a back-propagation network. *Proceedings of the Advances in Neural Information Processing Systems (NIPS)*, 396–404.

Lecun, Y., Bottou, L., Bengio, Y., & Haffner, P. (1998). Gradient-based learning applied to document recognition. *Proceedings of the IEEE*, *86*(11), 2278–2324. doi:10.1109/5.726791

Lee, C.-Y., S. X. (2015). Deeply supervised nets. *Proceedings of AISTATS.*

Lee, S. I., Celik, S., & Logsdon, B. A. (2018). A Machine Learning approach to integrate big data for precision medicine in acute myeloid leukemia. *Nature Communications*, *9*(42), 1–15. PMID:29298978

Leonardo de Oliveira, M., Silva, A. C., Cardoso de Paiva, A., & Gattass, M. (2009). Detection of breast masses in mammogram images using growing neural gas algorithm and ripley's K function. *J. Signal Processing Sys*, *55*(1), 77–90. doi:10.100711265-008-0209-3

Levin, A., Lischinski, D., & Weiss, Y. (2008). A closed-form solution to natural image matting. *IEEE Transactions on Pattern Analysis and Machine Intelligence*, *30*(2), 228–242. doi:10.1109/TPAMI.2007.1177 PMID:18084055

Levin, D. C., Parker, L., Halpern, E. J., & Rao, V. M. (2019). Coronary CT angiography: Reversal of earlier utilization trends. *Journal of the American College of Radiology*, *16*(2), 147–155. doi:10.1016/j.jacr.2018.07.022 PMID:30158087

Li, Y. H., Yeh, N. N., Chen, S. J., & Chung, Y. C. (2019). Computer-assisted diagnosis for diabetic retinopathy based on fundus images using deep convolutional neural network. *Mobile Information Systems, 2019.*

Li, Z. C., Lang, Y., Chen, J., Liew, J., & Feng. (2019). *Deep reasoning with multi-scale context for salient object detection.* arXiv preprint arXiv:1901.08362

Liao, L. (2019). A Survey of Deep Learning-Based Object Detection. *IEEE Access: Practical Innovations, Open Solutions*, *7*, 128837–128868.

LIDC. (n.d.). Retrieved from https://wiki.cancerimagingarchive.net/display/Public/LIDC-IDRI

Lin, T. Y. P., Dollár, R., Girshick, K., & He. (2017). *Feature pyramid networks for object detection*. openaccess.thecvf.com

Lindeberg, T., & Li, M.-X. (1997). Segmentation and classification of edges using minimum description length approximation and complementary junction cues. *Computer Vision and Image Understanding*, *67*(1), 88–98. doi:10.1006/cviu.1996.0510

Lin, M., Q. C. (2014). Network in network. *International Conference on Learning Representations*.

Li, Q., You, J., & Zhang, D. (2012). Vessel segmentation and width estimation in retinal images using multiscale production of matched filter responses. *Expert Systems with Applications*, *39*(9), 7600–7610. doi:10.1016/j.eswa.2011.12.046

Litjens, G., Kooi, T., Bejnordi, B. E., Setio, A. A. A., Ciompi, F., Ghafoorian, M., van der Laak, J. A. W. M., van Ginneken, B., & Sánchez, C. I. (2017). A survey on deep learning in medical image analysis. *Medical Image Analysis*, *42*, 60–88. doi:10.1016/j.media.2017.07.005 PMID:28778026

Liu, Cai, Pujol, Kikinis, & Feng. (2014). *Early Diagnosis of Alzheimer's Disease with Deep Learning*. IEEE.

Liu, S. S., De Mello, J., Gu, G., Zhong, M.H., & Yang. (2017). Learning affinity via spatial propagation networks. Advances in Neural.

Liu, I., & Sun, Y. (1993). Recursive tracking of vascular networks in angiograms based on the detection-deletion scheme. *IEEE Transactions on Medical Imaging*, *12*(2), 334–341. doi:10.1109/42.232264 PMID:18218423

Long, J. E., & Shelhamer, T. D. (2015). Fully convolutional networks for semantic segmentation. *Proceedings of the IEEE CVPR 2015*.

Long, J., E. S. (2017). Fully convolutional networks for semantic segmentation. *IEEE Transactions on Pattern Analysis and Machine Intelligence*, 640–651. PMID:27244717

Lundervold, A. S., & Lundervold, A. (2019). An overview of deep learning in medical imaging focusing on MRI. *Zeitschrift fur Medizinische Physik*, *29*(2), 102–127. doi:10.1016/j.zemedi.2018.11.002 PMID:30553609

Madani, A., Arnaout, R., Mofrad, M., & Arnaout, R. (2018). Fast and accurate view classification of echocardiograms using deep learning. *NPJ Digital Medicine*, *1*(6), 1–8. doi:10.103841746-017-0013-1 PMID:30828647

Mahapatra, D., Roy, P. K., Sedai, S., & Garnavi, R. (2016, October). Retinal image quality classification using saliency maps and CNNs. In *International Workshop on Machine Learning in Medical Imaging* (pp. 172-179). Springer. 10.1007/978-3-319-47157-0_21

Ma, K., Wang, J., Singh, V., Tamersoy, B., Chang, Y. J., Wimmer, A., & Chen, T. (2017). Multimodal image registration with deep context reinforcement learning. In *Proceedings of International Conference on Medical Image Computing and Computer-Assisted Intervention* (pp. 240-248). Springer. 10.1007/978-3-319-66182-7_28

Maninis, K. K., Pont-Tuset, J., Arbeláez, P., & Van Gool, L. (2016, October). Deep retinal image understanding. In *International conference on medical image computing and computer-assisted intervention* (pp. 140-148). Springer.

Mannil, M., Von Spiczak, J., Manka, R., & Alkadhi, H. (2018). Texture analysis and machine learning for detecting myocardial infarction in non contrast low-dose computed tomography: Unveiling the invisible. *Investigative Radiology*, *53*(6), 338–343. doi:10.1097/RLI.0000000000000448 PMID:29420321

Marín, D., Aquino, A., Gegúndez-Arias, M. E., & Bravo, J. M. (2010). A new supervised method for blood vessel segmentation in retinal images by using gray-level and moment invariants-based features. *IEEE Transactions on Medical Imaging*, *30*(1), 146–158. doi:10.1109/TMI.2010.2064333 PMID:20699207

Masotti, M. (2006). A ranklet –based image representation for mass classification in digital mammograms. *Journal of Medical Physics / Association of Medical Physicists of India*, *33*(10), 3951–3961. PMID:17089857

Matplotlib. (n.d.). *Matplotlibcontents.* Retrieved from https://matplotlib.org/

McPhee, S. J., Papadakis, M. A., & Tierney, L. M. (2017). *Current Medical Diagnosis & Treatment.* McGraw-Hill Medical New York.

Medical Futurist. (n.d.). *Top artificial intelligence companies in healthcare.* Retrieved from https://medicalfuturist.com/top-artificial-intelligence-companies-in-healthcare/

Medvedofsky, D., Addetia, K., Hamilton, J., Leon Jimenez, J., Lang, R. M., & Mor-Avi, V. (2015). Semi-automated echocardiographic quantification of right ventricular size and function. *The International Journal of Cardiovascular Imaging*, *31*(6), 1149–1157. doi:10.100710554-015-0672-4 PMID:25948160

Menegola, A., Fornaciali, M., Pires, R., Avila, S., & Valle, E. (2016). *Towards automated melanoma screening: Exploring transfer learning schemes.* arXiv preprint arXiv:1609.01228

Miao, S., Piat, S., Fischer, P., Tuysuzoglu, A., Mewes, P., Mansi, T., & Liao, R. (2018). Dilated fcn for multi-agent 2d/3d medical image registration. *Thirty-Second AAAI Conference on Artificial Intelligence.*

Miri, M. S., & Mahloojifar, A. (2010). Retinal image analysis using curvelet transform and multistructure elements morphology by reconstruction. *IEEE Transactions on Biomedical Engineering*, *58*(5), 1183–1192. doi:10.1109/TBME.2010.2097599 PMID:21147592

Moein, Monadjemi, & Moallem. (2009). A Novel Fuzzy-Neural Based Medical Diagnosis System. *International Journal of Biological & Medical Sciences*, *4*(3), 146–150.

Moeskops, P., Wolterink, J. M., van der Velden, B. H., Gilhuijs, K. G., Leiner, T., Viergever, M. A., & Išgum, I. (2016). Deep Learning for multi-task medical image segmentation in multiple modalities. In *Proceedings of International Conference on Medical Image Computing and Computer-Assisted Intervention* (pp. 478-486). Springer. 10.1007/978-3-319-46723-8_55

Moghaddasi, H., & Nourian, S. (2016). Automatic assessment of mitral regurgitation severity based on extensive textural features on 2D echocardiography videos. *Computers in Biology and Medicine*, *73*, 47–55. doi:10.1016/j.compbiomed.2016.03.026 PMID:27082766

Mohanasundaram, R., Malhotra, A. S., Arun, R., & Periasamy, P. S. (2019). Deep Learning and Semi-Supervised and Transfer Learning Algorithms for Medical Imaging. In *Deep Learning and Parallel Computing Environment for Bioengineering Systems* (pp. 139–151). Academic Press. doi:10.1016/B978-0-12-816718-2.00015-4

Monadjemi & Moallem. (2008). Automatic Diagnosis of Particular Diseases Using a Fuzzy-Neural Approach. *International Review on Computers & Software*, *3*(4), 406–411.

Motwani, M., Dey, D., & Berman, D. S. (2017). Machine learning for prediction of all-cause mortality in patients with suspected coronary artery disease: A 5-year multicentre prospective registry analysis. *European Heart Journal*, *38*, 500–507. PMID:27252451

Mozaffari, Emami, & Fathi. (2018). A comprehensive investigation into the performance, robustness, scalability and convergence of chaos-enhanced evolutionary algorithms with boundary constraints. *Artificial Intelligence Review*, ▪▪▪, 1–62.

Nair, V., G. E. (2010). Rectified linear units improve restricted boltzmann machines. *Proceedings of the International Con-ference on Machine Learning (ICML)*, 807–814.

Nakamoto, T., Taguchi, A., Ohtsuka, M., Suei, Y., Fujita, M., Tsuda, M., Sanada, M., Kudo, Y., Asano, A., & Tanimot, K. (2008). A computer-aided diagnosis system to screen for osteoporosis using dental panoramic radiographs. *J. Dento Maxillo Facial Radiology*, *37*(5), 274–281. doi:10.1259/dmfr/68621207 PMID:18606749

Narula, S., Shameer, K., Salem, O. A. M., Dudley, J. T., & Sengupta, P. P. (2016). Machine-learning algorithms to automate morphological and functional assessments in 2D echocardiography. *Journal of the American College of Cardiology*, *68*(21), 2287–2295. doi:10.1016/j.jacc.2016.08.062 PMID:27884247

National Cancer Institute. (2019). *Lung and bronchus cancer.* Retrieved from https://seer.cancer.gov/statfacts/html/lungb.html

Ngiam, J., Z. C. (2010). Tiled convolutional neural networks. *Proceedings of the Advancesin Neural Information Processing Systems (NIPS)*, 1279–1287.

Ngo, T. A., Lu, Z., & Carneiro, G. (2017). Combining deep learning and level set for the automated segmentation of the left ventricle of the heart from cardiac cine magnetic resonance. *Medical Image Analysis*, *35*, 159–171. doi:10.1016/j.media.2016.05.009 PMID:27423113

Nieman, K., Coenen, A., & Dijkshoorn, M. (2015). Computed tomography. In Advanced cardiac imaging. Woodhead. doi:10.1016/B978-1-78242-282-2.00005-6

Ning, X., Brian, P., Scott, C., Jimei, Y., Thomas, H. (2017). Deep GrabCut for Object Selection. *British Machine Vision Conference (BMVC)*.

Niu, X.-X., & Suen, C. Y. (2012). A novel hybrid cnn–svm classifier for recognizing handwritten digits. *Pattern Recognition, 45*(4), 1318–1325. doi:10.1016/j.patcog.2011.09.021

Noh, H., S. H. (2015). Learning deconvolution network for semantic segmentation. *Proceedings of the InternationalConference on Computer Vision (ICCV)*, 1520–1528.

NumPy. (2020). *NumPy*. Retrieved from https://numpy.org/

O'Regan, D. P. (2020). Putting machine learning into motion: Applications in cardiovascular imaging. *Clinical Radiology, 75*(1), 33–37. doi:10.1016/j.crad.2019.04.008 PMID:31079952

Obermeyer, Z., & Emanuel, E. J. (2016). Predicting the Future - Big Data, Machine Learning, and Clinical Medicine. *The New England Journal of Medicine, 375*(13), 1216–1219. doi:10.1056/NEJMp1606181 PMID:27682033

Otsu, N. (1979). A threshold selection method from gray-level histograms. *IEEE Transactions on Systems, Man, and Cybernetics, 9*(1), 62–66. doi:10.1109/TSMC.1979.4310076

Palani, D., & Venkatalakshmi, K. (2019). An IoT based predictive modelling for predicting lung cancer using fuzzy cluster based segmentation and classification. *Journal of Medical Systems, 43*(2), 21. doi:10.100710916-018-1139-7 PMID:30564924

Palanivel, M., & Duraisamy, M. (2012). Adaptive Color Texture Image Segmentation Using α-Cut Implemented Interval Type-2 Fuzzy C-Means. *Res. J. Appl. Sci, 7*(5), 258–265. doi:10.3923/rjasci.2012.258.265

Panch, T., Szolovits, P., & Atun, R. (2018). Artificial Intelligence, Machine Learning and health systems. *Journal of Global Health, 8*(2), 1–8. doi:10.7189/jogh.08.020303 PMID:30405904

Pandit, P., & Anand, A. (2016). *Artificial neural networks for detection of malaria in RBCs.* arXiv preprint arXiv:1608.06627

Pandya, M. D., Shah, P. D., & Jardosh, S. (2019). Medical image diagnosis for disease detection: A deep learning approach. In *U-Healthcare Monitoring Systems* (pp. 37–60). Academic Press. doi:10.1016/B978-0-12-815370-3.00003-7

Pashaei, S., & Jazayeri. (2018). Brain Tumor Classification via Convolutional Neural Network and Extreme Learning Machines. In *8th International Conference on Computer and Knowledge Engineering (ICCKE 2018)*. Ferdowsi University of Mashhad.

Pattanaik, P. A., & Swarnkar, T. (2018). Comparative analysis of morphological techniques for malaria detection. *International Journal of Healthcare Information Systems and Informatics, 13*(4), 49–65. doi:10.4018/IJHISI.2018100104

Pearce, Wong, Mirtskhulava, AlMajeed, Bakuria, & Gulua. (2016). Artificial Neural Network and Mobile Applications in Medical Diagnosis. *2015 17th UKSimAMSS International Conference on Modelling and Simulation.*

Plis, S. M., Hjelm, D. R., Salakhutdinov, R., Allen, E. A., Bockholt, H. J., Long, J. D., & Calhoun, V. D. (2014). Deep Learning for neuroimaging: A validation study. *Frontiers in Neuroscience*, *8*(229), 1–11. PMID:25191215

Polonsky, T., McClelland, R., & Jorgensen, N. (2010). Coronary artery calcium score and risk classification for coronary heart disease prediction. *Journal of the American Medical Association*, *303*(16), 1610–1616. doi:10.1001/jama.2010.461 PMID:20424251

Ponikowski, P., Voors, A. A., Anker, S. D., Bueno, H., Cleland, J. G. F., Coats, A. J. S., Falk, V., González-Juanatey, J. R., Harjola, V.-P., Jankowska, E. A., Jessup, M., Linde, C., Nihoyannopoulos, P., Parissis, J. T., Pieske, B., Riley, J. P., Rosano, G. M. C., Ruilope, L. M., Ruschitzka, F., ... van der Meer, P. (2016). The Task Force for the diagnosis and treatment of acute and chronic heart failure of the European Society of Cardiology (ESC). (2016) ESC Guidelines for the diagnosis and treatment of acute and chronic heart failure. *European Heart Journal*, *37*(27), 2129–2200. doi:10.1093/eurheartj/ehw128 PMID:27206819

Poostchi, M., Silamut, K., Maude, R. J., Jaeger, S., & Thoma, G. (2018). Image analysis and machine learning for detecting malaria. *Translational Research; the Journal of Laboratory and Clinical Medicine*, *194*, 36–55. doi:10.1016/j.trsl.2017.12.004 PMID:29360430

Porumb, Iadanza, Massarod, & Pecchia. (2020). A convolutional neural network approach to detect congestive heart failure. *Biomedical Signal Processing and Control*, *55*, 101597. doi:10.1016/j.bspc.2019.101597

Pradeep, K. R., & Naveen, N. C. (2018). Lung cancer survivability prediction based on performance using classification techniques of support vector machines, C4. 5 and Naive Bayes algorithms for healthcare analytics. *Procedia Computer Science*, *132*, 412–420. doi:10.1016/j.procs.2018.05.162

Precision. (2020). Retrieved May 18, 2020 from https://en.wikipedia.org/wiki/Precision_and_recall

Prentašić, P., & Lončarić, S. (2016). Detection of exudates in fundus photographs using deep neural networks and anatomical landmark detection fusion. *Computer Methods and Programs in Biomedicine*, *137*, 281–292. doi:10.1016/j.cmpb.2016.09.018 PMID:28110732

PyPI- Pandas. (2020). *Pandas 1.0.1*. Retrieved May 18,2020 from https://pypi.org/project/pandas/

Rachata, Charoenkwan, Yooyativong, Chamnongthal, Lursinsap, & Higuchi. (2008). Automatic prediction system of dengue haemorrhagic-fever outbreak risk by using entropy and artificial neural network. In *Proceedings of the International Symposium on Communications and Information Technologies*. IEEE.

Rajaraman, S., Candemir, S., Xue, Z., Alderson, P. O., Kohli, M., Abuya, J., Thoma, G. R., & Antani, S. (2018, July). A novel stacked generalization of models for improved TB detection in chest radiographs. In *2018 40th Annual International Conference of the IEEE Engineering in Medicine and Biology Society (EMBC)* (pp. 718-721). IEEE. 10.1109/EMBC.2018.8512337

Rajaraman, S., Antani, S. K., Poostchi, M., Silamut, K., Hossain, M. A., Maude, R. J., Jaeger, S., & Thoma, G. R. (2018). Pre-trained convolutional neural networks as feature extractors toward improved malaria parasite detection in thin blood smear images. *PeerJ*, *6*, e4568. doi:10.7717/peerj.4568 PMID:29682411

Raval, Bhatt, Kumhar, Parikh, & Vyas. (2016). Medical diagnosis system using machine learning. *International Journal of Computer Science & Communication*, *7*(1), 177–182.

Razzak, Naz, & Zaib. (2017). *Deep Learning for Medical Image Processing: Overview, Challenges and Future, DL for medical imaging*. Cornell university.

Razzak, Naz, & Zaib. (2017). *Deep Learning for Medical Image Processing: Overview, Challenges and Future*. arXiv:1704.06825v1

Ren, Fei, Liang, Ji, & Cheng. (2019). A hybrid neural network model for predicting kidney disease in hypertension patients based on electronic health records. *BMC Medical Informatics and Decision Making, 19*(Suppl 2), 51. doi:10.118612911-019-0765-4

RiyahiAlam, N., Younesi, F., & RiyahiAlam, M.S. (2009). Computer-Aided mass detection on digitized mammograms using a novel hybrid segmentation system. *Intl. J. Biol. & Biomedical Engg.*, *3*(4), 51–58.

Ronneberger, O. P., Fischer, T., & Brox. (2015). U-net: Convolutional networks for biomedical image segmentation. In *International Conference on Medical*. Springer.

Ronneberger, O., Fischer, P., & Brox, T. (2015). U-net: convolutional networks for biomedical image segmentation. In Lecture notes in computer science: Vol. 9351. *Medical Image Computing and Computer-Assisted Intervention e MICCAI 2015. MICCAI 2015*. Springer. doi:10.1007/978-3-319-24574-4_28

Rueckert, D. (2016). Engineering, Physical Sciences Research Council. *Smart Heart: next generation cardiovascular healthcare via integrated image acquisition, reconstruction, analysis and learning*. Available at: http://gow.epsrc.ac.uk/NGBOViewGrant.aspx?GrantRef1/4EP/P001009/1

Russakovsky, J. D. (2015). Magenetlarge scale visual recognition challenge. *International Journal of Conflict and Violence*, 211-252.

Russell, S., & Norvig, P. (2003). *Artificial Intelligence: A Modern Approach* (2nd ed.). Prentice Hall.

Sajjad, Khan, Muhammad, Wu, Ullah, & Baik. (2019). Multi-grade brain tumor classification using deep CNN with extensive data augmentation. *Journal of Computational Science*, *30*, 174–182.

Samad, M. D., Wehner, G. J., Arbabshirani, M. R., Jing, L., Powell, A. J., Geva, T., Haggerty, C. M., & Fornwalt, B. K. (2018). Predicting deterioration of ventricular function in patients with repaired tetralogy of Fallot using machine learning. *European Heart Journal Cardiovascular Imaging*, *19*(7), 730–738. doi:10.1093/ehjci/jey003 PMID:29538684

Schlegl, T., Waldstein, S. M., Vogl, W.-D., Schmidt-Erfurth, U., & Langs, G. (2015). Predicting semantic descriptions from medical images with convolutional neural networks. *Lecture Notes in Computer Science, 9123*, 437–448. 10.1007/978-3-319-19992-4_34

Schlemper, J., Caballero, J., & Hajnal, J.V. (2018). A deep cascade of convolutional neural networks for dynamic MR image reconstruction. *IEEE Trans Med Imaging*, *37*(2), 491-503.

Scikit Learn. (2020). *Scikit-Learn Machine learning in python.* Retrieved from https://scikit-learn.org/stable/

Sengupta, P. P., Huang, Y. M., Bansal, M., Ashrafi, A., Fisher, M., Shameer, K., Gall, W., & Dudley, J. T. (2016). Cognitive machine-learning algorithm for cardiac imaging; a pilot study for differentiating constrictive pericarditis from restrictive cardiomyopathy. *Circulation: Cardiovascular Imaging*, *9*(6), 1–10. doi:10.1161/CIRCIMAGING.115.004330 PMID:27266599

Sepehr, M. H., Jamarani, B. H., & Rezai rad, G. A. (2005). Multiwavelet based neural network for breast cancer diagnosis. *Proceedings of Intl. Conf. Graphics, Vision & Image Processing*, 29-34.

Sercu, V. G. (2016). Dense prediction on sequences with time-dilated convolutions for speech recognition. *Proceedings of the Advances in Neural Information Processing Systems (NIPS) Workshops.*

Serj, Lavi, Hoff, & Valls. (2018). *A Deep Convolutional Neural Network for Lung Cancer Diagnostic*. arXiv:1804.08170

Shah, S. J., Katz, D. H., Selvaraj, S., Burke, M. A., Yancy, C. W., Gheorghiade, M., Bonow, R. O., Huang, C.-C., & Deo, R. C. (2015). Heart failure phenomapping for novel classification of heart failure with preserved ejection fraction. *Circulation*, *131*(3), 269–279. doi:10.1161/CIRCULATIONAHA.114.010637 PMID:25398313

Shanmugam, V., & Banu, R. D. W. (2013, January). Retinal blood vessel segmentation using an extreme learning machine approach. In 2013 IEEE Point-of-Care Healthcare Technologies (PHT) (pp. 318-321). IEEE. doi:10.1109/PHT.2013.6461349

Shannon, C. E. (1948). A mathematical theory of communication. *The Bell System Technical Journal*, *27*(3), 379–423. doi:10.1002/j.1538-7305.1948.tb01338.x

Shimabukuro, D., Barton, C. W., Feldman, M. D., Mataraso, S. J., & Das, R. (2017). Effect of a Machine Learning-based severe sepsis prediction algorithm on patient survival and hospital length of stay: Randomised clinical trial. *BMJ Open Respiratory Research*, *4*(1), e000234. doi:10.1136/bmjresp-2017-000234 PMID:29435343

Shin, Tenenholtz, Rogers, Schwarz, Senjem, Gunter, Andriole, & Michalski. (2018). *Medical Image Synthesis for Data Augmentation and Anonymization using Generative Adversarial Networks*. arXiv:1807.10225v2

Siegersma, K. R., Leiner, T., Chew, D. P., Appelman, Y., Hofstra, L., & Verjans Neth, J. W. (2019). Artificial intelligence in cardiovascular imaging: State of the art and implications for the imaging cardiologist. *The Hearing Journal*, *27*, 403–413. PMID:31399886

Silberman, N., Ahrlich, K., Fergus, R., & Subramanian, L. (2010, March). Case for automated detection of diabetic retinopathy. *2010 AAAI Spring Symposium Series.*

Simonyan & Zisserman. (2014). *Very deep convolutional networks for large-scale image recognition.* arXiv preprint arXiv:1409.1556

Simonyan, K., A. Z. (2015). Very deep convolutional networks for large-scale image recognition. *Proceedings of the International Conference on Learning Representations (ICLR).*

Singh, N., & Hamde, S. (2019). Tuberculosis detection using shape and texture features of chest X-rays. In *Innovations in Electronics and Communication Engineering* (pp. 43–50). Springer. doi:10.1007/978-981-13-3765-9_5

Snaauw, G., Gong, D., & Maicas, G. (2019). End-to-end diagnosis and segmentation learning from cardiac magnetic resonance imaging. *2019 IEEE 16th International Symposium on Biomedical Imaging (ISBI 2019),* 802–5.

Soh, L. K., & Tsatsoulis, C. (1999). Texture analysis of SAR sea ice imagery using gray level co-occurrence matrices. *IEEE Transactions on Geoscience and Remote Sensing, 37*(2), 780–795. doi:10.1109/36.752194

Soille, P. (2013). *Morphological image analysis: principles and applications.* Springer Science & Business Media.

South Sudan Medical Journal. (n.d.). Retrieved from http://www.southsudanmedicaljournal.com/archive/february-2011/malaria-in-south-sudan-1.-introduction-and-pathophysiology.html

Srivastava, Hinton, Krizhevsky, Salakhutdinov, & Sutskever. (2014). Dropout: a simple way to prevent neural networks from overfitting. *JMLR.*

Starfield, B., Hyde, J., Gérvas, J., & Heath, I. (2008). The concept of prevention: A good idea gone astray? *Journal of Epidemiology and Community Health, 62*(7), 580–583. doi:10.1136/jech.2007.071027 PMID:18559439

Stöppler & Marks. (n.d.). *Lung cancer article.* Retrieved from https://www.medicinenet.com/lung_cancer/article.htm

Sudarshan, V., Ng, E. Y., & Acharya, U. R. (2015). Computer-aided diagnosis of myocardial infarction using ultrasound images with DWT, GLC Mand HOS methods: A comparative study. *Computers in Biology and Medicine, 62*, 86–93. doi:10.1016/j.compbiomed.2015.03.033 PMID:25912990

Suinesiaputra, A., Sanghvi, M. M., Aung, N., Paiva, J. M., Zemrak, F., Fung, K., Lukaschuk, E., Lee, A. M., Carapella, V., Kim, Y. J., Francis, J., Piechnik, S. K., Neubauer, S., Greiser, A., Jolly, M.-P., Hayes, C., Young, A. A., & Petersen, S. E. (2018). Fully-automated left ventricular mass and volume MRI analysis in the UK Biobank population cohort: Evaluation of initial results. *The International Journal of Cardiovascular Imaging, 34*(2), 281–291. doi:10.100710554-017-1225-9 PMID:28836039

Suk, H. I., & Shen, D. (2013). Deep learning-based feature representation for AD/MCI classification. In *Proceedings of International Conference on Medical Image Computing and Computer-Assisted Intervention* (pp. 583-590). Springer. 10.1007/978-3-642-40763-5_72

Summers, R. M. (2003). Road maps for advancement of radiologic computer-aided detection in the 21st century. *Radiology, 229*(1), 11–13. doi:10.1148/radiol.2291030010 PMID:14519863

Suradkar, P. T. (2013). Detection of malarial parasite in blood using image processing. *International Journal of engineering and innovative Technology, 2*(10), 124-126.

Szegedy, C., Liu, W., Jia, Y., Sermanet, P., Reed, S., Anguelov, D., . . . Rabinovich, A. (2014). *Going deeper with convolutions*. arxiv:1409.4842.

Szegedy, C., Sergey, I., Vincent, V., & Alexander, A. A. (2017). Inception-v4, inception-resnet and the impact of residual connections on learning. *Thirty-First AAAI Conference on Artificial Intelligence*.

Szegedy, C., Vincent, V., Sergey, I., Jon, S., and Zbigniew, W. (2016). Rethinking the inception architecture for computer vision. *Proceedings of the IEEE conference on computer vision and pattern recognition*, 2818-2826. 10.1109/CVPR.2016.308

Szegedy, C., W. L. (2015). Going deeper with convolutions. *Proceedings of the IEEE Conference on Computer Vision and Pattern Recognition (CVPR)*, 1-9.

Szegedy, C., Wei, L., Yangqing, J., Pierre, S., Scott, R., Dragomir, A., Dumitru, E., Vincent, V., Andrew, R. (2015). Going deeper with convolutions. *Proceedings of the IEEE conference on computer vision and pattern recognition*, 1-9.

Tabassian, M., Alessandrini, M., Herbots, L., Mirea, O., Pagourelias, E. D., Jasaityte, R., Engvall, J., De Marchi, L., Masetti, G., & D'hooge, J. (2017). Machine learning of the spatio-temporal characteristics of echocardiographic deformation curves for infarct classification. *The International Journal of Cardiovascular Imaging, 33*(8), 1159–1167. doi:10.100710554-017-1108-0 PMID:28321681

Tabassian, M., Sunderji, I., Erdei, T., Sanchez-Martinez, S., Degiovanni, A., Marino, P., Fraser, A. G., & D'hooge, J. (2018). Diagnosis of heart failure with preserved ejection fraction: Machine learning of spatiotemporal variations in left ventricular deformation. *Journal of the American Society of Echocardiography, 31*(12), 1272–1284. doi:10.1016/j.echo.2018.07.013 PMID:30146187

Tachibana, R., Näppi, J. J., Hironaka, T., Kim, S. H., & Yoshida, H. (2016). Deep learning for electronic cleansing in dual- energy ct colonography. *Proceedings of the SPIE Medical Imaging, 9785*.

Tamborini, G., Piazzese, C., Lang, R. M., Muratori, M., Chiorino, E., Mapelli, M., Fusini, L., Ali, S. G., Gripari, P., Pontone, G., Andreini, D., & Pepi, M. (2017). Feasibility and Accuracy of automated software for transthoracic three dimensional left ventricular volume and function analysis: Comparisons with two-dimensional echocardiography, three-dimensional transthoracic manual method, and cardiac magnetic resonance imaging. *Journal of the American Society of Echocardiography*, *30*(11), 1049–1058. doi:10.1016/j.echo.2017.06.026 PMID:28916243

Tang, A., Tam, R., Cadrin-Chênevert, A., Guest, W., Chong, J., Barfett, J., & Poudrette, M. G. (2018). Canadian Association of Radiologists white paper on Artificial Intelligence in radiology. *Canadian Association of Radiologists Journal*, *69*(2), 120–135. doi:10.1016/j.carj.2018.02.002 PMID:29655580

Tan, L. K., Liew, Y. M., Lim, E., & McLaughlin, R. A. (2017). Convolutional neural network regression for short-axis left ventricle segmentation in cardiac cine MR sequences. *Medical Image Analysis*, *39*, 78–86. doi:10.1016/j.media.2017.04.002 PMID:28437634

Taylor, C.A., Fonte, T.A., & Min, J.K. (2013). Computational fluid dynamics applied to cardiac computed tomography for noninvasive quantification of fractional flow reserve: scientific basis. *J Am Coll Cardiol*, *61*(22), 2233-41.

TensorFlow. (n.d.). *TensorFlow About.* Retrieved from https://www.tensorflow.org/about/

Tesche, C., De Cecco, C. N., & Albrecht, M.H. (2017). Coronary CT angiography derived fractional flow reserve. *Radiology*, *285*(1), 17-33.

Tesche, C., De Cecco, C. N., & Baumann, S. (2018). Coronary CT angiography derived fractional flow reserve: machine learning algorithm versus computational fluid dynamics modeling. *Radiology*, *288*(1), 64-72.

Tesche, C., Vliegenthart, R., Duguay, T. M., De Cecco, C. N., Albrecht, M. H., De Santis, D., Langenbach, M. C., Varga-Szemes, A., Jacobs, B. E., Jochheim, D., Baquet, M., Bayer, R. R. II, Litwin, S. E., Hoffmann, E., Steinberg, D. H., & Schoepf, U. J. (2017). Coronary computed tomographic angiography-derived fractional flow reserve for therapeutic decision making. *The American Journal of Cardiology*, *120*(12), 2121–2127. doi:10.1016/j.amjcard.2017.08.034 PMID:29102036

The cancer imaging archive. (2020). Retrieved from https://www.cancerimagingarchive.net/about-the-cancer-imaging-archive-tcia/

Tom, M. (1997). *Mitchell, Machine Learning*. McGraw-Hill.

Tong, W. (2020). Machine learning for spatiotemporal big data in air pollution. In *Spatiotemporal Analysis of Air Pollution and Its Application in Public Health* (pp. 107–134). Elsevier. doi:10.1016/B978-0-12-815822-7.00005-4

Toward Data Science Natasha Sharma. (2019). *Importance of distance Metrics in Machine learning modeling*. Retrieved 13 January, 2019 from https://towardsdatascience.com/importance-of-distance-metrics-in-machine-learning-modelling-e51395ffe60d

Toward Data Science. (n.d.). Retrieved from https://towardsdatascience.com/understanding-and-coding-a-resnet-in-keras-446d7ff84d33

Tsaneva, M. (2008). Texture features for segmentation of satellite images. *Cybernetics and Information Technologies*, *8*(3), 73–85.

Tuceryan, M., & Jain, A. K. (1998). The Handbook of Pattern Recognition and Computer Vision, chapter 2.1. Texture Analysis. World Scientific Co.

Vajda, S., Karargyris, A., Jaeger, S., Santosh, K. C., Candemir, S., Xue, Z., Sameer, A., & Thoma, G. (2018). Feature selection for automatic tuberculosis screening in frontal chest radiographs. *Journal of Medical Systems*, *42*(8), 146. doi:10.100710916-018-0991-9 PMID:29959539

Vala, H. J., & Baxi, A. (2013). A review on Otsu image segmentation algorithm. *International Journal of Advanced Research in Computer Engineering & Technology*, *2*(2), 387–389.

Van Den Boomgaard, R., & Van Balen, R. (1992). Methods for fast morphological image transforms using bitmapped binary images. *CVGIP. Graphical Models and Image Processing*, *54*(3), 252–258. doi:10.1016/1049-9652(92)90055-3

van Ginneken & S´anchez. (2017). *A Survey on Deep Learning in Medical Image Analysis*. arXiv,1702.05747v2

Van Grinsven, M. J., van Ginneken, B., Hoyng, C. B., Theelen, T., & Sánchez, C. I. (2016). Fast convolutional neural network training using selective data sampling: Application to hemorrhage detection in color fundus images. *IEEE Transactions on Medical Imaging*, *35*(5), 1273–1284. doi:10.1109/TMI.2016.2526689 PMID:26886969

van Rosendael, A. R., Maliakal, G., Kolli, K. K., Beecy, A., Al'Aref, S. J., Dwivedi, A., Singh, G., Panday, M., Kumar, A., Ma, X., Achenbach, S., Al-Mallah, M. H., Andreini, D., Bax, J. J., Berman, D. S., Budoff, M. J., Cademartiri, F., Callister, T. Q., Chang, H.-J., ... Min, J. K. (2018). Maximization of the usage of coronary CTA derived plaque information using a machine learning based algorithm to improve risk stratification; insights from the CONFIRM registry. *Journal of Cardiovascular Computed Tomography*, *12*(3), 204–209. doi:10.1016/j.jcct.2018.04.011 PMID:29753765

Vedaldi, A., & Lenc, K. (2015). MatConvNet - Convolutional Neural Networks for MATLAB. *Proc. of the ACM Int. Conf. on Multimedia*.

Visin, F., K. K. (2015). A recurrent neural network for object segmentation. *Proceedings of the IEEE Conference on Computer Vision and Pattern Recognition (CVPR) Workshops*.

Wang, He, & Liu. (2018). Intelligent optimal control with critic learning for a nonlinear overhead crane system. *IEEE Transact. Ind. Inf.*, *14*(7), 2932-2940.

Wang, Z. T. O. (2015). Encoding time series as images for visual inspection and classification using tiled convolutional neural networks. *Proceedings of the Association for the Advancement of Artificial Intelligence (AAAI) Workshops*.

Wang, S., Yin, Y., Cao, G., Wei, B., Zheng, Y., & Yang, G. (2015). Hierarchical retinal blood vessel segmentation based on feature and ensemble learning. *Neurocomputing*, *149*, 708–717. doi:10.1016/j.neucom.2014.07.059

Wolterink, J. M., Leiner, T., DeVos, B. D., van Hamersvelt, R. W., Viergever, M. A., & Išgum, I. (2016). Automatic coronary artery calcium scoring in cardiac CT angiography using paired convolutional neural networks. *Medical Image Analysis*, *34*, 123–136. doi:10.1016/j.media.2016.04.004 PMID:27138584

Wolterink, J. M., Leiner, T., Takx, R. A. P., Viergever, M. A., & Išgum, I. (2015). Cardiac CT with ambiguity detection. *IEEE Transactions on Medical Imaging*, *34*(9), 1867–1878. doi:10.1109/TMI.2015.2412651 PMID:25794387

Wolterink, J. M., Leiner, T., Viergever, M. A., & Isgum, I. (2017). Generative adversarial networks for noise reduction in low-dose CT. *IEEE Transactions on Medical Imaging*, *36*(12), 2536–2545. doi:10.1109/TMI.2017.2708987 PMID:28574346

World Health Organization. (2013). *Global tuberculosis report 2013*. World Health Organization.

World Health Organization. (n.d.). *Malaria*. https://www.who.int/news-room/fact-sheets/detail/malaria

Worrall, D. E., Wilson, C. M., & Brostow, G. J. (2016). Automated retinopathy of prematurity case detection with convolutional neural networks. In *Deep Learning and Data Labeling for Medical Applications* (pp. 68–76). Springer. doi:10.1007/978-3-319-46976-8_8

Wu, A., Xu, Z., Gao, M., Buty, M., & Mollura, D. J. (2016, April). Deep vessel tracking: A generalized probabilistic approach via deep learning. In *2016 IEEE 13th International Symposium on Biomedical Imaging (ISBI)* (pp. 1363-1367). IEEE. 10.1109/ISBI.2016.7493520

Wu, G., Kim, M., Wang, Q., Munsell, B. C., & Shen, D. (2015). Scalable high-performance image registration framework by unsupervised deep feature representations learning. *IEEE Transactions on Biomedical Engineering*, *63*(7), 1505–1516. doi:10.1109/TBME.2015.2496253 PMID:26552069

Xie, S. (2016). R. G. Aggregated Residual Transformations for Deep Neural Networks. Academic Press.

Xie, J., Girshick, R., & Farhadi, A. (2016). Unsupervised deep embedding for clustering analysis. *Proceedings of the 33rd international Conference on international Conference on machine learning*, 48, 478-87.

Xu, N. B., Price, S., & Cohen. (2017). Deep image matting. *Proceedings of the IEEE, CVPR, 2017*. openaccess.thecvf.com

Xu, Y., Wang, Y., Yuan, J., Cheng, Q., Wang, X., & Carson, P. L. (2019). Medical breast ultrasound image segmentation by Machine Learning. *Ultrasonics*, *91*, 1–9. doi:10.1016/j.ultras.2018.07.006 PMID:30029074

Yang, D., Subramanian, G., Duan, J., Gao, S., Bai, L., Chandramohanadas, R., & Ai, Y. (2017). A portable image-based cytometer for rapid malaria detection and quantification. *PLoS One*, *12*(6), e0179161. doi:10.1371/journal.pone.0179161 PMID:28594960

Yang, H., & Chen, Y. P. P. (2015). Data mining in lung cancer pathologic staging diagnosis: Correlation between clinical and pathology information. *Expert Systems with Applications*, *42*(15-16), 6168–6176. doi:10.1016/j.eswa.2015.03.019

Yu, Wang, Ng, Ma, Mo, Li, Fong, Xing, Song, Xie, Si, Wee, Welsch, So, & Yu. (2018). Deep learning enables automated scoring of liver fibrosis stages. *Scientific Reports*, *8*(16016). Advance online publication. doi:10.103841598-018-34300-2

Yu, F., V. K. (2016). Multi-scale context aggregation by dilated convolutions. *Proceedings of the International Conference onLearning Representations (ICLR).*

Zana, F., & Klein, J. C. (2001). Segmentation of vessel-like patterns using mathematical morphology and curvature evaluation. *IEEE Transactions on Image Processing*, *10*(7), 1010–1019. doi:10.1109/83.931095 PMID:18249674

Zeiler, M. D., D. K. (2010). Deconvolutional networks. *Proceedings of the IEEE Conference onComputer Vision and Pattern Recognition (CVPR)*, 2528-2535.

Zeiler, M. D., G. W. (2011). Adaptive deconvolutional networks for mid and high level feature learning. *Proceedings of the International Conference on Computer Vision (ICCV)*, 2018–2025. 10.1109/ICCV.2011.6126474

Zeiler, M. D., R. F. (2014). Visualizing and understanding convolutional networks. *Proceedings of the European Conference onComputer Vision (ECCV)*, 818–833.

Zhang, J., Z. L. (2016). Top-down neural attention by excitation backprop. *Proceedings of theEuropean Conference on Computer Vision (ECCV)*, 543-559.

Zhang, J., Gajjala, S., Agrawal, P., Tison, G. H., Hallock, L. A., Beussink-Nelson, L., Lassen, M. H., Fan, E., Aras, M. A., Jordan, C. R., Fleischmann, K. E., Melisko, M., Qasim, A., Shah, S. J., Bajcsy, R., & Deo, R. C. (2018). Fully automated echocardiogram interpretation in clinical practice. *Circulation*, *138*(16), 1623–1635. doi:10.1161/CIRCULATIONAHA.118.034338 PMID:30354459

Zhang, L., Li, Q., You, J., & Zhang, D. (2009). A modified matched filter with double-sided thresholding for screening proliferative diabetic retinopathy. *IEEE Transactions on Information Technology in Biomedicine*, *13*(4), 528–534. doi:10.1109/TITB.2008.2007201 PMID:19389699

Zhang, Y. E. K. (2016). Augmenting supervised neural networks with unsupervised objectives for large-scaleimage classification. *Proceedings of the International Conference on Machine Learning (ICML)*, 612-621.

Zhang, Y., Hsu, W., & Lee, M. L. (2009). Detection of retinal blood vessels based on nonlinear projections. *Journal of Signal Processing Systems for Signal, Image, and Video Technology*, *55*(1-3), 103–112. doi:10.100711265-008-0179-5

Zhao, Y. Q., Wang, X. H., Wang, X. F., & Shih, F. Y. (2014). Retinal vessels segmentation based on level set and region growing. *Pattern Recognition*, *47*(7), 2437–2446. doi:10.1016/j.patcog.2014.01.006

Zheng, Q. L. (2014). Time series classification using multi-channels deep convolutional neural networks. *Proceedings of the International Conference on Web-Age Information Management (WAIM)*, 298–310. 10.1007/978-3-319-08010-9_33

Zheng, Q., Delingette, H., Duchateau, N., & Ayache, N. (2018). 3-D consistent and robust segmentation of cardiac images by deep learning with spatial propagation. *IEEE Transactions on Medical Imaging*, *37*(9), 2137–2148. doi:10.1109/TMI.2018.2820742 PMID:29994087

Zhou, B. A. K. (2016). Learning deep features for discriminative localization. *Proceedings of the IEEE Conference on Computer Vision and Pattern Recognition (CVPR)*, 2921–2929.

Zhou, X., Shen, Q., & Liu, L. (2008). New two-dimensional fuzzy C-means clustering algorithm for image segmentation. *J.Central South Univ. Technol*, *15*(6), 882–887. doi:10.100711771-008-0161-1

Ziabari, M. K. (2018). *Mobile Self-Triage Applications: A Usability Perspective* (Doctoral dissertation). University of Ottawa.

Zilly, J., Buhmann, J. M., & Mahapatra, D. (2017). Glaucoma detection using entropy sampling and ensemble learning for automatic optic cup and disc segmentation. *Computerized Medical Imaging and Graphics*, *55*, 28–41. doi:10.1016/j.compmedimag.2016.07.012 PMID:27590198

Zreik, M., Leiner, T., & de Vos, B. D. (2016). Automatic segmentation of the left ventricle in cardiac CT angiography using convolutional neural networks. *IEEE 13th International Symposium on Biomedical Imaging (ISBI)*, 40–43. 10.1109/ISBI.2016.7493206

Zreik, M., Lessmann, N., vanHamersvelt, R. W., Wolterink, J. M., Voskuil, M., Viergever, M. A., Leiner, T., & Išgum, I. (2018). Deep learning analysis of the myocardium in coronary CT angiography for identification of patients with functionally significant coronary artery stenosis. *Medical Image Analysis*, *44*, 72–85. doi:10.1016/j.media.2017.11.008 PMID:29197253

Zreik, M., van Hamersvelt, R. W., Wolterink, J. M., Leiner, T., Viergever, M. A., & Isgum, I. (2019). A Recurrent CNN for Automatic Detection and Classification of Coronary Artery Plaque and Stenosis in Coronary CT Angiography. *IEEE Transactions on Medical Imaging*, *7*(38), 1588–1598. doi:10.1109/TMI.2018.2883807 PMID:30507498

About the Contributors

Sanjay Saxena is an Assistant Professor in Department of Computer Science & Engineering, International Institute of Information Technology, Bhubaneswar, India. He has completed Ph.D. from Indian Institute of Technology (BHU), Varanasi, India in High Performance Medical Image Processing. Also, he completed Post Doctorate Research from Perelman School of Medicine, University of Pennsylvania, United States of America and worked on Brain Tumor (Glioblastoma) segmentation and analysis. He has published several research papers in peer reviewed international journals and conferences.

Sudip Paul is currently an Assistant Professor and Head (I/C) in Department of Biomedical Engineering, School of Technology, North-Eastern Hill University (NEHU), Shillong, India. He completed his Post-doctoral research at School of Computer Science and Software Engineering, The University of Western Australia, Perth. He was one of the most prestigious fellowship awardee (Biotechnology Overseas Associateship for the Scientists working in North Eastern States of India: 2017-18 supported by Department of Department of Biotechnology, Government of India. He received his Ph.D degree from Indian Institute of Technology (Banaras Hindu University), Varanasi with specialization in Electrophysiology and brain signal analysis. He has many credentials in his credit out of which his First Prize in Sushruta Innovation Award 2011 sponsored by Department of Science and Technology, Govt. of India and also he also organized many workshops and conferences out of which most significant are the 29th Annual meeting of the Society for Neurochemistry, India and IRBO/APRC Associate School 2017. Dr. Sudip published more than 90 International journal and conference papers and also filled four patents. Recently he completed six book projects and six are ongoing as editor. Dr. Sudip is a member of different Societies and professional bodies, including APSN, ISN, IBRO, SNCI, SfN, IEEE, IAS. He received many awards specially World federation of Neurology (WFN) travelling fellowship, Young Investigator Award, IBRO Travel Awardee and ISN Travel Awardee. Dr. Sudip also contributed his knowledge in different international journals as editorial board members. He has presented his research accomplishments in USA, Greece, France, South Africa, and Australia.

* * *

Hmidi Alaeddine received his Master's degree in embedded electronic systems from the University of Sousse, Tunisia, in 2017. He is currently pursuing a Ph.D. degree at the Faculty of Sciences, Monastir University, Monastir, Tunisia. His research interests are related to, deep neural network, Classification, reconfigurable architectures, network on chip, and image processing.

Nikita Banerjee received B.Tech in Computer Science and Engineering from Gandhi Institute for Technology, BPUT, Odiaha, India and perusing M.Tech in Computer Science and Engineering from College of Engineering and Technology, Odisha, India. Her special field of interest includes Machine Learning, Digital image process, Data Mining. Her major strength lies in Algorithm, Machine learning, Internet of web Technology.

Subhalaxmi Das received B.Tech in Computer Science and Engineering from Biju Patnaik University of Technology, Odisha, India and M.Tech in computer Science and Engineering from KIIT University, Odisha, India. She is currently working as lecturer in Dept of Computer Science and Engineering, College of Engineering and Technology, a constituent college of Biju Patnaik University of Technology, Odisha, India. She has 10 years of teaching experience. She has published some innovative ideas in International journal and Conference in the area of Spatial Data Mining. Her major strength lies in Algorithms, Data mining, Database Systems, Soft Computing.

J. Jane Rubel Angelina received the B.E degree in Computer Science and Engineering from Madurai Kamaraj University, India. She received the M.E degree in Computer Science and Engineering from Anna University, India. She received the PhD degree in Information and Communication Engineering from Anna University, India. She is currently working as an Assistant Professor at Thiagarajar College of Engineering, India. Her research interests include Storage Systems and Data Deduplication

Malek Jihene was born in Tunis, on Feburay 1 1973. She received the B.S. degree in Physics from Monastir University, in 1994; the M.S. and the the Ph.D. degree in Electronics and Microelectronics from Faculte des Sciences de Monastir in 1996 and 2002 respectively. Since 2002 she has been maitre-assistant in Electronics and

Microprocessors with the Electronics department, Institut Supérieur des Sciences Appliquées et de Technologie de Sousse. Her current research interests include: biomedical engineering, medical image processing and visualization.

Bohang Li received Bachelor's degree in Huazhong University of Science and Technology(HUST), majored in Electronic Engineering(EE) in 2016. After that, he received Master's degree in Peking University, majored in Electronic Engineering (EE). Currently, he works as a full-time data scientist mainly focus on Image Processing Algorithms.

Sudhir Kumar Mohapatra is an Associate Professor in Department of Software Engineering, Addis Ababa Science & Technology University, Ethiopia. He has completed Ph.D. from SOA University, India in Software Testing. He has published several research papers in peer reviewed international journals and conferences. He is also reviewer in international journals of high repute.

Alli P. received BE degree in Electronics and communication Engineering from Madras university and M.S degree in Software Systems from BITS Pilani Rajasthan . She received the PhD degree in Information and Communication Engineering from Madurai Kamaraj University.. She is currently working as Dean and Head of the Department of CSE at Velammal College of Engineering and Technology, Madurai, India. She has published several papers in International Journals / Conferences. Her current areas of interest include Medical Image Processing and Network and Information Security. She has guided 9 research scholars and 2 research scholars are pursuing currently. She is acting as a principal investigator for research projects received from DST and IEI.

Selene Pirola is a Research Associate in the Xu Group in the Department of Chemical Engineering at Imperial College London. She completed her BSc and MSc in Biomedical Engineering at Politecnico di Milano (Milan, Italy) in 2012 and 2015, respectively, with a master thesis project in which she developed a platform for the analysis of 4D flow MRI data for the evaluation of the fluid-dynamic alterations induced in the ascending aorta by bicuspid aortic valve (BAV) disease. Her PhD was awarded in 2019 by Imperial College London. Her PhD research focused on the evaluation of the aortic haemodynamics after aortic valve replacement using image-based computational fluid dynamics. Her current research focuses on thoracic aortic aneurysm development and progression, transcatheter aortic valve implantation (TAVI), and on haemodynamics in aortic dissection and after thoracic endovascular repair.

Yousuf Salmasi is a Resident in Cardiothoracic Surgery, Clinical Research Fellow in the Department of Surgery, Imperial College London, UK. His academic interests include 4D-flow MRI of the cardiovascular system, aortic biomechanics, misdiagnosis of aortic dissection, gene mutations in aortopathies and meta analysis.

Sumesh Sasidharan is Australia Awards Endeavour postdoctoral fellow, working as Research Associate in the Department of Bioengineering at Imperial College London. His research interests are in finite element analysis, cardiovascular biomechanics and tissue engineering.

S. Sasikala is currently working as a Associate Professor in Department of Computer Science and Engineering, Velammal College of Engineering and Technology, Madurai. She received doctorate in faculty of Information and Communication Engineering from Anna University India, 2016. She has published more than 18 Journal and 30 Conference papers in the area of Data mining and Big Data Analytics with Elsevier Science Direct, Springer and IEEE publishers. She has published two International Scientific books in KDD and Data mining and Data warehousing. She is serving as an Editorial Board Member and Reviewer for many reputed journals like IEEE, ELSEVIER and SPRINGER. She has 19 years experience in teaching and Research. Prior to joining Velammal College of Engineering and Technology, she served at Velammal College of Engineering and Technology, K.L.N. College of Information Technology Madurai, Velammal College of Engineering and Technology Madurai, P.S.N.A Engineering college Dindigul and Sethu Institute of technology Madurai. Her research interests include Data Mining, Internet of Things, Machine Learning Paradigms and Optimizations.

S. J. Subhashini is working as Assistant Professor of CSE Department in Velammal College of Engineering and Technology, Tamilnadu, India. She received B.E degree in Computer Science and Engineering from Madurai Kamaraj university and M.E degree in Computer Science and Engineering from Anna university, Chennai. She has completed her Ph.D in Anna University Chennai. She has more than 15 years of experience. Her areas of interest include data mining, image processing, wireless networks and cloud computing.

Janani Viswanathan is an Assistant Professor in Department of Biomedical Engineering, Sri Ramakrishna Engineering College.

Index

I

K

L

M

N

P

S

T

Purchase Print, E-Book, or Print + E-Book

IGI Global's reference books can now be purchased from three unique pricing formats:
Print Only, E-Book Only, or Print + E-Book.
Shipping fees may apply.

www.igi-global.com

Recommended Reference Books

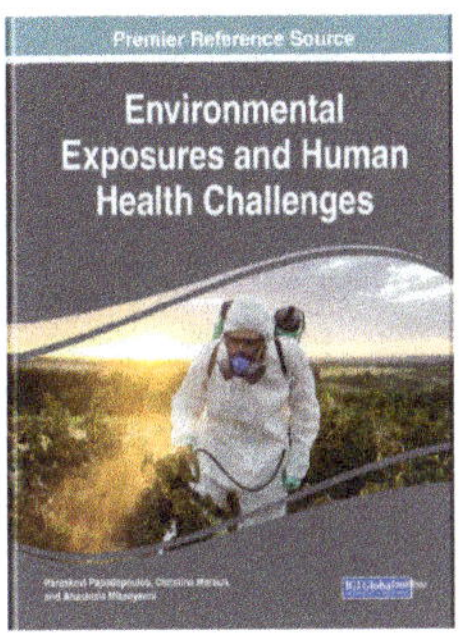

ISBN: 978-1-5225-7635-8
© 2019; 449 pp.
List Price: $255

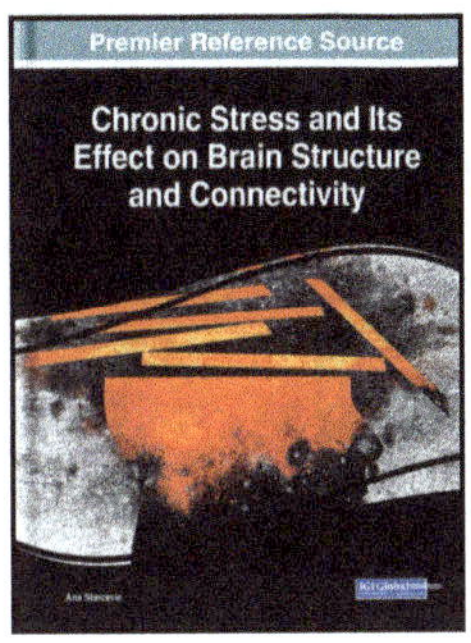

ISBN: 978-1-5225-7513-9
© 2019; 318 pp.
List Price: $225

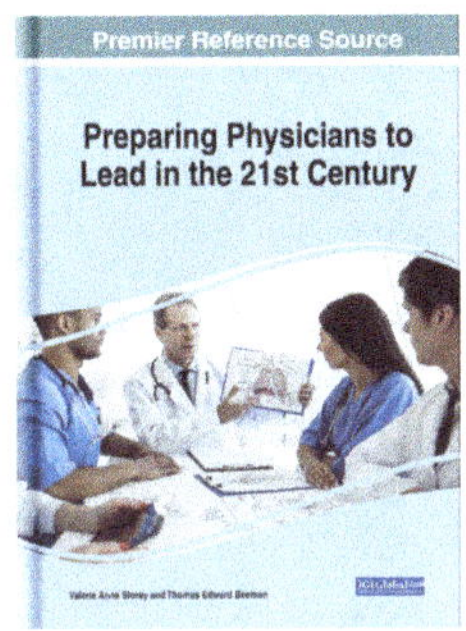

ISBN: 978-1-5225-7576-4
© 2019; 245 pp.
List Price: $245

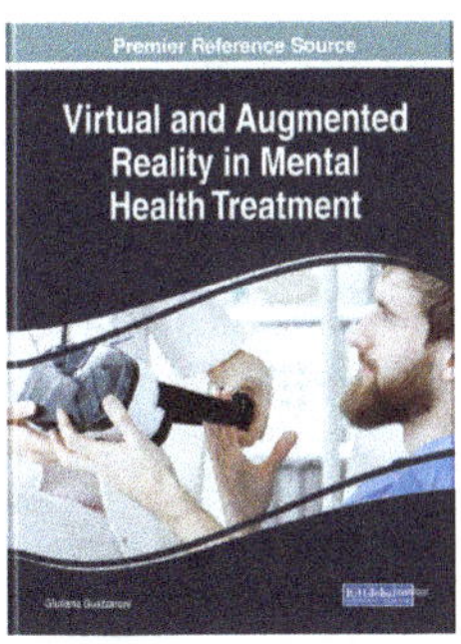

ISBN: 978-1-5225-7168-1
© 2019; 329 pp.
List Price: $265

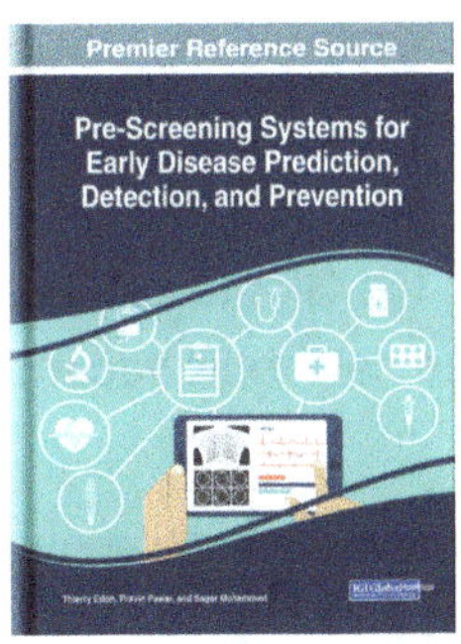

ISBN: 978-1-5225-7131-5
© 2019; 395 pp.
List Price: $245

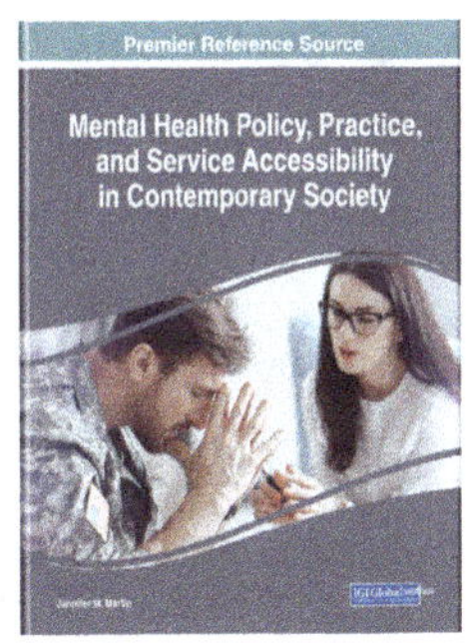

ISBN: 978-1-5225-7402-6
© 2019; 323 pp.
List Price: $245

Looking for free content, product updates, news, and special offers?
Join IGI Global's mailing list today and start enjoying exclusive perks sent only to IGI Global members.
Add your name to the list at **www.igi-global.com/newsletters.**

Publisher of Peer-Reviewed, Timely, and Innovative Academic Research

IGI Global
DISSEMINATOR OF KNOWLEDGE

www.igi-global.com Sign up at www.igi-global.com/newsletters facebook.com/igiglobal twitter.com/igiglobal

Ensure Quality Research is Introduced to the Academic Community

Become an IGI Global Reviewer for Authored Book Projects

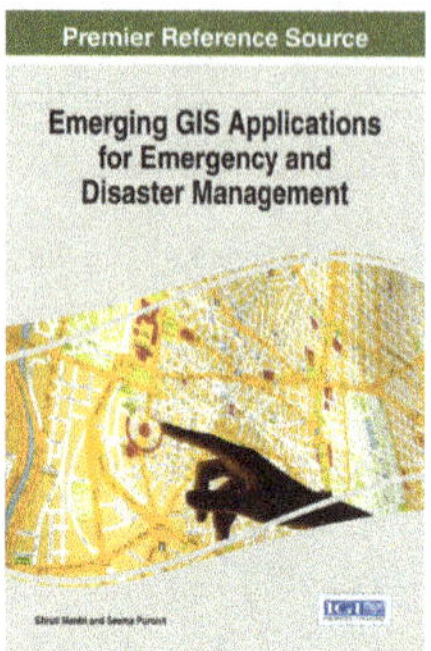

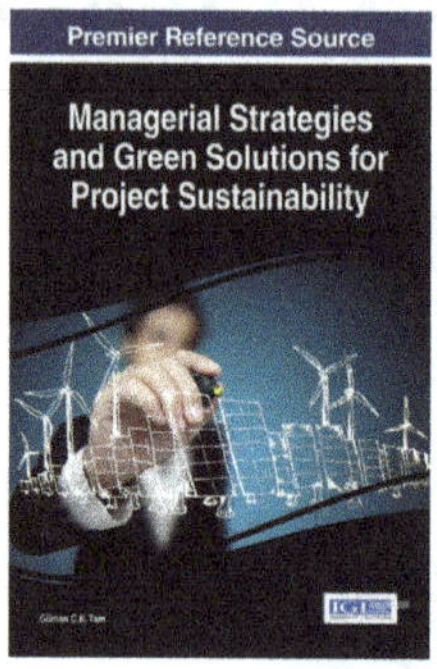

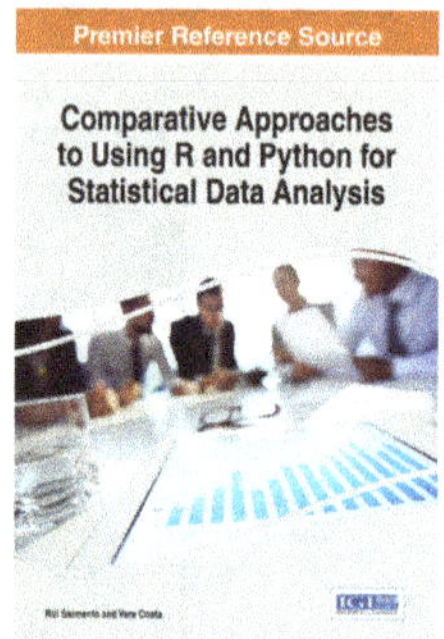

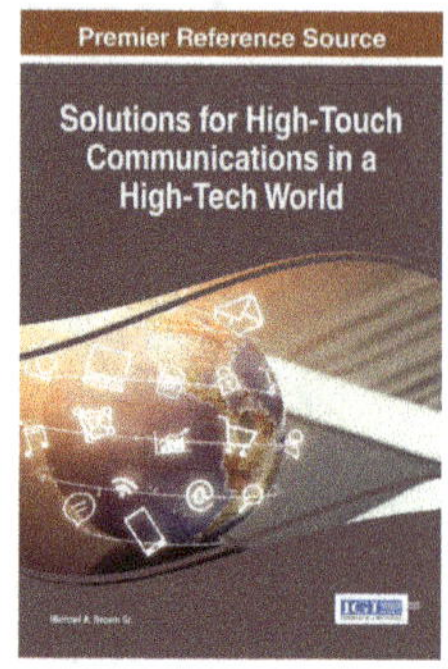

The overall success of an authored book project is dependent on quality and timely reviews.

In this competitive age of scholarly publishing, constructive and timely feedback significantly expedites the turnaround time of manuscripts from submission to acceptance, allowing the publication and discovery of forward-thinking research at a much more expeditious rate. Several IGI Global authored book projects are currently seeking highly-qualified experts in the field to fill vacancies on their respective editorial review boards:

Applications and Inquiries may be sent to:
development@igi-global.com

Applicants must have a doctorate (or an equivalent degree) as well as publishing and reviewing experience. Reviewers are asked to complete the open-ended evaluation questions with as much detail as possible in a timely, collegial, and constructive manner. All reviewers' tenures run for one-year terms on the editorial review boards and are expected to complete at least three reviews per term. Upon successful completion of this term, reviewers can be considered for an additional term.

If you have a colleague that may be interested in this opportunity, we encourage you to share this information with them.

IGI Global Proudly Partners With eContent Pro International

Receive a 25% Discount on all Editorial Services

Editorial Services

IGI Global expects all final manuscripts submitted for publication to be in their final form. This means they must be reviewed, revised, and professionally copy edited prior to their final submission. Not only does this support with accelerating the publication process, but it also ensures that the highest quality scholarly work can be disseminated.

English Language Copy Editing

Let eContent Pro International's expert copy editors perform edits on your manuscript to resolve spelling, punctuaion, grammar, syntax, flow, formatting issues and more.

Scientific and Scholarly Editing

Allow colleagues in your research area to examine the content of your manuscript and provide you with valuable feedback and suggestions before submission.

Figure, Table, Chart & Equation Conversions

Do you have poor quality figures? Do you need visual elements in your manuscript created or converted? A design expert can help!

Translation

Need your documjent translated into English? eContent Pro International's expert translators are fluent in English and more than 40 different languages.

Hear What Your Colleagues are Saying About Editorial Services Supported by IGI Global

"The service was very fast, very thorough, and very helpful in ensuring our chapter meets the criteria and requirements of the book's editors. I was quite impressed and happy with your service."

– Prof. Tom Brinthaupt, Middle Tennessee State University, USA

"I found the work actually spectacular. The editing, formatting, and other checks were very thorough. The turnaround time was great as well. I will definitely use eContent Pro in the future."

– Nickanor Amwata, Lecturer, University of Kurdistan Hawler, Iraq

"I was impressed that it was done timely, and wherever the content was not clear for the reader, the paper was improved with better readability for the audience."

– Prof. James Chilembwe, Mzuzu University, Malawi

Email: customerservice@econtentpro.com **www.igi-global.com/editorial-service-partners**

IGI Global
DISSEMINATOR OF KNOWLEDGE
www.igi-global.com

Celebrating Over 30 Years of Scholarly Knowledge Creation & Dissemination

InfoSci®-Books

A Database of Over 5,300+ Reference Books Containing Over 100,000+ Chapters Focusing on Emerging Research

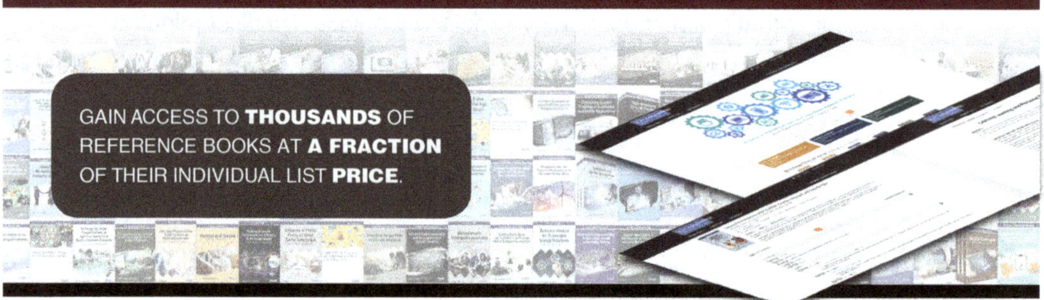

InfoSci®-Books Database

The **InfoSci®-Books** database is a collection of over 5,300+ IGI Global single and multi-volume reference books, handbooks of research, and encyclopedias, encompassing groundbreaking research from prominent experts worldwide that span over 350+ topics in 11 core subject areas including business, computer science, education, science and engineering, social sciences and more.

Open Access Fee Waiver (Offset Model) Initiative

For any library that invests in IGI Global's InfoSci-Journals and/ or InfoSci-Books databases, IGI Global will match the library's investment with a fund of equal value to go toward **subsidizing the OA article processing charges (APCs) for their students, faculty, and staff** at that institution when their work is submitted and accepted under OA into an IGI Global journal.*

INFOSCI® PLATFORM FEATURES

- No DRM
- No Set-Up or Maintenance Fees
- A Guarantee of No More Than a 5% Annual Increase
- Full-Text HTML and PDF Viewing Options
- Downloadable MARC Records
- Unlimited Simultaneous Access
- COUNTER 5 Compliant Reports
- Formatted Citations With Ability to Export to RefWorks and EasyBib
- No Embargo of Content (Research is Available Months in Advance of the Print Release)

**The fund will be offered on an annual basis and expire at the end of the subscription period. The fund would renew as the subscription is renewed for each year thereafter. The open access fees will be waived after the student, faculty, or staff's paper has been vetted and accepted into an IGI Global journal and the fund can only be used toward publishing OA in an IGI Global journal. Libraries in developing countries will have the match on their investment doubled.*

To Learn More or To Purchase This Database:
www.igi-global.com/infosci-books
eresources@igi-global.com • Toll Free: 1-866-342-6657 ext. 100 • Phone: 717-533-8845 x100

IGI Global
DISSEMINATOR OF KNOWLEDGE
www.igi-global.com

IGI Global
DISSEMINATOR OF KNOWLEDGE
www.igi-global.com

Publisher of Peer-Reviewed, Timely, and Innovative Academic Research Since 1988

IGI Global's Transformative Open Access (OA) Model: **How to Turn Your University Library's Database Acquisitions Into a Source of OA Funding**

In response to the OA movement and well in advance of Plan S, IGI Global, early last year, unveiled their OA Fee Waiver (Offset Model) Initiative.

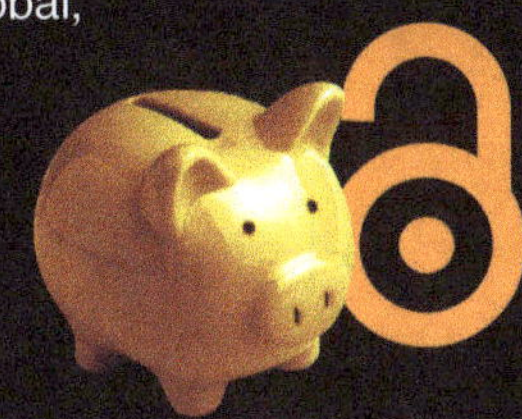

Under this initiative, librarians who invest in IGI Global's InfoSci-Books (5,300+ reference books) and/or InfoSci-Journals (185+ scholarly journals) databases will be able to subsidize their patron's OA article processing charges (APC) when their work is submitted and accepted (after the peer review process) into an IGI Global journal.*

How Does it Work?

1. When a library subscribes or perpetually purchases IGI Global's InfoSci-Databases including InfoSci-Books (5,300+ e-books), InfoSci-Journals (185+ e-journals), and/or their discipline/subject-focused subsets, IGI Global will match the library's investment with a fund of equal value to go toward subsidizing the OA article processing charges (APCs) for their patrons.

   Researchers: Be sure to recommend the InfoSci-Books and InfoSci-Journals to take advantage of this initiative.
2. When a student, faculty, or staff member submits a paper and it is accepted (following the peer review) into one of IGI Global's 185+ scholarly journals, the author will have the option to have their paper published under a traditional publishing model or as OA.
3. When the author chooses to have their paper published under OA, IGI Global will notify them of the OA Fee Waiver (Offset Model) Initiative. If the author decides they would like to take advantage of this initiative, IGI Global will deduct the US$ 1,500 APC from the created fund.
4. This fund will be offered on an annual basis and will renew as the subscription is renewed for each year thereafter. IGI Global will manage the fund and award the APC waivers unless the librarian has a preference as to how the funds should be managed.

Hear From the Experts on This Initiative:

"I'm very happy to have been able to make one of my recent research contributions, 'Visualizing the Social Media Conversations of a National Information Technology Professional Association' featured in the *International Journal of Human Capital and Information Technology Professionals*, freely available along with having access to the valuable resources found within IGI Global's InfoSci-Journals database."

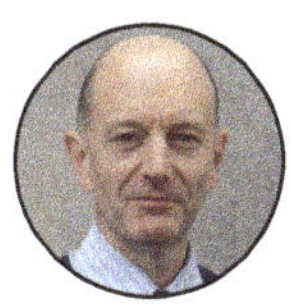

– **Prof. Stuart Palmer**, Deakin University, Australia

For More Information, Visit: www.igi-global.com/publish/contributor-resources/open-access or contact IGI Global's Database Team at eresources@igi-global.com

ARE YOU READY TO PUBLISH YOUR RESEARCH?

IGI Global
DISSEMINATOR OF KNOWLEDGE

IGI Global offers book authorship and editorship opportunities across 11 subject areas, including business, computer science, education, science and engineering, social sciences, and more!

Benefits of Publishing with IGI Global:

- Free, one-on-one editorial and promotional support.
- Expedited publishing timelines that can take your book from start to finish in less than one (1) year.
- Choose from a variety of formats including: Edited and Authored References, Handbooks of Research, Encyclopedias, and Research Insights.
- Utilize IGI Global's eEditorial Discovery® submission system in support of conducting the submission and blind review process.
- IGI Global maintains a strict adherence to ethical practices due in part to our full membership with the Committee on Publication Ethics (COPE).
- Indexing potential in prestigious indices such as Scopus®, Web of Science™, PsycINFO®, and ERIC – Education Resources Information Center.
- Ability to connect your ORCID iD to your IGI Global publications.
- Earn royalties on your publication as well as receive complimentary copies and exclusive discounts.

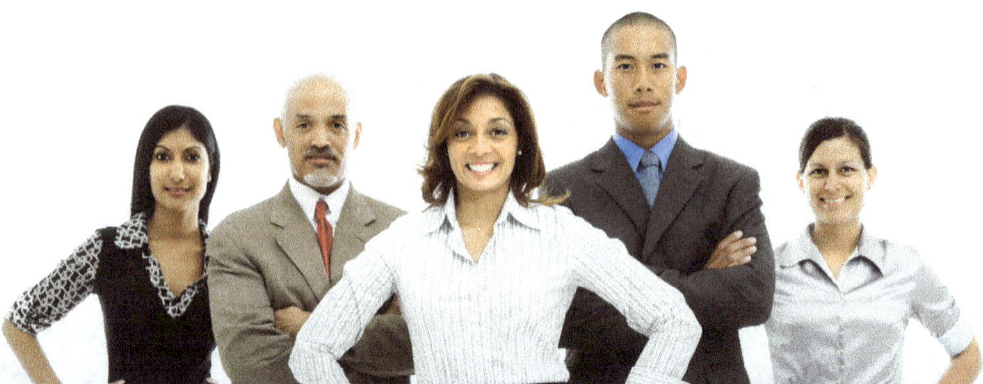

Get Started Today by Contacting the Acquisitions Department at:

acquisition@igi-global.com

www.igi-global.com/infosci-ondemand

InfoSci®-OnDemand

Continuously updated with new material on a weekly basis, InfoSci®-OnDemand offers the ability to search through thousands of quality full-text research papers. Users can narrow each search by identifying key topic areas of interest, then display a complete listing of relevant papers, and purchase materials specific to their research needs.

Comprehensive Service

- Over 125,000+ journal articles, book chapters, and case studies.
- All content is downloadable in PDF and HTML format and can be stored locally for future use.

No Subscription Fees

- One time fee of $37.50 per PDF download.

Instant Access

- Receive a download link immediately after order completion!

"It really provides an excellent entry into the research literature of the field. It presents a manageable number of highly relevant sources on topics of interest to a wide range of researchers. The sources are scholarly, but also accessible to 'practitioners'."

- Lisa Stimatz, MLS, University of North Carolina at Chapel Hill, USA

"It is an excellent and well designed database which will facilitate research, publication, and teaching. It is a very useful tool to have."

- George Ditsa, PhD, University of Wollongong, Australia

"I have accessed the database and find it to be a valuable tool to the IT/IS community. I found valuable articles meeting my search criteria 95% of the time."

- Prof. Lynda Louis, Xavier University of Louisiana, USA

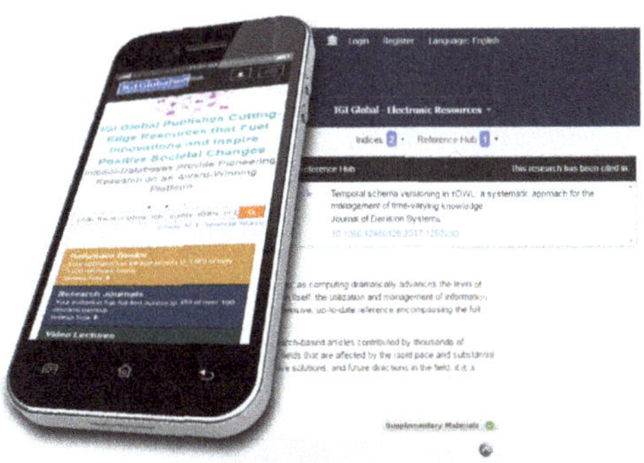

Recommended for use by researchers who wish to immediately download PDFs of individual chapters or articles.

www.igi-global.com/e-resources/infosci-ondemand

IGI Global
DISSEMINATOR OF KNOWLEDGE
www.igi-global.com

www.ingramcontent.com/pod-product-compliance
Lightning Source LLC
LaVergne TN
LVHW080856300926
849162LV00003B/443